Community-based Animal Healthcare

Vetwork UK

Vetwork UK is a non-government organization focussing on primary-level animal health and welfare issues in developing and industrialized countries. Our activities include collation and dissemination of information related to community-based veterinary services, with a view to informing workers at all levels from field level through to policy level. Veterinary UK also conducts action-oriented research and provides technical support to a range of donors, community groups, governmental and non-government organizations.

For further information write to:
Vetwork UK
35D Beach Lane
Musselburgh EH21 6JX
Scotland, United Kingdom

or visit us at http://www.vetwork.org.uk

FEINSTEIN INTERNATIONAL FAMINE CENTER

The Feinstein International Famine Center of Tufts University has been established to effect changes in the international community dealing with famine, disaster relief and refugees. It was created as a response to failed emergency and relief efforts in times of famine and complex emergencies. The Center is premised on the conviction that famine can be better prevented and that emergency response can be altered to improve success in building sustainable societies. The Center directs a one-year training professional Master Degree program in Humanitarian Assistance jointly offered by the School of Nutrition Science and Policy and the Fletcher School of Law and Diplomacy at Tufts University. It also provides training, evaluation and technical assistance to agencies involved in emergency response, while also managing community-based innovative programs in complex emergencies.

For further information write to:
Feinstein International Famine Center
96 Packard Avenue
Medford
Massachusetts 02155
USA

Telephone + 617 627 3423
or visit the website at http://www.tufts.edu/nutrition/famine

Community-based Animal Healthcare

A Practical Guide to Improving Primary Veterinary Services

Compiled by

Andy Catley, Stephen Blakeway and Tim Leyland

Practical
ACTION
PUBLISHING

Practical Action Publishing Ltd
25 Albert Street, Rugby, CV21 2SD, Warwickshire, UK
www.practicalactionpublishing.com

© Vetwork UK 2002

First published 2002

ISBN 10: 1 85339 485 8
ISBN 13 Paperback: 9781853394850
ISBN Library Ebook: 9781780441078
Book DOI: https://doi.org/10.3362/9781780441078

Since 1974, Practical Action Publishing has published and disseminated books and
information in support of international development work throughout the world.
Practical Action Publishing is a trading name of Practical Action Publishing Ltd
(Company Reg. No. 01159018), the wholly owned publishing company of Practical
Action. Practical Action Publishing trades only in support of its parent charity objectives
and any profits are covenanted back to Practical Action (Charity Reg. No. 247257, Group
VAT Registration No. 880 9924 76).

Reasonable efforts have been made to publish reliable data and information, but the
author and publisher cannot assume responsibility for the validity of all materials or for
the consequences of their use.

Typeset by Wyvern 21, Ltd

The manufacturer's authorised representative in the EU for product safety is
Lightning Source France, 1 Av. Johannes Gutenberg, 78310 Maurepas, France.
compliance@lightningsource.fr

Contents

Acknowledgements

Many people contributed advice and ideas during the production of this book. Where possible, we have tried to add names to specific contributions. In addition, we would also like to thank Catherine Robinson, Darlington Akabwai, Bob Wagner, Suzan Bishop, Nitya Ghotge of ANTHRA, Bob Hott, Ashford Gichohi, Maximillian Baumann, Bryony Jones, Mesfin Ayele, Lex Ross and Penny Rogers. Vincent Nyalick drew the cartoons.

Much of the experience described in the book arose from projects run by ActionAid, FARM Africa, Intermediate Technology Development Group, Oxfam United Kingdom/Ireland, Pan African Rinderpest Campaign (OAU/IBAR), Save the Children UK, UNICEF-Operation Lifeline Sudan (Southern Sector) Livestock Programme, VetAid, VSF-Belgium and VSF-Switzerland. This list is by no means exhaustive and many other organizations have contributed to the development of community-based animal health services. Technical support to OAU/IBAR and UNICEF was provided by the Section of International Veterinary Medicine, Tufts University and the Feinstein International Famine Centre, Tufts University.

The Tanzania case study in Chapter 8 is published with the kind permission of the Director of the Division of Veterinary Services within the Ministry of Water and Livestock Development, The United Republic of Tanzania. The authors are grateful to Dr Adela Kondela for contributing to the case study.

Funding for the writing of the book was made available from the Office for Foreign Disaster Assistance, United States Agency for International Development via the Participatory Community-based Animal Health and Vaccination (PARC-VAC) Project, Organization of African Unity/Interafrican Bureau of Animal Resources. The PARC-VAC Project was recently superceded by the establishment of the Community-based Animal Health and Participatory Epidemiology (CAPE) Unit, also with OAU/IBAR.

Abbreviations

AHA	animal health assistant
AHT	animal health technician
ALIN	Arid Lands Information Network
ALRMP	Arid Lands Resource Management Project
CAH	community animal healthcare
CAHW	community-based animal health worker
CBO	community-based organization
CBPP	contagious bovine pleuropneumonia
CLW	community livestock worker
CRDP	Central Rangelands Development Project
DCA	Dutch Committee for Afghanistan
DFID	Department for International Development (United Kingdom)
DRF	drug revolving fund
EVK	ethnoveterinary knowledge
FAO	Food and Agriculture Organization
GTZ	Gesellschaft für Technische Zusammenarbeit (German Development Agency)
IIED	International Institute for Environment and Development
ITDG	Intermediate Technology Development Group
KVAPS	Kenya Veterinary Privatization Scheme
MCF	malignant catarrhal fever
NAHA System	Nomadic Animal Health Auxiliary System
NGO	non-government organization
OAU/IBAR	Organization of African Unity/Interafrican Bureau for Animal Resources
OIE	Office International des Epizooties (World Organization for Animal Health)
PA	participatory appraisal
PACE	Pan African Programme for the Control of Epizootics
PARC	Pan African Rinderpest Campaign
PDS	participatory disease search
PLA	participatory learning and action
PRA	participatory rural appraisal
rp	rinderpest
RRA	rapid rural appraisal
RMC	resource management committee
SCF(UK)	Save the Children, (UK)
SERP	South East Rangelands Project
SPS Agreement	Agreement on the Application of Sanitary and Phytosanitary Measures
SSI	semi-structured interview
TNA	training needs assessment
VRTI	Vivekanand Research and Training Institute (India)
WHO	World Health Organization
WTO	World Trade Organization

Introduction to the guide

Andy Catley

CONTENTS

1.1 A brief history of community-based approaches to animal healthcare

In the 1980s, various organizations noted the poor development of veterinary services in some areas of the world where livestock were highly valued, both socially and economically. Lack of veterinary services was a particular problem in more remote areas, with harsh environments, difficult terrain and poor infrastructure. In some regions, these problems were compounded by civil war and the breakdown of veterinary services and infrastructure. The dryland regions of Africa and India, the mountains of Nepal and Afghanistan, and the forests of south-east Asia demanded new approaches to veterinary care in places where veterinarians where either unable or unwilling to venture.

Non-government organizations (NGOs) such as the Intermediate Technology Development Group (ITDG), Oxfam UK/Ireland and FARM Africa began to look at these problems from an Appropriate Technology perspective, which aimed to make

On the move in northern Eritrea

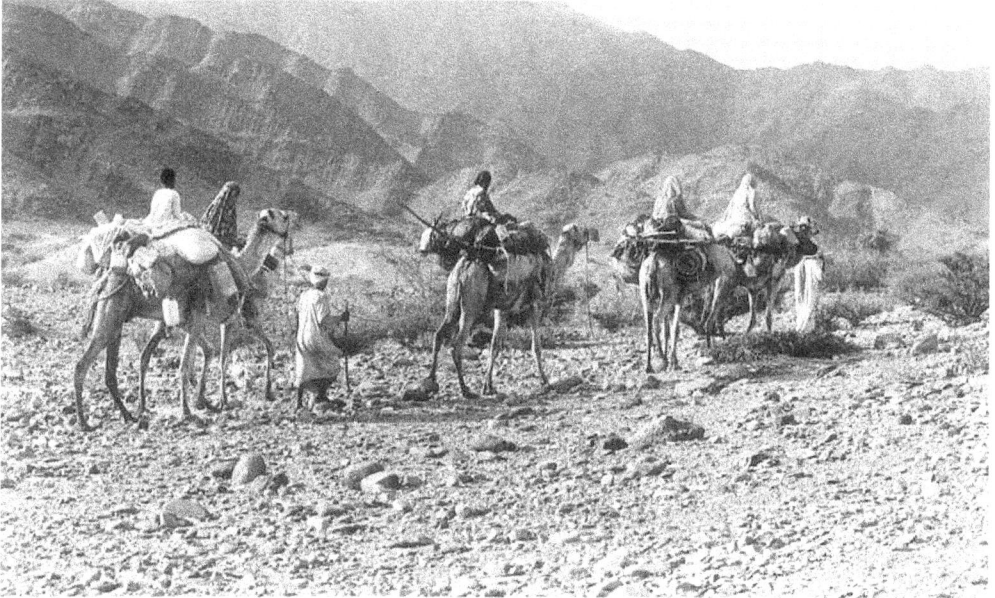

Plate 1.1 Mobile communities, such as these pastoralists in a remote area of northern Eritrea, are difficult to reach using conventional approaches to veterinary service delivery. (*Andy Catley*)

A remote well in Somaliland

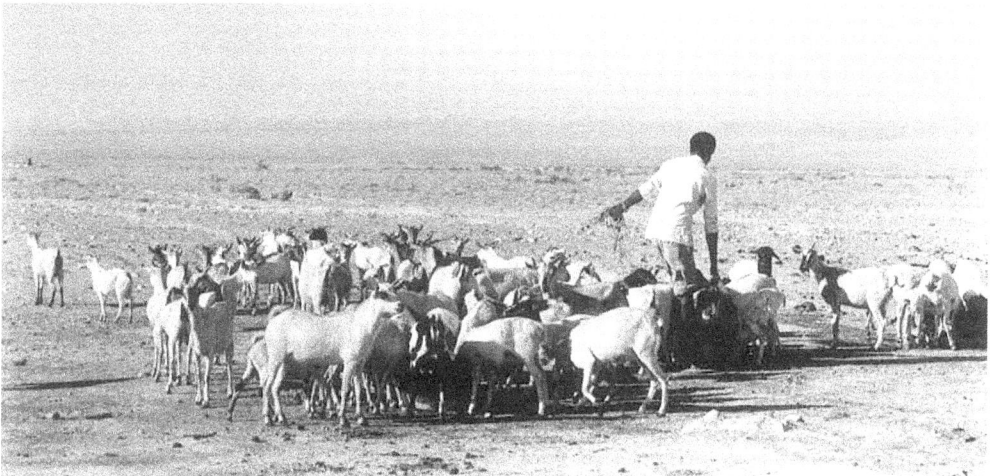

Plate 1.2 This kind of area is often suited to community-based delivery systems. (*Andy Catley*)

best use of local livestock knowledge and husbandry skills. An important principle here was to build upon what people already knew and were already doing. Typically, communities selected people for basic animal health and husbandry training, and these workers became known as 'paravets', 'barefoot vets', 'basic veterinary workers' and other names in local languages. Other development agencies, particularly Deutsche Gesellschaft für Technische Zusammenarbeit (GTZ), established programmes using primary-level veterinary workers in Thailand and Somalia. Around the same time, community participation was emerging as an important approach in rural development. The arrival of community participation was accompanied by a family of data collection, learning and facilitation methods and approaches such as rapid rural appraisal (RRA), participatory rural appraisal (PRA) and participatory learning and action (PLA).

As interest in community-based approaches grew, non-government and government agencies began to experiment. Numerous projects began to appear in African, Asian and Latin American countries and, in Africa, experiences were reviewed regularly through events such as ITDG's annual workshops in Kenya. Gradually, the ideas of community participation began to feature more clearly, and, in some places, attempts were made to improve local ownership and management of projects. More vets began to use participatory approaches and methods to work with communities to identify and analyse local animal health problems, and work out solutions to these problems.

1.2   About the guide

This book uses the term 'community-based animal health worker' (CAHW) to encompass a range of names for primary-level veterinary workers. By 'community-

Where there are no roads

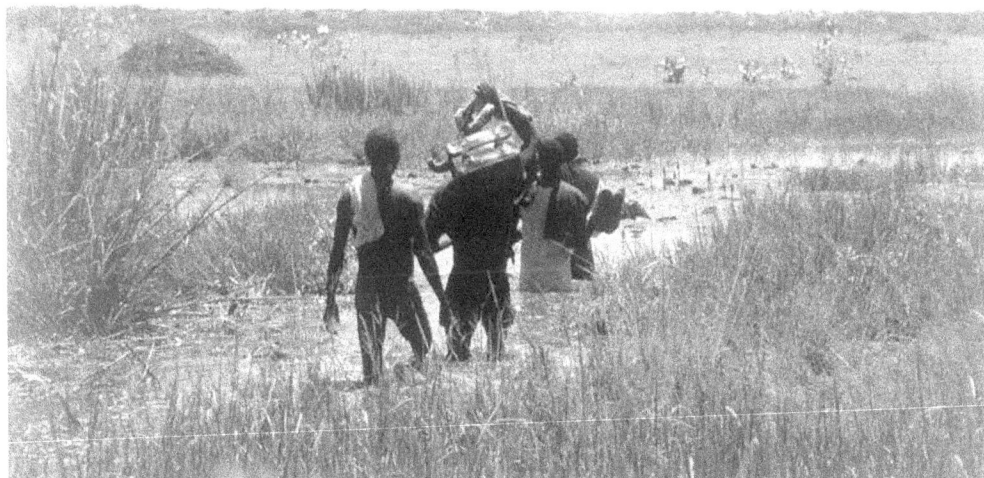

Plate 1.3 Community-based animal health workers (CAHWs) wading through swamps in southern Sudan. Few veterinarians are willing to work in these conditions.
(*Tim Leyland*)

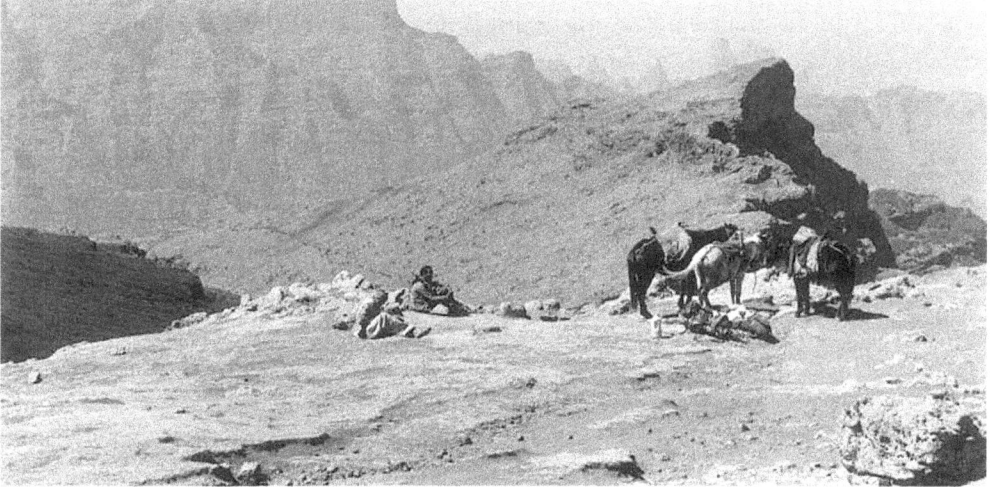

Plate 1.4 Millions of people living in the mountainous areas of Ethiopia can be reached only on foot or by mule. Can CAHWs provide a basic veterinary service to these people? (*Andy Catley*)

CAHWs in Afghanistan

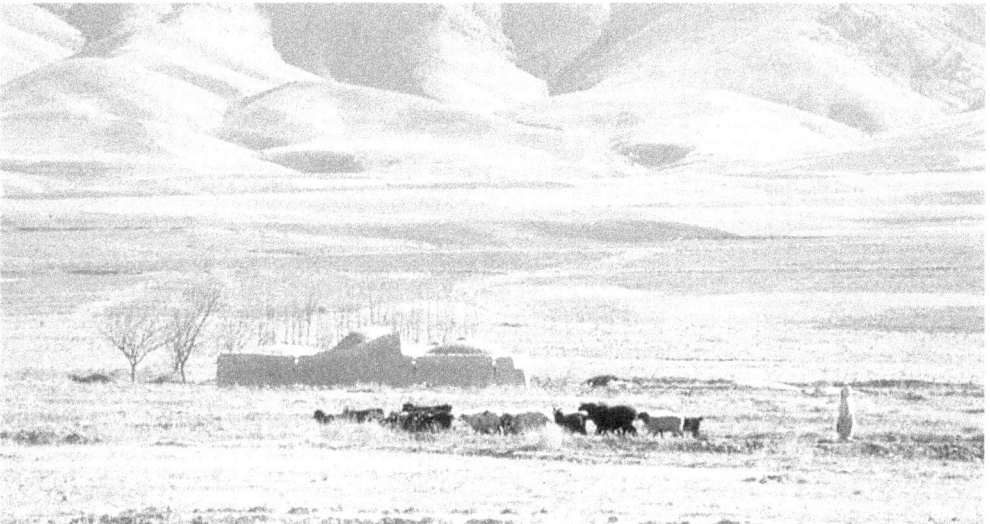

Plate 1.5 Afghanistan has been developing CAHWs for over ten years. This approach is increasingly recognized by government as an important component of the national veterinary service. (*Stephen Blakeway*)

based', we mean that the CAHWs live and probably grew up in the community concerned. The CAHW is known and respected in the community, is recognized as a knowledgeable livestock keeper, and was selected for training by the community. The CAHW provides a preventive, diagnostic and curative service that is limited to important animal health problems, as identified by livestock keepers in the community concerned.

In the late 1990s, interest in community-based animal healthcare was growing rapidly. Many NGOs, often with limited in-house veterinary expertise, were setting up projects. Some government veterinary departments were also trying to develop community-based projects, but lacked knowledge or experience of the approach. In many cases, both government vets and NGOs attempted to start projects without really understanding the key issues or recognizing the new attitudes and skills they needed to acquire.

Box 1.1 A practical guide

◆ This book provides vets and others with practical information on how to establish and sustain community-based animal health systems.
◆ Primarily, the book is targeted at veterinary professionals with no, or limited, experience of CAHWs but who wish to establish a project. These readers include private practitioners who want to develop links with communities that are not reached by a private clinic or pharmacy.
◆ The book details the various stages of a CAHW project. It describes participatory data collection, training needs for veterinary personnel, financial systems, training of CAHWs, monitoring and assessment, and ways to share information with others. The guide provides advice on variations in project design and implementation according to local requirements and policy environment.

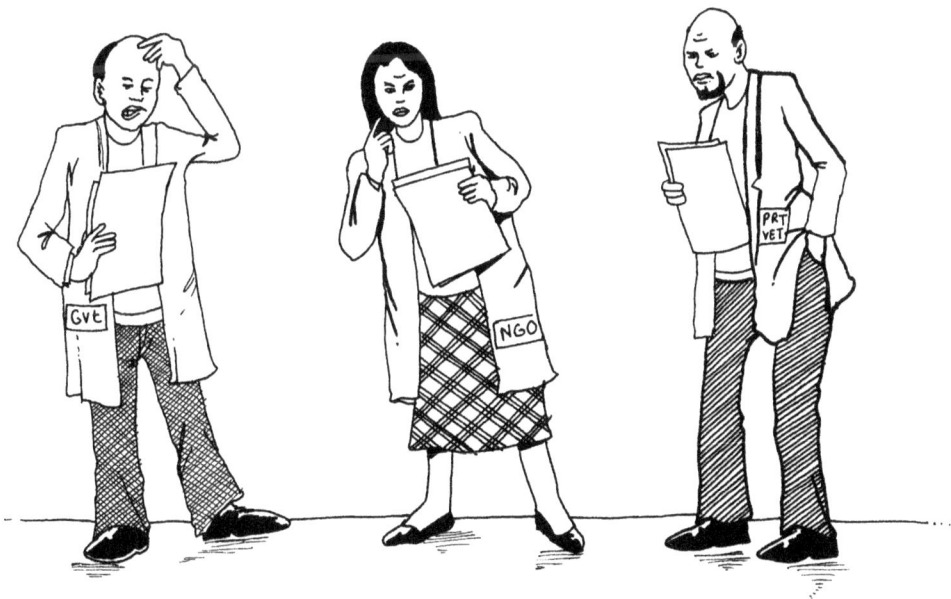

This community-based approach looks very interesting, but where can I find more information?

An important feature of the book is that it does not focus only on how to train CAHWs, but looks more broadly at the wider environment in which CAHWs operate and at the factors that encourage sustainable services. In many countries, policies and laws are being revised in order to incorporate basic animal health workers into the official veterinary workforce. However, policy and legislative reform takes place in capital cities, far away from those areas where community-based approaches have been tried and tested.

Box 1.2 A reference for policy makers

The book is also a point of reference for policy makers. It describes the key theories behind community-based services, and the 'nuts and bolts' needed to make these services function.

Other books cover policy aspects of community-based veterinary care and therefore this guide focuses on the 'how-to-do-it' practicalities and the process of using field experiences to influence appropriate policy change.

The book is also aimed at other readers such as:

◆ government or project staff who are already involved with CAHW projects and who would like to learn about the experiences and systems used by other projects;

◆ PRA trainers who are involved in training veterinary professionals;

◆ veterinary professionals who are responsible for training CAHWs or training others to train CAHWs;

◆ extension staff, agriculturalists and project managers;

◆ government veterinarians who are responsible for collecting official data on livestock disease incidence and prevalence.

1.3   Where to find the information you need

Summary of the chapters in the guide

Chapter 2: Getting started

A community-based approach means working with local people and livestock keepers right from the start. If you are about to begin work, Chapter 2 describes how to build relationships with communities and embark on joint analysis of animal health problems and solutions. The use of participatory approaches and methods is central to this process, and often requires veterinary staff to receive training in PRA. Ideally, all stakeholders should be involved in these early stages of the project, and particular attention should be paid to those things that people are already doing to improve the health of their animals. This includes developing a thorough understanding of indigenous livestock knowledge and reviewing the strengths and weaknesses of the veterinary care options that already exist. Participatory approaches should also enable the project workers to listen and learn from those people who tend to be overlooked. These people include women and less wealthy livestock keepers.

Chapter 3: Taking a long-term perspective

As experience with CAHWs has developed, a number of strengths and weaknesses have emerged. On the positive side, people with basic training and strong indigenous know-how were able to provide a service that was highly valued by livestock keepers. However, many projects suffered from poor sustainability because the CAHWs depended on veterinary medicines that were provided by government or NGOs, often at subsidized rates. In government systems, drug procurement and delivery were often bureaucratic and subject to the 'diminishing revolving fund' syndrome. In NGOs, lack of technical support sometimes resulted in inappropriate drug procurement. Even NGO projects which started successfully collapsed when funding was withdrawn or the NGO closed the project for other reasons. Therefore, sustainability is a key issue in CAHW systems. Ways to support CAHWs *in the long term* need to be considered and built-in to projects at the outset. Links to a support mechanism – including private vets, pharmacists and trainers – need to be developed for efficient drug supply, monitoring and refresher training. Links with government and official certification of CAHWs are also important. These and other sustainability issues are described in Chapter 3.

Chapters 4 and 5: Participative and practical training for effective learning

Participative and practical training methods are the most effective way of training CAHWs. These methods respect the existing knowledge of the trainees, and use this knowledge as the basis for new learning. Specific training tools enable trainees to share and discuss their knowledge, while also acquiring knowledge from each other and the trainer. Participative training with practical, hands-on exercises can be used with both literate and illiterate trainees. As this approach differs markedly from lecturing and classroom teaching, trainers of CAHWs usually need training before training others. This is sometimes called 'Training of Trainers' and, together with other training issues, is described in Chapters 4 and 5.

Chapter 6: How to monitor and evaluate community-based animal health projects

When community-based animal health projects are being implemented it is important to follow the progress of project activities, find out if the project has provided benefits and, if so, to whom, how and why. Regular monitoring and good impact assessments help to identify weaknesses that can then be resolved. Although monitoring and evaluation are important management tools and learning opportunities, they are often among the weakest components of a CAHW system. Chapter 6 describes approaches and methods for assessing projects from the perspectives of both local people (including the intended project beneficiaries) and 'outsiders' (project staff, government vets, donors and others).

Chapter 7: Community-based disease surveillance

Due to their presence in remote areas, their indigenous knowledge and their basic veterinary training, CAHWs are well-placed to take part in national disease surveillance. Contributions can include early warning reports, routine written or verbal reports of disease outbreaks, collection of samples and assisting disease investigation teams. When action is taken in response to a disease event, CAHWs can also be useful, front-line workers for organizing communities and treating or vaccinating animals. Although community-based disease surveillance systems are relatively new, there is an increasing need for state veterinary services to improve disease information flow from remote areas.

Chapter 8: How to change policies and laws

Appropriate policies and legislation are important for the long-term sustainability of community-based systems. Ideally, successful field experiences should influence the development of supportive policy and legislation. Therefore, there is a need to develop links between remote field-level stakeholders and central policy makers. Small-scale pilot projects and events such as workshops and study tours can be useful ways of introducing CAHW projects to vets in central government or academic institutions. By reference to real life examples, ways to change policy are described in Chapter 8.

Chapter 9: Sharing experiences and learning from others

Knowledge and understanding of community-based animal health services will develop if people write up their work and share experiences with others. At field level, it can be useful to learn from the ideas, successes and mistakes of other workers, while also contributing towards the growing body of knowledge on this important mode of animal health service provision. There are also many topics that are closely linked to community-based approaches, and networking promotes discussion and the emergence of new ideas. The role of sharing information and networking is discussed in Chapter 9, together with ideas on how to network.

Where to find information on participatory methods

The guide includes examples of specific participatory methods for use during the various stages of CAHW projects. Some readers may be particularly interested in these methods, which can be found on pages with an arrow alongside.

1.4　Further reading

At the end of the guide, a 'Further reading' section lists books, reports and published papers drawn from both the animal health sector and broader areas of participatory development work.

1.5　Developing and improving the guide

The guide is a first attempt at helping vets to design and implement successful community-based projects. Inevitably, there may be mistakes and omissions, or you may disagree with some of the advice offered. Perhaps you also have useful information that could be included in future versions of the guide: this might be an experience of ways to select CAHWs, a new training or monitoring method, or a useful approach for facilitating policy development. Whatever you have to say, we would like the guide to be an organic book that will grow into something better. Contacting Vetwork UK will help ensure that your views are taken into account. We very much look forward to hearing from you.

Getting started

David Hadrill, Andy Catley and Karen Iles

2.1   Introduction

This chapter describes the first stages of setting up a community-based animal health worker (CAHW) system. The chapter focuses on ways for veterinary staff to understand the most important animal health problems from the perspective of livestock keepers. During this process, technical staff can work closely with communities to consider the different options for improving basic veterinary care according to local conditions and existing services. CAHW systems are not the only way of improving primary animal healthcare and the decision to embark on a community-based approach can be reached only after all the main problems and ideas have been thoroughly discussed. CAHW systems work best when they are supported by both veterinary staff and livestock keepers in the community.

Different people within communities have their own perspectives, needs and ideas for improving veterinary services and it is important to include all these people in the initial stages of a community-based system. The various interest groups within a system are sometimes called 'stakeholders' because all these people have a 'stake' in what happens and will be affected, either positively or negatively, by the new service. Some common stakeholder groups in CAHW services are outlined in Box 2.1. This list is not exhaustive and each project will have its own stakeholder groups.

In addition to recognizing and working with different stakeholders, project staff involved in community animal healthcare (CAH) systems will need to review their own skills and capacity during the early stages of a project. Experience from around the world shows that training in participatory approaches and methods is particularly useful for veterinary staff involved in CAHW services and this chapter makes frequent reference to these methods. However, it should be noted that participatory assessment is not only about methods and tools, but also requires professionals to adopt a respectful, sensitive and open approach to working with communities. In community-based programmes, veterinary staff need to recognize their own limitations and be willing to learn in partnership with local people.

Box 2.1 Common stakeholder groups in community-based animal health services

The following groups will all be affected by the development of a new type of animal health service. A key question to ask during the initial stages of a CAH project is: 'How will each of these different groups benefit or suffer from the project'?

Livestock owners and carers

People who own or look after animals. This stakeholder group includes a wide range of people who may vary from a woman who rears a few chickens in her backyard to a wealthy farmer or pastoralist who owns hundreds of cattle.

Veterinary personnel

Including veterinarians, veterinary assistants, vaccinators and any other type of worker who has an official, recognized qualification or role. This stakeholder group includes government veterinary staff at both field level and centrally, and private veterinarians.

Traditional practitioners

Including herbalists, bone setters, religious healers and others.

Unofficial suppliers of veterinary drugs

Including traders, merchants and black-market dealers who might sell drugs directly to livestock keepers.

Project staff

Who may be employed by the government or a development agency.

2.2 Learning with communities about their animals: the use of participatory surveys and workshops

The first stage of establishing a CAHW system is for the community and project staff to learn more about the proposed project area by compiling and analysing background information together. This process helps the veterinary staff to learn more about local needs and is the beginning of a working relationship between the project and the community. As mentioned above, participatory learning approaches can be very useful during the initial assessment of the animal health situation in a particular area. There

---

Box 2.2 Names and abbreviations for participatory approaches and methods

AEA	Agroecosystem Analysis
BA	Beneficiary Assessment
DELTA	Development Education Leadership Teams
D&D	Diagnosis and Design
DRP	Diagnostico Rural Participativo
FPR	Farmer Participatory Research
FSR	Farming Systems Research
GRAAP	Groupe de recherche et d'appui pour l'auto-promotion paysanne
MARP	Méthode Accéléré de Recherche Participative
PA	Participatory Appraisal
PALM	Participatory Analysis and Learning Methods
PAR	Participatory Action Research
PD	Process Documentation
PLA	Participatory Learning and Action
PRA	Participatory Rural Appraisal
PRAP	Participatory Rural Appraisal and Planning
PRM	Participatory Research Methods
PTD	Participatory Technology Development
RA	Rapid Appraisal
RAAKS	Rapid Assessment of Agricultural Knowledge Systems
RAP	Rapid Assessment Procedures
RAT	Rapid Assessment Techniques
RCA	Rapid Catchment Analysis
REA	Rapid Ethnographic Assessment
RFSA	Rapid Food Security Assessment
RMA	Rapid Multi-perspective Appraisal
ROA	Rapid Organizational Assessment
RRA	Rapid Rural Appraisal

---

is a large and growing family of participatory methods with various names and acronyms (see Box 2.2), but this book uses the term 'participatory appraisal' (PA) to encompass the general philosophy and ideas behind participatory ways of working.

Some important reasons for using PA are:

◆ The process of gathering information is carried out in a spirit of cooperation and mutual learning. Provided that the whole community has the opportunity to participate in gathering information, at the end of the experience all community members know it is accurate. When participative learning has gone well, community members are pleased to have been able to help outsiders learn about their animals. Livestock owners will also share ownership of the data and, therefore, have confidence in the decisions that are made using the information that has been collected.

◆ In many countries there is a lack of technical data on livestock disease in less wealthy or remote areas. Although conventional livestock disease surveys produce scientific data, these surveys are often time-consuming and costly to implement. In these situations, participatory methods produce sufficient information on animal health problems and services for the purpose of making decisions about basic clinical care.

◆ Many livestock-owning communities know a great deal about their animals and have rational strategies for preventing and treating livestock diseases. This indigenous knowledge, including local names for livestock diseases and parasites, is a valuable resource for CAHW systems and tends to feature prominently in participatory animal health surveys. Indigenous knowledge can be used during the design of CAHW training courses and, to some extent, the training curriculum and training methods will depend on how much local trainees already know about animal diseases and treatments (see Chapters 4 and 5).

◆ The people who control this early stage of the project are usually local or expatriate development workers, or national veterinary staff. These people can be viewed as 'outsiders' who often come from very different cultural, wealth and educational backgrounds to the livestock keepers (see Box 2.3). Many veterinarians prefer to live in a town rather than in rural areas where most livestock are kept. The use of PA helps to break down cultural barriers and limits professional biases, but still provides much useful information that is relevant to the area in question.

Training for project veterinary staff

Given the value of participatory methods in CAHW systems, it is usually beneficial for project staff to receive training in PA from a local agency. Although there are many excellent PA training manuals now available (see Further reading), there is no substitute for staff taking time to learn new skills in a well-organized training course

Box 2.3 Cultural and professional differences between livestock keepers and veterinary professionals: the example of pastoralists in African drylands

In many dryland areas of eastern Africa, pastoral livestock-rearing communities have been isolated from development activities and, typically, are still regarded as uncivilized and ignorant by the educated elite who live in the towns. As education services are usually poor in pastoral areas, there are few students from pastoral societies enrolling in university courses, including veterinary medicine, and therefore most of the vets working in pastoral areas are not pastoralists themselves.

In countries such as Kenya, Ethiopia, Eritrea, Uganda and Tanzania it is usual to find government vets in pastoral areas who:
- are not of the same ethnic group and do not share the same language, religion or customs of the local people;
- are not accustomed to the harsh, hot climatic conditions in pastoral areas;
- have not received much technical training on livestock diseases or management in dryland areas because veterinary courses are geared towards highland areas and more intensive production systems.

In this situation, it is easy to see why so many government veterinarians in dryland areas describe their postings as a punishment.

that allows opportunity to practise approaches and methods in the field. In some countries there are specialized training institutes that focus on development issues and offer short training courses in participatory methods. Sometimes these courses can be adapted to suit the particular needs of veterinary staff working with CAHW projects. When searching for an appropriate course, it is useful to seek opinions from previous attendants because the quality of training courses can vary. Training in PA should be for a minimum of ten days divided between class work and fieldwork.

An alternative to sending staff away on a PA course is to recruit a trainer who provides training in the project area. Sometimes it is possible to arrange the fieldwork component of the training to take place during a participatory survey, the results of which will influence the design of the CAHW system. However, this requires careful thought because project staff may need to practise rather than apply PA at this stage of the project.

Another useful form of training to consider during the early stages of a CAHW project is a study tour for project staff. A study tour involves visits to CAHW projects in other areas and exposes project staff to alternative ways of working and practical experiences. When study tours can be arranged in-country they can be a relatively inexpensive learning and confidence-building tool for CAH projects. They

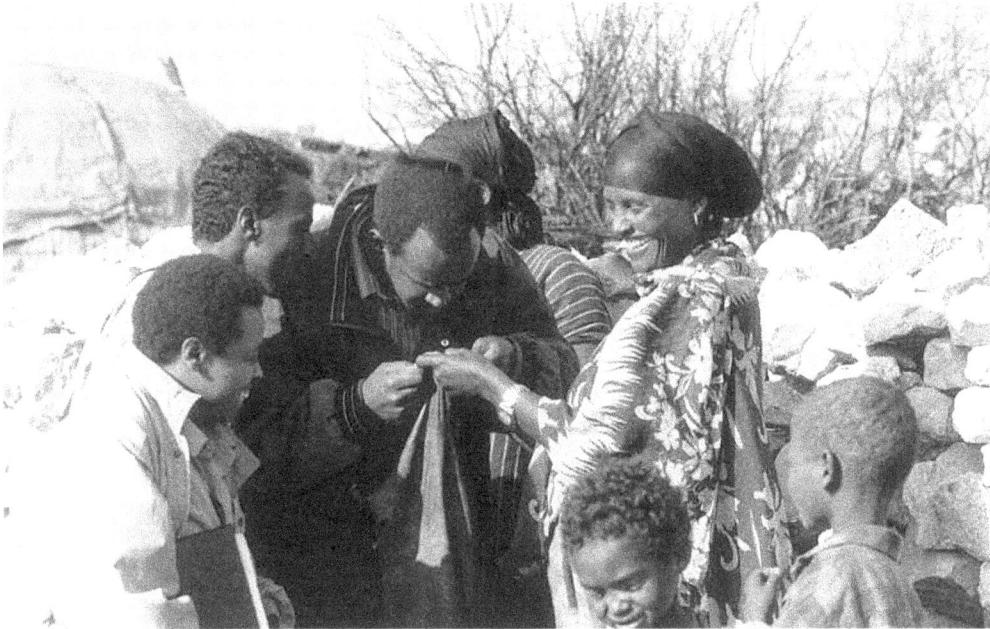

Plates 2.1 and 2.2 Participatory appraisal is not just about using tools to collect information. Outsiders need to take an active interest in learning with local people about how they live. (*Andy Catley*)

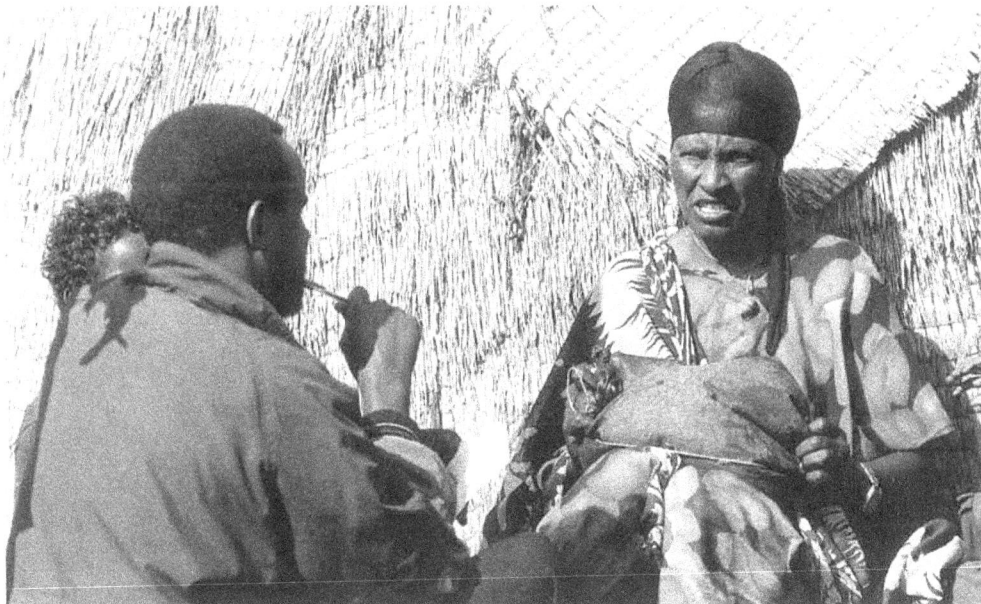

also enable technical staff to develop links with professional colleagues who might act as sources of advice or provide training inputs to the project.

Handing over the stick during a participatory appraisal (PA) training session for veterinary workers

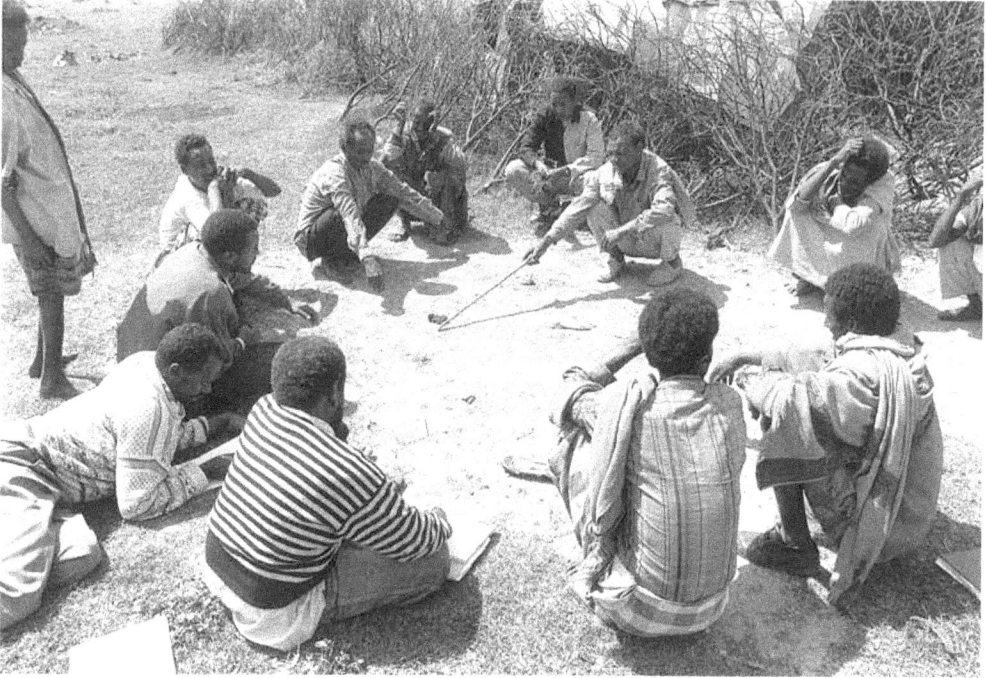

Plate 2.3 Taking time to listen to local people's opinions and ideas is central to participatory analysis. (*Andy Catley*)

Survey design and key issues to investigate

Once project veterinary staff have been trained in participatory approaches and methods, a participatory survey of animal healthcare and constraints in the proposed project area should be designed and implemented. When designing a survey, the two key questions are: 'What information do we need?' and 'How are we going to obtain the information?' The information required can normally be listed under headings such as socio-political, livelihoods, livestock management and diseases, existing animal health services, and options for improving animal health services.

Before conducting work at community level, project staff should seek information from secondary sources such as government livestock records (livestock census data, animal health reports), research institute reports and any scientific publications that relate to the project area. These documents will probably provide useful background information on livestock facilities and problems in the area and will help the survey team to develop checklists for the participatory survey. It might also be possible to talk to other development workers, see reports prepared by development agencies and meet government vets or other livestock workers in local offices. Whatever the source of this secondary information, it is important that the project's technical staff are familiar with the views and writing of other workers.

Meet a range of wealth, power and gender groups during a participatory assessment

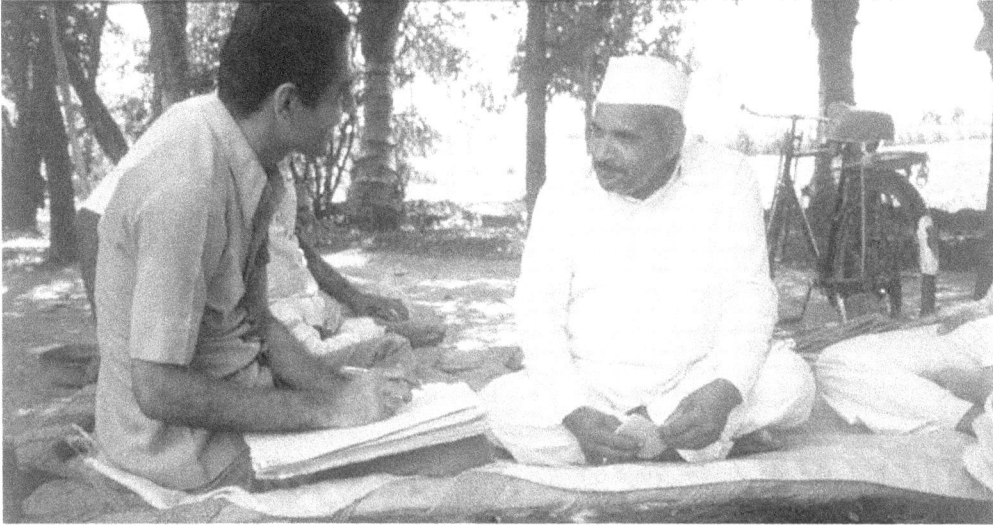

Plate 2.4 Meeting local leaders and dignitaries for the official view on your project is an important part of working at community level. (*David Hadrill*)

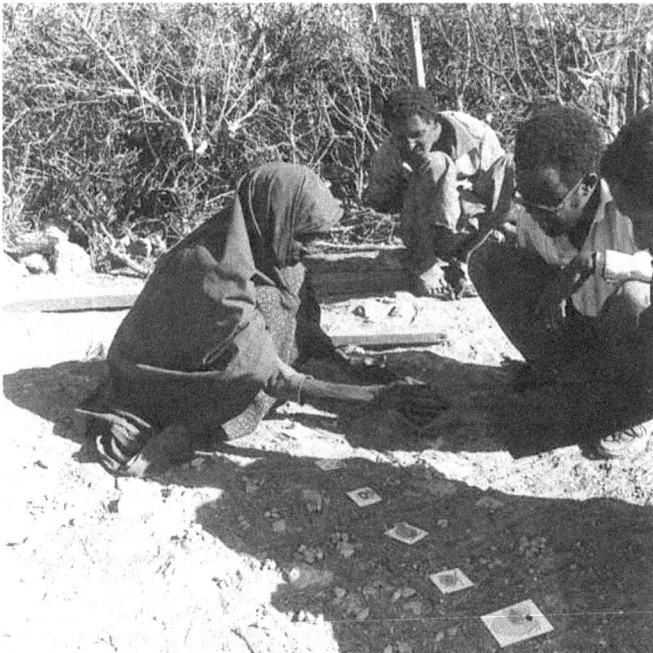

Plate 2.5 Make sure that less powerful people have a chance to contribute their views as well. For example, women often know as much, if not more, about livestock than men. This woman in Somaliland explains the links between different types of ticks and livestock health problems. (*Andy Catley*)

During the design of CAHW systems, some key issues and information requirements that need to be considered in participatory survey are as follows:

Be aware of inequalities due to wealth, status and gender

For reasons of diplomacy and official endorsement of project activities, it is important to meet those who hold power locally. Wealthy individuals, politicians or senior government officers can also provide useful background information on an area and give details of official policy on veterinary service delivery. However, it is important to realize that influential leaders may not be the best source of information on animal health services and the participatory survey proper should seek opinions from a range of people who are involved in livestock rearing. It is also important to make a special effort to reach those people who are disadvantaged or marginalized, perhaps through reasons of wealth or gender. There may be local leaders demanding action to solve a problem with their cows, but the majority of poorer people may own only chickens and goats. The whole system needs investigation and analysis.

Use indigenous leadership and social structures in remote communities

In some areas, communities have very little contact with government structures and they organize themselves along traditional lines. To work effectively with these communities it is necessary to understand the traditional social units and leadership and, where necessary, use these structures and individuals as entry points into communities.

Box 2.4 Entry points for community-based animal health services: examples of indigenous institutions and structures in pastoralist communities

Misrepresentation of communities is a common problem in CAHW systems. In pastoralist areas of eastern Africa, outsiders such as veterinarians or project staff tend to meet people in the main urban centres. The authorities in these centres, although important, are often government personnel, traders, educated people or elders who are no longer living with their animals on the range. The views of these people are not always representative of the true pastoralist communities who are living in remote areas with their livestock.

The experience of many CAHW projects is that, in order to work effectively with pastoralists, their traditional forums, leaders and representatives should be identified and used as entry points. This means travelling into the remote areas, staying with the people and finding out how their communities are functioning and how decision making takes place.

Turkana, northern Kenya

The Turkana of northern Kenya have well-organized, mobile groups of family units

---

called *adakars* which, traditionally, move together under the leadership of a *general* or *seer*. Each *adakar*, consisting of 10–20 families, has its own parliament called the *ekitoingikiliok* (tree of men) where the heads of families meet each day to discuss important issues. The *adakar* leaders are the crucial entry points for community-based animal health work with Turkana communities. These people are very effective at passing messages to the other *adakar* members and can mobilize communities rapidly.

Dinka, southern Sudan

In the Dinka areas of southern Sudan, dry season grazing of cattle involves the formation of cattle camps. Traditionally, the cattle camps have different levels of leadership and these leaders, such as *wot* and *gol* leaders, are responsible for making key decisions regarding the management of the camps. Within each *gol*, herders are linked by kinship ties and are accustomed to reaching decisions by consensus. The main entry points for understanding animal health issues in Dinka communities are the cattle camps.

Somali herders

Somali pastoral society is based on kinship ties and a highly segmented, patrilineal clan system. The smallest and most stable clan unit is called a *dia*-paying group. The members of the *dia*-paying group have collective responsibility for the payment of *dia* (blood money compensation) and it is as a member of a *dia*-paying group that a Somali herder is most commonly involved in joint decision making. *Dia*-paying groups vary in size from a few hundred to a few thousand members but each has a traditional home territory, sometimes called a *deegaan*. The whole of Somalia can be mapped out according to the traditional boundaries of the *dia*-paying group and it is this unit rather than any government-appointed body or individual that represents the interests of herders on the range.

(contributions from Darlington Akabwai of PARC-VAC and William Mogga of UNICEF-OLS)

Learn from indigenous services

In many rural areas there are traditional healers and herbalists who have provided a service to livestock keepers for many years. Even today, most modern pharmaceuticals are derived from plant remedies. Many veterinarians are wary of traditional practices because usually they have not been validated by scientists. However, people are often paying either in cash or in kind for the services of a traditional healer or similar worker. Consequently, when discussing ways to improve animal health services the existence of privately operating indigenous workers is a reflection of people's willingness to use a service that they perceive to be beneficial. This is often a useful lesson for CAHW systems and discussions about indigenous services should not be overlooked.

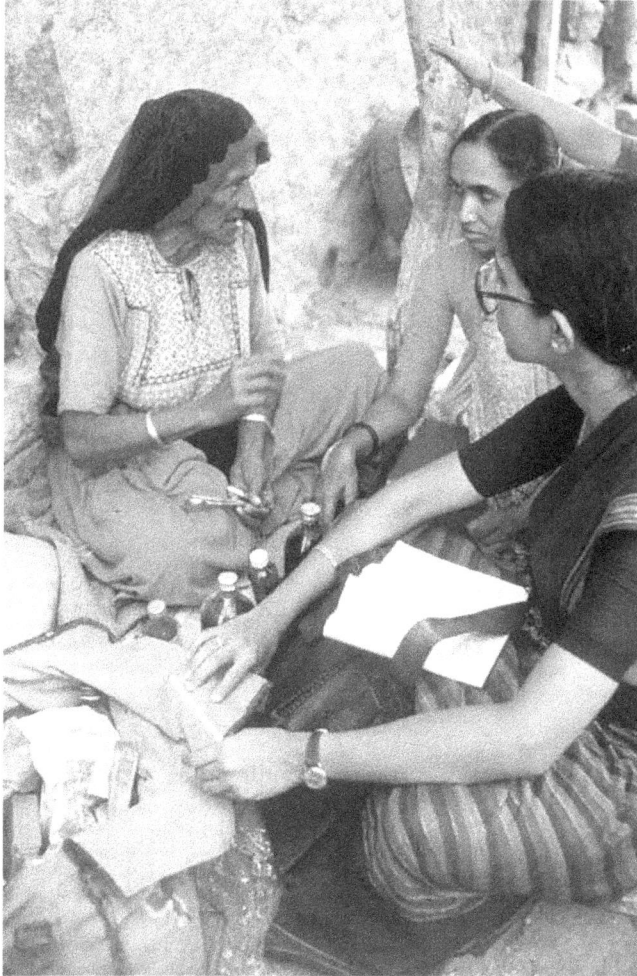

Plate 2.6 In Gujarat, India, many semi-structured interviews with livestock owners and traditional healers built up the VRTI's understanding of the work of the *deshi* doctors. In the photograph, Hasbaima talks about her knowledge of helping with difficult births and her use of local plants for treating a range of problems. Hasbaima was later trained to recognize and treat some other diseases by ITDG and VRTI and equipped with a primary animal healthcare kit. (*David Hadrill*)

Identify deficits in local knowledge

Information is needed on local animal management and who owns the animals. Livestock keepers know a great deal about their animals. However, sometimes they also believe that weak or dying animals could be saved if they had 'modern' medicines to cure diseases. This may be true, but it is essential to learn more about how the animals are kept because the way animals are looked after can cause disease. For example, under-nutrition or overcrowded, dirty pens could be significant factors and it could be more worthwhile improving animal management than treating disease.

20

Discuss willingness and ability to pay

During the survey, when the community and project staff are learning about the system, it is also necessary to discuss how animal health services will be paid for. For any service to continue, costs have to be covered. An outside funding agency may be willing to buy medicines or other materials for the project but this type of donation needs to be very carefully considered. Experience from many CAHW projects indicates that free donations of drugs or any form of subsidized drug supply system is not sustainable and, when the project closes, the system collapses. It is often better to involve existing private drug suppliers in the project or seek ways of encouraging small-scale private activities such as veterinary pharmacies to supply CAHWs. Essentially, a CAHW should be a private operator.

If people say: 'But we are so poor, we need outsiders to pay for the medicines for us', then it is necessary to discuss with them what would happen after, if outside funding is withdrawn. Discuss whether it is better to have two years of free service and then no supplies, or to have trained animal health workers able to continue to work for many years in the community. The subject of making sure the project is able to survive without outside assistance is dealt with in more detail in Chapter 3.

It is vital to consider this issue during the participatory survey and subsequent project planning. The community is going to have to pay for the project's inputs eventually, and discussions must be held to make this concept clear.

Consider incentives for CAHWs

It is not only the procurement of project inputs such as medicines that needs to be considered at a very early stage in relation to project sustainability. If a CAHW system seems to attract approval during a participatory survey, project staff must also think about incentives for CAHWs and raise this issue as soon as possible with the community. In many cases, CAHWs have been expected to provide their services free of charge but, in those projects where this has happened, the CAHWs have often dropped out of the system. Examples of incentives include:

- *cash;*
- *raised status and more respect from the community in which they work;*
- *payment in kind (for example, exchanging milk or live animals for services rendered);*
- *the chance to go away to training courses;*
- *a combination of these things.*

It is usually necessary to reward the CAHWs with cash payments to keep them doing the job – cash rather than credit is the norm. However, communities can discuss this and agree a system which keeps both livestock owners and CAHWs happy. The important point is that this discussion must take place during the 'getting started' stages of the project.

Planning and conducting the survey

With knowledge of some of the important information which needs to be collected in the participatory survey, the survey team can begin to plan its work and conduct the survey. Advice on planning participatory surveys can be found in many of the PA manuals listed in the 'Further reading' section. However, some important points to remember are:

- Inform the community well in advance that you are planning to visit and would like to spend time discussing livestock issues. Give an idea of the time period that you intend to stay in the area and, preferably, stay at least one night in the village. Avoid visits during busy periods (e.g. harvest time) or holidays.
- Recognize local customs regarding outsiders' access to women. Always try to include trained female facilitators in your survey team and be aware that women and other groups are only available for discussion at certain times of day.
- Clarify the arrangements for accommodation and food for the survey team, including payment.
- Draw up a work plan with the survey team so that all team members are clear about their roles; think carefully about how the team will be introduced and how the purpose of the visit will be explained to the community. Be open and do not raise expectations about future assistance.
- Leave time for proper analysis and discussion of the survey findings towards the end of the survey.

Some useful participatory methods

Looking more closely at participatory methods, as mentioned previously there are many useful manuals and guides already available (see Further reading) and the need to train veterinary staff is discussed in this chapter (see *Training for project veterinary staff*). Participatory methods that are particularly useful for understanding and analysing livestock health and husbandry issues are listed in Table 2.1.

This list is intended as a guide and should not necessarily be followed rigorously in every situation. Project staff can adapt the information needs and methods of data collection according to local conditions and, if possible, previous experience of using participatory tools in different areas. For example, while some informants respond well to visual tools such as mapping and diagrams, others prefer oral communication and interview-type methods.

The following section provides more details about some of the participatory methods listed in Table 2.1. Again, readers should consult general PA manuals or attend training courses in order to learn about and practise the use of participatory methods.

Table 2.1 *The design of a participatory survey: information needs and tools for understanding community perceptions of animal healthcare needs*

Information needed	Useful participatory tools
Socio-political	
• system boundary from the community perspective and official perspective	social maps
• social organization e.g. clans, castes, religious and wealth groups	Venn diagrams
• local leaders in the community; are they government appointed or traditional leaders? How are they elected and what is their role?	semi-structured interviews (SSI)
• existing modes for collective decision making and action	SSI
Livelihoods	
• relative importance of different food production and income-generation methods for households of different wealth and location in the project area	natural resource maps, ranking, proportional piling and wealth ranking
• seasonal variations in the above	seasonal calendars
• household-level division of labour and ownership of assets	labour calendars
Livestock husbandry and health	
• types of livestock reared; relative importance/uses/value for different wealth and gender groups including both economic and socio-cultural benefits of livestock	livestock species scoring
• approximate livestock holdings	proportional piling
• livestock management, seasonal tasks, division of labour and decision making roles of different family members	grazing maps, movement maps and seasonal calendars
• constraints to livestock ownership and production, relative importance of constraints	scoring
• important animal health problems	livestock disease scoring, progeny histories
• seasonal variations in disease incidence	disease calendars
Existing animal health services	
• options for treating sick animals	service maps
• use of traditional medicines and healer	SSI
• existing levels of payment for different types of service	SSI
• relative importance of options according to user wealth and type of health problem	proportional piling, scoring
• constraints facing existing services, relative importance of constraints	SSI, scoring
Options for improving animal health services	
• community perceptions of the value of treatments for different animal health problems	SSI
• community perceptions of need to develop services by type of service	SSI, scoring
• relative importance of different service characteristics e.g. cost, availability, accessibility, personal relations with health worker	SSI, scoring

Box 2.5 Participatory mapping

Some of the benefits of participatory mapping are as follows:

◆ Some types of information are best expressed using a diagram. For example, it is usually easier to explain the geography of an area using a map rather than a verbal description alone.

◆ When a large map is constructed on the ground, many people can see what is going on and can contribute to the map. Therefore, many people can participate.

◆ People do not need to be literate to construct a map.

◆ The process of map-making requires action and discussion among the participants. Therefore, participatory mapping is a useful method to use at the beginning of a survey. The method acts as a kind of 'ice-breaker'.

◆ Maps can illustrate a considerable amount of information e.g. the boundaries of a community, types of natural resources, grazing areas, location of services, roads, footpaths, wells, areas infested with biting flies or ticks, and so on.

◆ Maps can also show movement of livestock e.g. seasonal movements to grazing areas.

Method

◆ Ask the groups of informants to construct maps on the ground using simple, locally available materials.

◆ Explain to the informants the types of information they might show on the map.

◆ It is often useful to ask different age or gender groups to construct their own maps, and then compare the maps. This can show how different people perceive and prioritize different issues.

◆ Leave the informants sufficient time to complete the map, say 45 minutes to one hour. Do not interfere, but be available to provide advice if requested.

◆ When the map is completed, ask the informants to explain the map to you. Use open or probing questions to follow up interesting features of the map and cross-check information.

Examples of participatory mapping are shown in Figures 2.1 and 2.2

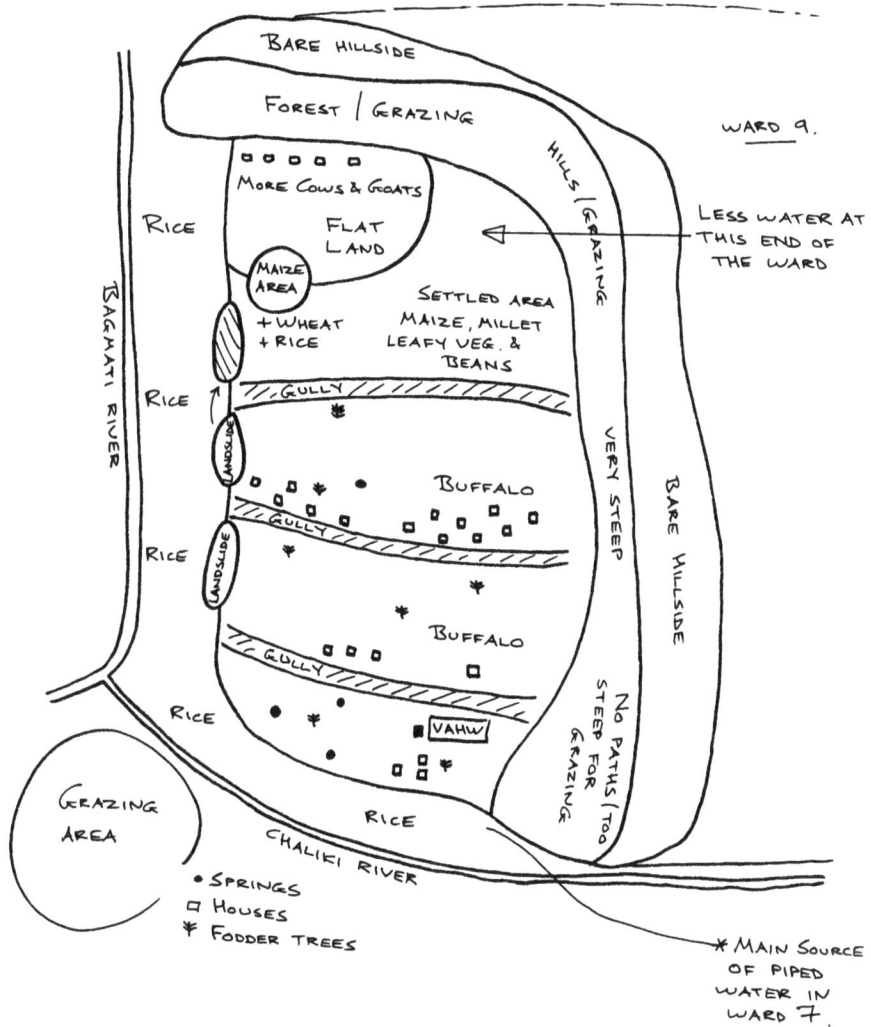

Figure 2.1 Map of Pyutar Village Development Committee area, Ward 9 by Krishna Bahadur Thing and Iman Singh Ghale. (Source: RRA Notes 20 IIED)

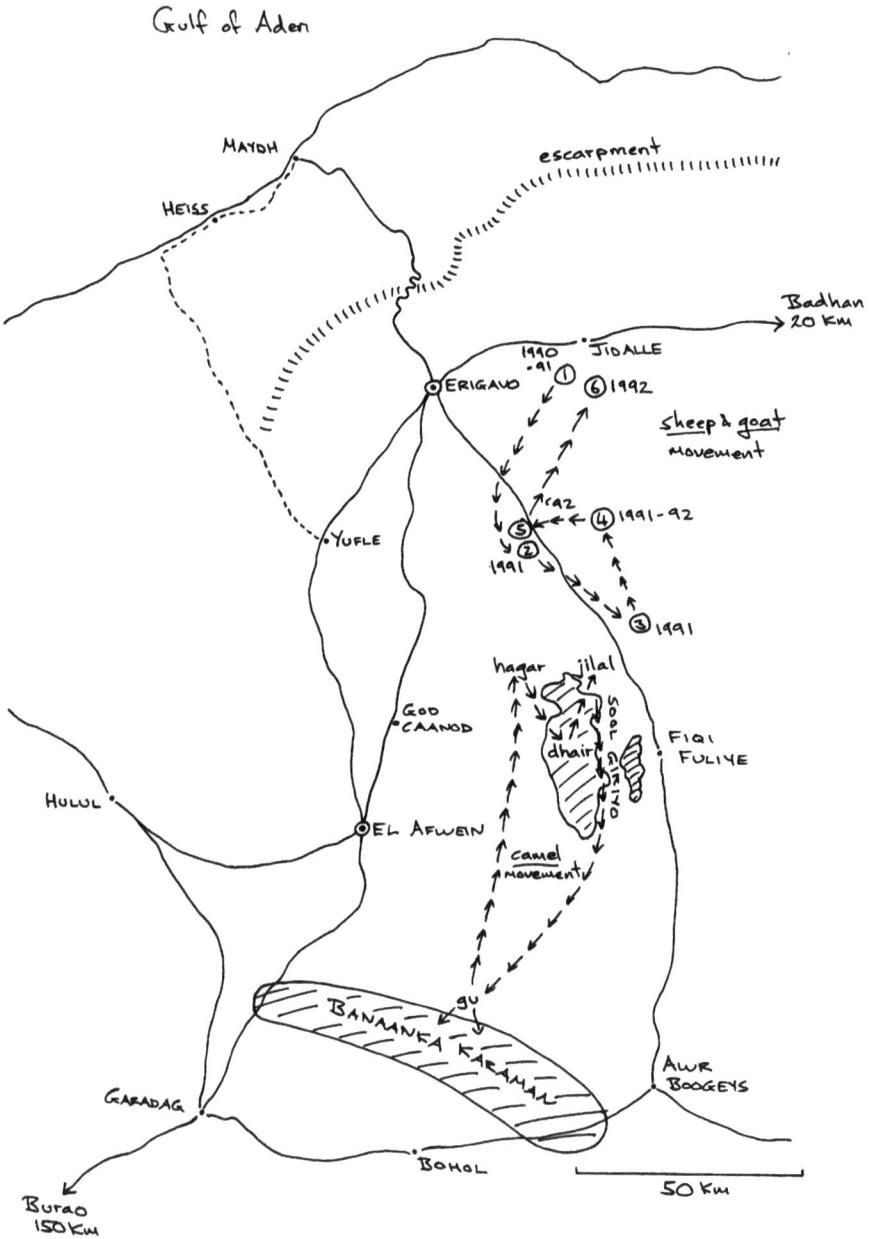

Gulf of Aden

MAYDH

HEISS

escarpment

Badhan
→ 20 Km

ERIGAVO

1990 -91 ① JIDALLE

⑥ 1992

sheep & goat movement

YUFLE

gu2

⑤ ④ 1991-92

② 1991

③ 1991

hagar   jilal

SOOL DIRIYO

dhair

FIQI FULIYE

GOD CAANOD

HULUL

EL AFWEIN

camel movement

gu

BANAANKA KARAMAN

AWR BOOGEYS

GARADAG

BOHOL

50 Km

Burao
150 Km

Figure 2.2 Mapping livestock movements in Sanaag region, Somaliland.

Table 2.2 Seasonal movements of livestock in Sanaag region, Somaliland

Season	Description of movement	
	Camels	Sheep and goats
Gu (spring rain)	They often go down to the plains at Karaman (south of El Afwein) if it is peaceful; otherwise to Sool Giriyo.	When it rains, they move to the south of the district (e.g. Sool Giriyo).
Hagar (hot, summer)	They stay on the plains, remaining close to water sources such as Gof.	Towards the escarpment and windy close to the water points (Madare, Erigavo area).
Dhair (autumn rain)	If there is plenty of rain they move to Sool Giriyo.	To the plains (Sool Giriyo, Qaarey).
Jilaal (long, dry winter)	Stay near water sources around Sool Giriyo e.g. Gof.	To the nearest water source, especially towards the escarpment.

Box 2.6 The question list from the ethnoveterinary interview guide

The ethnoveterinary question list is intended for use during informal, semi-structured interviews. The list can easily be memorized and each question is more of a prompt for opening up discussion than a rigid question in a questionnaire. More guidance on the use of the ethnoveterinary question list can be found in the publications listed in the 'Further reading' section.

1. What species, breeds, ages and sexes of animals are affected by this disease?
2. Is there seasonality or other timing to the appearance of the disease?
3. Does it usually affect one animal or a group of animals at the same time? Does it spread from animal to animal (i.e. is it contagious or infectious)?
4. What causes the disease: natural/physical causes, supernatural/non-physical causes or both? Describe.
5. Are there ways to prevent/avoid this disease? If so, what are they?
6. Describe the main symptoms, if possible in order of progression and timing. What is the first symptom seen and when? Also, what is the symptom, if any, which makes you decide it is this specific disease?
7. Are traditional treatments available? Basically what are they? Where/how are they obtained? What happens when they are used? (Please be as specific as possible.)
8. Are modern treatments available? What are they? Where/how are they obtained? What happens when they are used? (Please be as specific as possible.)
9. What usually happens if the animal is not treated?
10. When did you last have, or hear of, an animal with this disease? What did you do and what happened to the animal?

Box 2.7 The progeny history method

Many people who are highly dependent on livestock can provide detailed historical information on specific animals in a herd. For example, pastoralists in Africa often name each of their cattle or camels, and can describe the performance of each animal and even its mother or grandmother. Progeny histories are livestock genealogies which detail the fate of all the offspring of particular female animals. The method uses a brief question list which is applied to animals showing varying performance as perceived by the livestock keeper and described as 'good', 'average' and 'poor'. The key questions of the progeny history method are detailed below:

1. Ask the livestock owner to give the names of six bloodlines of animals and from them choose two good adult females, two average ones and two bad ones.
2. For one good animal, write down the name of the animal and ask:
   ◆ Where did it come from?
   ◆ How many pregnancies?
   ◆ How many abortions?
   ◆ If still in herd, is she pregnant, dry or barren?
3. Then, for each birth ask:
   ◆ Was it a single or a twin? (Record twins separately)
   ◆ What happened to it?
   ◆ Why?
   ◆ Age now, or age when left herd?
   If it was female, still in the herd and had given birth, record the name of the animal.
4. When you have finished all the births of the original animal, repeat questions 2 and 3 for each of the female offspring.
5. Repeat questions 2 and 3 for at least one average and one poor animal and, time permitting, for another good, average and poor animal.

When repeated with animals in different herds, the results of various progeny histories can be summarized quantitatively and presented as pie charts. An example from Samburu District, Kenya is shown in Figure 2.3.

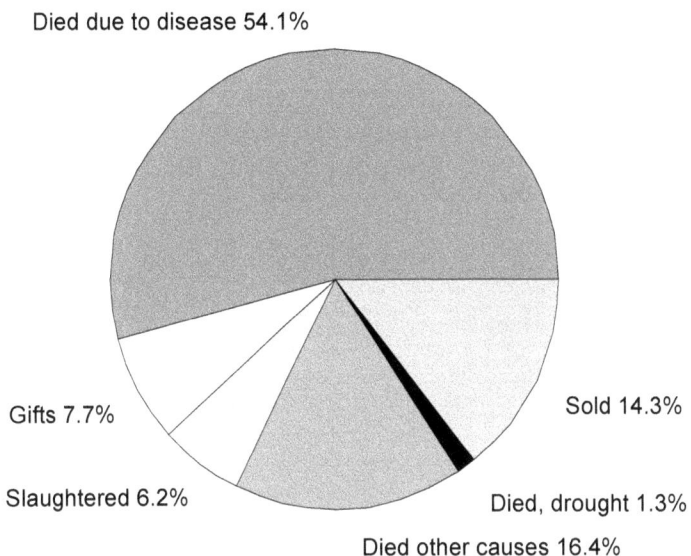

Figure 2.3 Results from the progeny history method. The pie chart summarizes the fate of sheep and goats leaving 121 Samburu flocks in Kenya.

Box 2.8 Pair-wise ranking of livestock problems

Pair-wise ranking of livestock problems is used to understand the relative importance of different problems affecting livestock. The method requires informants to produce a list of problems which are then written onto individual pieces of card or paper, or represented using everyday objects. The problems are then compared in pairs, and the most important problem identified.

The results are summarized in a table and an overall rank for each problem can be calculated by adding the number of times each problem is named. The example below is drawn from work by the Kenya Agricultural Research Institute in Nyatike Division, Migori District, Kenya. The overall ranks were found by adding up the number of times a particular problem appears in the table. For example, rinderpest appears six times in the table whereas foot and mouth appears only once. Note that the higher the rank, the more important the problem.

	SND	rabies	fleas	fmd	anaplas.	rp	ticks	drought	overall rank
drought	drought	rabies	drought	drought	drought	rp	drought	x	5
ticks	SND	rabies	fleas	fmd	anaplas.	rp	x		0
rp	rp	rabies	rp	rp	rp	x			6
anaplas.	SND	rabies	anaplas.	anaplas.	x				3
fmd	SND	rabies	fleas	x					1
fleas	SND	rabies	x						2
rabies	rabies	x							7
SND	x								4

Note:
anaplas. = anaplasmosis
rp = rinderpest
fmd = foot and mouth disease
SND = swollen neck and diarrhoea

Box 2.9 Livestock disease scoring

This scoring method is a more detailed analysis of livestock disease than simple pair-wise ranking. It not only prioritizes livestock diseases, but also gives reasons behind the choices that people make and shows the relative importance of these reasons against each disease.

Step 1: Identification of diseases to be scored

Ask people to name between five and ten important animal health problems using questions such as: 'What are the six most important livestock diseases in your animals throughout the year?' Write the diseases named by the informants onto separate pieces of card using the local language. Check that at least one informant is literate. If all informants are illiterate use different everyday objects to represent each named disease e.g. a stone could represent worms, a leaf could represent foot and mouth disease, and so on.

Step 2: Pair-wise comparison of the named items

First, choose two of the named diseases (represented as name cards or objects) and ask the question: 'Which of these two diseases is most important and why?' The informants will prioritize the two diseases and provide reasons for their decision. These reasons are called 'indicators'. Record all the responses and repeat the question until each disease has been compared with every other disease. At the end of the pair-wise comparisons of all the diseases, there will be a list of indicators that the informants used to compare the diseases.

Step 3: Scoring of diseases against indicators

Place the disease name cards or objects in a row on the ground. Collect a pile of stones using five stones per disease, for example if six diseases are being scored, 30 stones are required. Remind the informants of the first indicator mentioned during the pair-wise comparison; ask them to distribute the stones to show the relative importance of each disease against that indicator. All 30 stones must be used. After the stones have been allocated to each item, check the scoring with the informants and allow them to alter the scoring if they wish. Record the final number of stones allocated to each item, collect the stones and then repeat the scoring for each of the indicators.

Table 2.3 shows the results of livestock disease scoring from the ActionAid-Somaliland programme. Informants selected six diseases and pair-wise comparison of these diseases produced 25 indicators for scoring. Each indicator was scored against each disease using 30 stones.

Table 2.3 Results of livestock disease scoring with pastoralists in Sanaag region, Somaliland

	Diseases					
Indicators	Nairobi sheep disease	Coughing in camels	Worms, all species	Surra	Ulcerative balano-posthitis, sheep	Pox diseases
reduced local sale value	0	4	4	5	7	10
reduced export value	0	0	0	0	11	19
disease causes poverty	19	0	3	0	0	8
animal dies	15	0	6	0	0	9
animal lies down	7	0	23	0	0	0
animal becomes thin	0	0	17	13	0	0
animal aborts	0	24	0	0	0	6
skin is damaged	0	0	0	0	0	30
disease spread by ticks	30	0	0	0	0	0
disease in different species	0	0	0	0	0	30
milk yield falls	0	12	6	12	0	0

Table 2.3 *Continued*

Indicators	Diseases					
	Nairobi sheep disease	Coughing in camels	Worms, all species	Surra	Ulcerative balano post-hitis, sheep	Pox diseases
meat is inedible	4	0	8	0	0	18
disease cannot be treated	0	0	0	15	0	15
disease occurs in hot time	10	0	0	0	0	20
disease is contagious	0	11	0	2	4	13
disease spread by worms	0	0	30	0	0	0
disease affects sheep	22	0	0	0	8	0
causes subcutaneous oedema	0	0	16	0	6	8
disease causes diarrhoea	8	0	22	0	0	0
causes bloody diarrhoea	9	0	21	0	0	0
disease causes coughing	11	19	0	0	0	0
disease affects breeding	0	0	0	0	30	0
black lymph nodes after death	21	0	0	0	0	9
thin watery blood after death	0	6	6	11	0	7
congested meat after death	15	0	15	0	0	0

Box 2.10 Seasonal calendars of livestock diseases and disease vectors

In order to use seasonal calendars, project staff should understand and use local names for seasons, livestock diseases and biting flies, ticks or other vectors. With the participants, select important diseases, vectors or other indicators to be shown in the seasonal calendar.

Step 1

Draw a horizontal line on the ground to represent one full year. The line should be at least 1 metre in length. Divide the line according to local definitions of season and 'label' the seasons using common everyday items.

Step 2

It is useful (though not essential) to choose rainfall as the first indicator to be illustrated on the calendar. Take a set number of counters, for example 20 seeds. Ask the group to distribute the seeds among the seasons to show the relative proportion of rainfall by season.

Step 3

Take a second set of 20 seeds. For one of the diseases selected by the group, represent the disease using an object or simple line drawing. Ask the group to distribute the seeds according to the number of cases of that disease seen in each season.

Step 4

Repeat this procedure until all diseases, vectors or other indicators have been scored against each season.

Step 5

Ask the informants to explain the diagram. Use probing questions (e.g. Why? How?) to follow up interesting results.

The seasonal calendar shown in Figure 2.4 was produced by groups of Dinka livestock keepers in southern Sudan. It shows the seasonal pattern of rainfall, cattle diseases, biting flies, ticks and snails. The black dots represent the number of seeds that were used during the construction of the seasonal calendar.

It is important to 'interview' the seasonal calendar by asking the informants questions about it. For example:

◆ 'You've shown me that, for most diseases, most sick animals are seen during the season called *ruil*. Why is this?'
◆ 'Which diseases do the flies called *rum* transmit?'
◆ 'From the diagram, I can see that many of the flies, ticks and snails are most numerous during the rainy seasons. Why is this?'
◆ 'When is the best time of year to treat cattle with the disease called *jong acom*?'

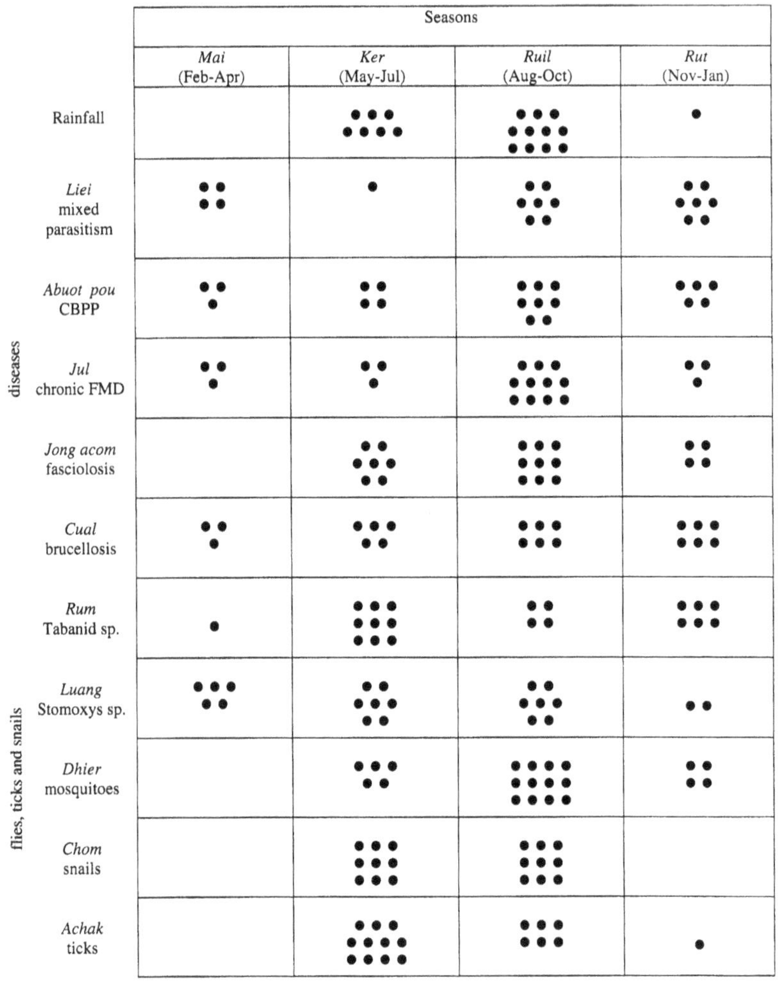

	Seasons			
	Mai (Feb-Apr)	*Ker* (May-Jul)	*Ruil* (Aug-Oct)	*Rut* (Nov-Jan)
Rainfall		••• ••••	••• ••• ••••	•
Liei mixed parasitism (diseases)	•• ••	•	•• ••• ••	•• •• ••
Abuot pou CBPP (diseases)	•• •	•• ••	••• ••• ••	••• ••
Jul chronic FMD (diseases)	•• •	•• •	••• ••••• •••••	•• •
Jong acom fasciolosis (diseases)		•• •• ••	••• ••• •••	•• ••
Cual brucellosis (diseases)	•• •	••• ••	••• •••	••• •••
Rum Tabanid sp. (flies, ticks and snails)	•	••• ••• •••	•• ••	••• •••
Luang Stomoxys sp. (flies, ticks and snails)	••• ••	•• •• ••	•• •• ••	••
Dhier mosquitoes (flies, ticks and snails)		••• ••	•••• ••• ••••	••
Chom snails (flies, ticks and snails)		••• ••• •••	••• ••• •••	
Achak ticks (flies, ticks and snails)		••• •••• ••••	••• •••	•

Figure 2.4 Seasonal calendar for cattle disease, biting flies, ticks and snails produced by Dinka herders from southern Sudan.

Analysing the information and making decisions

When using a community-based approach, it is important that the analysis of survey findings takes place within the community and becomes an integral part of the participatory survey process. This approach allows information to be cross-checked and, if necessary, action can be taken to follow up contradictory or confusing findings. As survey information is collated and summarized, copies of diagrams, maps, tables and important notes can be provided to community representatives almost immediately. This allows people to see that their views are an important part of the analysis and, by receiving their own copies of the information, they have clear ownership of the information. These aspects of participatory assessment contrast markedly with conventional surveys in which data is taken away from communities and analysed by researchers alone. In many cases, community representatives never receive a copy of the survey report.

When the analysis of findings is complete, project staff hold further discussion with the community to decide if a CAHW system is appropriate, practical and sustainable. In this process, meetings are held between the community and project staff at which the information is shared and used to answer the key questions outlined below. Facilitators (helpers from outside the community or project staff) have an important role in ensuring that everyone has a voice and that the meetings deal with the key questions in the time available without straying too far from the subject.

It will be necessary to hold a lot of meetings, taking care that all community groups are represented. The outside helpers must be very sensitive to local customs here. For example, if may be necessary to have separate meetings for women with female facilitators. Poorer groups must be given as much opportunity to state their case as the wealthier, who are often more powerful. Outside facilitators need to help all community members agree that the resulting plans are based on their needs, which have been learnt together by the outsiders and community during the information-gathering process.

Key question: Are animal health problems a major constraint for poorer livestock owners?

Are there other more important constraints? For example, marketing or animal management practices? If so, would a CAHW project be a practical solution to these problems for the livestock owners targeted by the project? Would animal management training be more useful?

Experience from the field

In India, cattle owners wanted antibiotics to treat infections in young calves. The calves were commonly born in houses where the floors were not cleaned and so infections entered the calves' bodies via the umbilical cord soon after birth. The appropriate solution was to clean the floors and to dip the cords in iodine solution. This was cheaper and more effective than trying to cure disease with antibiotics.

In Pakistan, working donkeys carrying loads of bricks at brick kilns were being treated regularly for pressure sores on their backs. However, a more appropriate intervention was to improve the padding and design of the harness and to improve the nutrition of the animals.

Key question: What are the main animal health problems to be addressed?

Is CAHW an appropriate response? Are major animal health concerns part of a bigger, national disease control programme? Can the two be combined? How should the government veterinary service be involved?

In some projects, government veterinarians have assisted with participatory surveys, training of CAHWs and drug supply. In most areas, government policy and legislation on CAHWs should also be considered (see Chapter 8).

Key question: What are the practical considerations for establishing a project?

Which groups most need community animal healthcare? Women, children, young men or older people? Are the needs of all groups the same?

> #### Experience from the field
> *In parts of south-west Uganda, men look after cattle, but women and children look after chickens, goats and sheep. In Somaliland, only young men look after the camels in the dry season when they move far from the camp looking for forage.*

Key question: Would any local interest groups make it difficult for CAHWs to function?

Would the government be co-operative? Which local, influential people are unhappy about the proposal (for example, local leaders or government vet staff)? What needs to be done to convince them to support the project?

Key question: How would a CAHW service be able to continue (be sustained) after the end of the project?

Consider how the service is to be paid for by the livestock owners. Consider the possibility of opening shops (preferably run by veterinary professionals) to supply medicines.

If most of the above key questions can be satisfactorily answered, a CAHW project may be appropriate and practical. However, there may still be important stakeholders who do not agree with the project and might even try to prevent the project starting. For example, private drug traders or government vets might hear rumours that the project is planning to give free drugs to CAHWs and this activity would disrupt their own business interests.

In order to prevent misunderstandings and make sure that all stakeholders agree with the proposal to start a CAHW project, the various stakeholders can be invited to a workshop to discuss all the issues and possible solutions. This type of workshop is an opportunity for community representatives to work with the project to present their ideas to other stakeholders and obtain feedback. Plans must be discussed with all sectors.

2.3 The first stages of project implementation

Defining roles and responsibilities

Assuming that there is agreement that a CAHW system is feasible in the project area, the next stage is to define *and document* the roles and responsibilities of the different

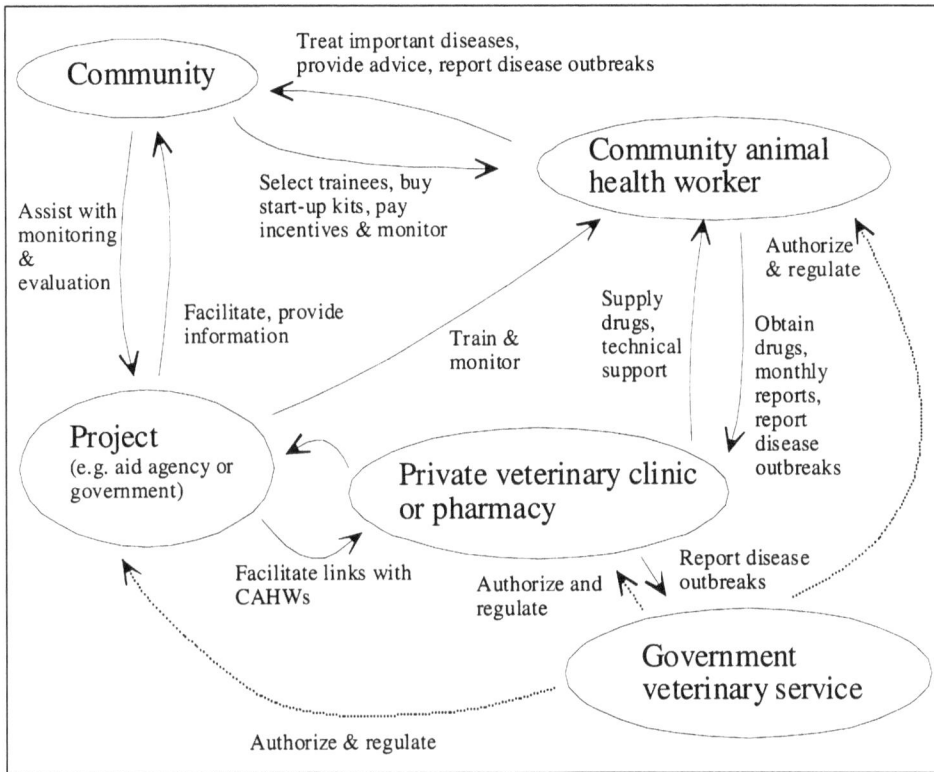

Figure 2.5 Examples of roles and responsibilities in a community-based animal health system.

players and prepare written agreements or memoranda of understanding. These agreements can prove to be very useful in the event of future misunderstanding and claims that groups or individuals were not aware of their responsibilities. An example of the types of roles and responsibilities in a CAHW project is provided in Figure 2.5. In this example, it can be seen that there are a number of key actors and organizations with a stake in the project, and the various linkages between these groups can be quite complicated. In part, this is one reason for ensuring that roles and responsibilities are clearly defined and written down.

Relationships between the different players will vary from project to project. In some cases, a private veterinary clinic or pharmacy will be absent at the beginning of a project but may develop as the project progresses. For example, in some countries the veterinary privatization process is supporting private facilities to develop in areas where government formerly provided all services. In the example above, the system has been designed so that the external agency (project) can leave the system after a relatively short time period. In this scenario, either private veterinarians or government can take over the role of providing training or refresher training for CAHWs. The most important aspect of the system is that communities take responsibility for selecting CAHWs and working with the project to monitor CAHW activities.

Looking at the specific roles of the CAHWs

The roles of the CAHWs should be discussed with the community during the participatory survey and when formulating agreements between the project's stakeholders. The role of the CAHWs depends on many factors, including which

---

Box 2.11 Examples of the roles of CAHWs

Wasaidizi wa Mifugo **(Helpers of Livestock), ITDG, Kenya**

◆ Treat animal health problems using unscheduled drugs, for example helminths, ticks, foot-rot, eye problems, mange and skin problems, fleas and lice, wounds, foot trimming, bloat, constipation, coccidiosis.
◆ Assist with difficult births.
◆ Refer difficult cases and diseases requiring the use of scheduled drugs such as antibiotics to a vet or other animal health professional.
◆ Vaccinate chickens against Newcastle disease.
◆ Sell unscheduled drugs to farmers for routine treatments e.g. deworming.
◆ Advise farmers on feeding and husbandry e.g. improved housing.

Operation Lifeline Sudan Livestock Programme, southern Sudan

◆ Diagnose and treat common diseases, for example helminths, pneumonia, trypanosomiasis, ticks and mange.
◆ Sell drugs to livestock keepers for routine treatments.
◆ Monitor and report diseases.
◆ Vaccinate cattle and carry out active surveillance for rinderpest (depending on area).

Basic Veterinary Workers, FAO, Afghanistan

◆ Treat common animal health problems, for example helminths, ticks, mange and other skin problems, bloat, stomach problems, pneumonia, tick-borne diseases, dystocia, foot-rot, foot trimming.
◆ Treat common poultry problems, for example coccidiosis, fleas and lice.
◆ Assist the vet in vaccination campaigns e.g. enterotoxaemia.
◆ Sell drugs to livestock keepers for routine treatments.
◆ Provide advice on improved husbandry methods.

Community-based animal health workers, SCF(UK), Regional Bureau of Agriculture, Region 3, Ethiopia

◆ Treat external and internal parasites.
◆ Castrate livestock.
◆ Refer difficult cases to government veterinary clinics or subclinics.

---

animal health problems the project is attempting to address, the needs of the community for animal health services, and government policy on disease control and drug use. CAHWs may be involved in such activities as treating animals, providing advice on animal husbandry, vaccination, improving drug supply to livestock keepers, and disease surveillance and monitoring. Some roles of CAHWs in different projects are summarized in Box 2.11.

The various roles that CAHWs can play means that they need a wide range of skills and knowledge. In addition to knowing how to treat animals, they also need to manage and replenish their drug kits, know how to charge livestock keepers for their services, how to provide advice on animal husbandry, how to keep records, and how to store drugs and vaccine. Some important issues to consider about the role of the CAHWs are discussed below.

a. Which diseases should CAHWs be trained to treat?

The decision about which diseases to train the CAHWs to treat depends on several factors, which must be discussed carefully with the community, veterinarian and government staff. The factors include:

- which diseases the community would like to be addressed;
- national policy on disease control;
- disease control strategies;
- drug use regulations.

Surveys will have identified diseases of most concern to livestock keepers in the area. It is unlikely that CAHWs will be able to tackle all animal health problems, so it important that the community prioritizes which diseases it would like the CAHWs to be trained to treat. This should be done in consultation with the project veterinarian(s).

Discussions with government during the survey will have highlighted national policy on disease control. For example, control of contagious bovine plueropneumonia (CBPP) may form part of government policy and CAHWs may be required to vaccinate against this disease. Another example is the control and eradication of rinderpest in certain regions of Africa, being co-ordinated by Pan African Rinderpest Campaign (PARC) in collaboration with governments and NGOs. In these areas one role of the CAHWs may also be to help organize and carry out vaccination campaigns with the community.

Decisions will have to be made concerning the strategy for dealing with certain disease problems. For example, for helminth control, should the project adopt a policy of strategic deworming for livestock? If so, CAHWs will need to be trained on when to advise livestock owners to deworm animals and which groups of animals should be treated. Another example is tick and tick-borne disease control. Depending on the breeds of cattle present, epidemiology of important tick-borne diseases, and tick challenge, the project staff may either advise minimal dipping or spraying to strengthen animals' natural immunity, or they may advocate a strategic tick control regime.

In some projects, CAHWs may also be required to provide vaccination services, for example against enterotoxaemia in small stock, or Newcastle disease in chickens. In these cases they require specific training in vaccine storage, transport, how to mix up the vaccine and how to administer it to the animals. Most countries have regulations regarding the use of veterinary drugs, and this affects which medicines the CAHWs are permitted to handle (see below).

b. Which drugs should CAHWs be trained to use?

The drugs that CAHWs will be trained to use depends on several factors including:

- the diseases CAHWs will treat;
- government regulations on drug use;
- availability of drugs;
- strategy for dealing with drug resistance.

There are many brands and types of drugs available on the market, and the project needs to make a decision about which drugs to use for dealing with disease problems prioritized by the community. The CAHWs should only be trained to use a limited range of drugs so as to avoid confusion. Obviously they should only be trained to use drugs to treat diseases that the project has prioritized.

Government and national veterinary bodies' regulations regarding the use of certain drugs will determine which drugs the CAHWs can be trained to use. For example, in some countries the treatment for payment of animals with drugs such as antibiotics is restricted to use by livestock professionals only. In these cases CAHWs are by law only allowed to use unscheduled drugs such as anthelmintics. It is important the project is aware of the national regulations concerning drug use. However, in some cases, CAHWs are permitted to use certain scheduled drugs under the supervision of a veterinarian and in agreement with government and regulatory bodies.

Another factor to consider is the strategy for dealing with potential drug resistance. The project will need to make a decision about how this is done, for example the use of different trypanocides in alternate years.

Availability of drugs also affects the decision about which drugs CAHWs are trained to use. CAHWs should be trained to use drugs that are readily available, and not drugs that have to be constantly imported by the project. (See *Free or subsidized veterinary drugs* in Chapter 3.)

c. What livestock issues will CAHWs discuss with the community?

In many instances CAHWs will be working in areas where livestock owners have already been using some western drugs. A common problem with this is that many people underdose, or use the wrong drug for a disease, and yet have strong opinions and beliefs about how to use these drugs. CAHWs need good communication and diplomatic skills in order to persuade livestock keepers in the correct treatment of animals.

In other cases, livestock owners may have been purchasing drugs from market traders. These drugs may not have been stored in suitable conditions (e.g. they have been kept out in the sun for extended periods) or their use-by date may have passed. The advice given by such traders in the use of drugs may also be inaccurate because of, for example, a lack of knowledge. The end result is that sometimes livestock owners are buying drugs unsuitable for the treatment of their animals and are consequently wasting their money. Again, CAHWs need good communication skills in order to make both livestock owners and traders aware of these issues.

It is vital that the project does not just focus on the technical skills and knowledge of the CAHWs. Their communication skills, behaviour and attitudes are just as important. The aim of a community-based animal health project is to develop a long-term sustainable service to livestock keepers. CAHWs therefore need to build a good working relationship with their clients – the livestock keepers – which takes time. Building trust and rapport means they must be able to deal with livestock keepers in an open, respectful and friendly manner. Training sessions that examine these issues should be planned into the CAHW course. It may be that some of the CAHWs' attitudes should be challenged, for example if they are disrespectful towards traditional knowledge and experience such as herbal treatments.

Selecting CAHWs

Another very important stage at the beginning of a CAHW project is the selection of people to be trained. This process is central to the success or failure of the project. Remember that CAHWs are usually part-time workers who live in the community and keep their own animals. In mobile communities, the CAHWs should also be moving with the herds. Issues of incentives for CAHWs and payment for drugs should already have been discussed so that people are aware that the CAHW service will be a private service. Depending on the size of the community and the system boundary, more than one CAHW might be required or perhaps one female and one male CAHW would be appropriate. The number of CAHWs to be trained should be one of the discussion points during meetings.

a. Who makes the selection?

The community, including all future users of the CAH service, should have a major say in the selection of CAHW trainees. In some projects, meetings are organized with the whole community in order to discuss how the selection will take place and the criteria for selection. Large meetings like this, which involve many people, have the advantage of openness and ensuring that as many people as possible know what is happening. A common problem in CAHW systems is that a small group of influential leaders – such as community elders or local administrators – select the CAHWs without proper consultation with the community. In these situations, the leaders often select their relatives for training and the problem is made worse if project staff are trying to rush the selection process.

b. Ensuring that women participate

The project should also be sure that women's opinions on trainee selection are heard. The participatory survey should have allowed opportunities for women to discuss their roles in livestock keeping and their options for treating sick livestock. Together with the women in the community, the project will need to decide whether female CAHWs should be trained and, if so, who will be responsible for selecting the trainees. It is unlikely that men alone will opt to select female CAHWs.

In some projects, the implementing agency defines how many female CAHWs should be selected relative to male CAHWs. For example, in the Oxfam UK/Ireland project in Kotido District, Uganda, a ratio of 50 female: 50 male CAHW trainees was

---

Box 2.12 The selection of community-based animal health workers: an example of women's involvement in Karamoja, Uganda

The people living in Kotido District – a remote semi-arid area of northern Uganda – include the Dodoth ethnic group. These people are agropastoralists and for many years they were isolated from effective development activities. The Dodoth were reliant on their cattle but they did not have access to basic veterinary services. Another feature of the Dodoth community was the low status of women compared with men. Women were not allowed to speak in public meetings, and in fact it was considered shameful for them to do so. Women had little control over household assets such as livestock, and violence against women was considered to be normal. As a result, women had very low self-esteem and believed that only men had knowledge.

The Oxfam UK/Ireland Kotido Livestock Development Project aimed to improve the food security of the Dodoth community by establishing a system of CAHWs. However, one of Oxfam's main beliefs was that sustainable development could only occur if women were equally involved in development processes. Therefore the project actively sought to include women whenever possible. A number of village-level cattle crush committees were established and the project insisted that at least two women should be included on each committee. Also, an equal number of men and women were selected and trained as CAHWs.

During a review of the project, it was evident that women were taking a very active role. They were speaking openly and effectively in meetings, and the men were listening. This work shows that, even in cultures where there are strong traditional taboos regarding the role of women in society, it is possible to include women in community-based animal health services. The female CAHWs in this project were able to show that they could contribute towards improved animal health as effectively as the men. As one woman said during the project review: 'Now we have voice too.'

Box 2.13 Learning from experience: why women can perform better than men in CAHW systems

ANTHRA is an organization of women veterinary scientists working primarily on issues of livestock development in the wider context of sustainable natural resource use. Over the years we have trained over 100 community-based animal health workers – both women and men – in different states in India. Our programmes lay a major emphasis on:

◆ low-cost management options for poor and marginal farmers, particularly women;
◆ preventive healthcare and immunizations for animals;
◆ use of household and indigenous treatments;
◆ first-aid skills.

Many of our CAHWs are young and therefore village people are often doubtful about their skills, and more so in the case of a woman CAHW. Over time, however, they have been able to gain the confidence of the village community. Often this has happened when they have launched a successful preventive healthcare programme such as vaccinations and proven that diseases are successfully controlled through such intervention. The women CAHWs were initially apprehensive about their ability to administer vaccinations. However, following the training programme these women are administering vaccinations responsibly and capably.

Many young men tend to drop out of a training process because they are constantly on the look-out for more attractive 'employment options', many times outside their villages . The reality of our experience is that in extremely resource-poor regions, these CAHWs cannot expect to sustain themselves economically through just this skill alone. Interestingly, women have a far better track record in terms of post-training service to their community than young men.

(contributed by ANTHRA, India)

used (see Box 2.12). In other parts of the world, experience is beginning to show that, despite profound gender biases, women can play valuable roles in CAH systems and can outperform their male colleagues (Box 2.13).

c. How many CAHWs to train?

A frequently asked question is: 'How many CAHWs should be trained for a particular community or to cover a given area?' Unfortunately, there is no simple formula for deciding how many CAHWs are required because this will vary according to livestock population, types of livestock management, types of animal health services already in place and other factors. Although ideal veterinary staffing levels have been proposed – such as the required number of workers per Tropical Livestock Unit – these measures are very approximate and are not helpful when planning a CAHW system.

Probably the most useful approach to deciding how many CAHWs to train is to discuss the issue with the community. By reference to the number of animals and the geographical area to be covered by the CAHW, it should be possible to arrive at a reasonable estimate for the number of CAHWs needed. These estimates can be very accurate if traditional leaders are consulted because they know the numbers of animals in particular areas and the social groupings that influence the coverage of the CAHWs. (See Box 2.4 for traditional entry points.)

Despite the many advantages of using local knowledge to inform discussion on how many CAHWs to train, it is not uncommon for communities to propose more CAHWs than are necessary. This situation can arise because training in animal health topics can be very popular and many people wish to attend. Also, when communities are characterized by specific social groups (e.g. clans), each group may prefer to select one of its own as a CAHW. While this approach is socially appropriate, if there are too many CAHWs the amount of work available to each CAHW will be relatively small. Consequently, the financial and other incentives required by some CAHWs will be insufficient for them to continue working.

In some countries, the issue of how many CAHWs to train will also be influenced by trends towards the private delivery of clinical services. Ultimately, if CAHWs are linked to private outlets for veterinary medicines such as clinics or pharmacies, then the principles of private business will determine how many CAHWs are needed. Ideally, business plans for veterinary clinics or pharmacies in these areas should use market surveys to predict the demand for services. In part, the number of CAHWs trained by a private veterinarian (perhaps supported by an NGO or other agency) will be calculated from the business plan.

When considering these points about CAH systems, it should be remembered that a participatory survey can be conducted by a private vet when drawing up a business plan and credit application. Although experience with this approach is only just emerging, it offers the potential to combine the approaches and methods of participatory assessment with the community, with a sustainable system for supplying veterinary medicines to CAHWs. The involvement of the private vet also ensures adequate professional supervision of the CAHWs and technical support. These issues are discussed more fully in Chapter 3.

For new projects with no or limited experience of CAH systems, a 'pilot project' approach can be used which aims to test CAHWs on a small scale before embarking on a larger project. With this approach, learning how to design and implement CAH work is a specific objective of the project. A relatively small number of CAHWs are trained and monitored and the system is fine-tuned according to how the CAHWs perform. If the system works well, more CAHWs can be trained to fill gaps in the existing target area or to expand into new areas.

d. Selection criteria

For communities to have a clear stake in the system and feel that the CAHWs are 'their CAHWs' it is important that they have a major say in determining the criteria for selecting CAHWs. Project staff will have their own views on what makes a good CAHW, and these views can inform but should not dominate the selection process. Project staff can guide the selection and make suggestions regarding the characteristics of a suitable candidate. However, ultimately it is up to the members of the community to decide what type of person they prefer.

The project should also be aware that both the community and the project might make mistakes during the selection process. This is not always a bad thing and sometimes cannot be avoided. During monitoring and evaluation of projects (see Chapter 6), weaknesses in the system will be identified and corrected. This is part of learning how to design and manage CAHW systems. Different projects have different criteria. Box 2.14 provides some examples.

Box 2.14 Selection criteria for CAHWs

FARM Africa, Ethiopia

Ideally, the trainees should be selected by the community itself. They should be willing to serve the community, be responsible and respected members of the community. They should be successful livestock keepers themselves. They should be prepared to serve for a reasonable period and be unlikely to leave soon after training has been completed. It is not essential that they are able to read or write, although it is an added bonus if they can. Illiteracy should not prevent otherwise suitable candidates from being trained. Ideally, at least two trainees per community should be trained so that if one is sick or leaves the community then there is still one remaining.

Intermediate Technology Development Group, Kamujine, Kenya

They should:
◆ have demonstrated a commitment to helping their communities;
◆ be honest;
◆ be established, married with children and have livestock of their own;
◆ be healthy and able and willing to walk long distances.

GTZ (German Development Agency), Central Rangelands Development Project, Somalia

NAHAs (Nomadic Animal Health Assistants) ought to be:
◆ innovative, receptive and young (preferably between 20 and 30 years);
◆ well accepted by and integrated in their nomadic community;
◆ able to read, write and calculate on a basic level;

◆ willing to travel over some distance without a vehicle.

Exceptions are possible, especially over the educational level, if a *sacoyaqan* (traditional healer) is proposed for the training.

United Nations Development Programme, Community Development for Remote Township Project, Myanmar, Burma

Livestock Volunteer Workers should be:
◆ educated (at least secondary education);
◆ have spirit for community;
◆ supported by the majority of villagers;
◆ wealthy;
◆ ready to serve the community all the time;
◆ aged 25 to 40 years.

Vétérinaires sans frontières-Belgium, southern Sudan

The trainees should:
◆ be cattle owners;
◆ have grown up among cattle and their livelihood should revolve around cattle;
◆ be known by the people;
◆ be young, healthy and energetic;
◆ be obedient;
◆ be respectful;
◆ not be a thief or drunkard;
◆ not be a town-dweller;
◆ be literate or illiterate.

When people are proposed as candidates for CAHW training, it is important that they are fully aware of the tasks expected of them and the incentives they might receive. In particular, in some projects CAHWs have a misconception that they are government or NGO employees and will receive a salary from the veterinary services. It should be made very clear during the CAHW selection process that these workers are part-time, private operators who will receive incentives from the community. Incentives can take various forms (cash, food, livestock and others) and will be defined by the community and CAHWs.

e. The issue of literacy when selecting CAHWs

When discussing selection criteria, an important and often contentious point is whether CAHWs need to be literate. Experience from the field shows that there are both advantages and disadvantages to literate and illiterate CAHWs, as summarized in Box 2.15. While literacy is useful during training and reporting, it is not difficult to train illiterate CAHWs in basic animal healthcare and pictorial formats can be used for reporting (see Chapters 4, 5 and 6). In some projects, literate CAHWs are selected but these people have usually received some kind of formal education and can sometimes use their position as a CAHW as a 'stepping-stone' to better employment opportunities. In other words, educated and literate CAHWs are more likely to leave the community when better work comes along. This issue needs careful consideration during the selection of CAHWs.

Box 2.15 Some advantages and disadvantages of literate and illiterate CAHWs

Illiterate CAHWs are:

◆ more likely to have spent long periods caring for livestock and therefore possess stronger indigenous knowledge;
◆ more likely to be acceptable to livestock keepers, because livestock keepers may also be illiterate;
◆ more likely to be acceptable to livestock keepers because illiterate CAHWs are often older than literate CAHWs;
◆ less likely to use their position as a CAHW as a 'stepping-stone' to another job;
◆ less able to understand written instructions or provide written reports – *but*, effective training methods for illiterate CAHWs are well-established and pictorial reporting formats have been widely used.

Literate CAHWs are:

◆ able to use written training materials and make written reports on their activities;
◆ less likely to be acceptable to livestock keepers because, in some communities, people who have attended school are regarded as 'foreign' or corrupted with values different from those of the people in the community;
◆ more likely to have experience of, and preference for, an urban lifestyle than a rural, livestock-rearing way of life.

Note that a CAHW project that includes literacy as a criteria for trainee selection will tend to favour the selection of men over women. This is because boys' attendance at school usually exceeds girls' attendance at school.

---

f. Should traditional healers be selected as CAHWs?

As discussed previously in this chapter, in many rural communities there are traditional practitioners who treat sick livestock. The service provided by these practitioners varies enormously but can include herbal remedies, cautery, bone-splinting and assistance with difficult births. In some communities, spiritual or religious practices are also used. In addition to the type of service available, the numerous forms of payment for the use of traditional healers and the wide range of relationships between individuals in the community and the healer must be considered. Therefore, it is difficult to recommend hard and fast guidelines for the selection of local healers as CAHWs. The golden rule, if any, is to let members of the community decide. They will know about the behaviour of the traditional healers in their own area and will also hold opinions regarding the effectiveness of the service on offer. In other places, traditional veterinary knowledge is widespread and not restricted to a small number of local specialists. In these areas, it is likely that a knowledgeable livestock keeper will be aware of common traditional veterinary practices. This information should form part of the participatory survey.

Box 2.16 How can traditional healers be involved in CAHW programmes? An example from India

In India, it is ANTHRA's experience that traditional healers still play a very important role in most villages. They are 'store houses' of information on traditional knowledge, practices and remedies. At ANTHRA we have encouraged our Community Animal Health Workers to actively interact with healers and assist them on their rounds. In turn, traditional healers attend our training programmes to upgrade their own knowledge and skills. Gradually, healers have been organized into active healers' forums – and ANTHRA has provided a platform for discussion and exchange between different healer groups and farmers.

Apart from administering different modern medicines we have also trained our CAHWs to make different remedies for simple diseases using locally available materials. These medicines have become exceedingly popular with local people and this further helps in the acceptance of the CAHW by the village community.

(contributed by ANTHRA, India)

2.4   Summary

This chapter has outlined some of the important first steps in establishing a CAHW system. The main points to note are as follows:

◆ When deciding whether a CAHW system is appropriate, identify all stakeholders and start to think about how they might benefit or suffer from the project.

◆ Develop experience in using PA methods and, during animal health surveys, be sure to seek the views of women and less wealthy livestock keepers.

- Remember to refer to technical reports if these are available; if resources allow, consider combining a participatory survey with conventional disease investigation work in the project area.
- Learn from existing indigenous services and understand how these services function. How do traditional livestock healers benefit from the services they provide?
- Understand local animal health practices and language. Identify those things that people are doing well and aim to build on this knowledge. Also recognize weaknesses in traditional knowledge and prompt discussions on how these weaknesses might be overcome.
- Financial sustainability is a crucial issue in CAHW systems. Introduce concepts like payment for services and CAHW incentives as soon as possible during dialogue with livestock keepers (see Chapter 3).
- Stakeholder workshops can be a useful way to bring all the key players together and identify 'best bet' options for improving basic animal health services. Community representatives can present their views directly to other stakeholders.
- Selection of CAHWs requires careful facilitation and patience. Try not to rush and allow plenty of time for people to select their CAHWs. Do not allow a small group of elders or government officials to dominate the selection process and ensure that women are properly represented.

These stages form the basis of a CAH system and, when conducted well, allow local people to have a big say in deciding how a new service will develop. Ultimately, CAHWs should be responsible to the communities they serve and therefore the responsibility for selecting and supporting CAHWs should lie with the community.

Trust and open working relationships between projects and livestock keepers do not happen overnight and the project should be willing to invest much time during the early stages to listen to people's views and understand local decision-making processes. This time factor, together with adequate resources for training project staff in participatory methods, should feature in project proposals to funding agencies. In the past, many projects have tended to rush to train CAHWs without thinking about how the system will function in the long term. CAHWs are of little use if they cannot be properly selected, monitored or supplied with veterinary drugs.

In Box 2.17, a methodology for establishing CAHW systems is outlined which has evolved from the experiences of various projects from around the world. This methodology has proven to be very successful but note that many months can pass before CAHWs are even selected. Although there is sometimes pressure from donors or government to train CAHWs as quickly as possible, this approach often results in problems that require much time and effort to correct later on.

Box 2.17 Initial stages in the PARC-VAC approach to community-based animal health in eastern Africa

Feasibility study/site selection

The study is carried out using simple rapid appraisal tools in order to convince the facilitating project or private veterinarian of the importance of livestock and the perceived problems of the area. In order for livestock owners to share in any animal health activities they have to prioritize animal health as a problem. If other problems are more pressing then these problems cannot be disregarded.

PA/community dialogue/social contract or community action plan

Once a decision to become more involved in a given location has been made, the work of establishing a community-based service begins. People participate in joint analysis, development of action plans and formation or strengthening of local institutions. As groups take control over local decisions and determine how available resources are used, so they have a stake in maintaining structures or practices. Important aspects of PA are:

◆ Build on what people already know.
◆ Develop people's abilities and skills to analyse and evaluate their surroundings and problems.
◆ Reveal whether human and material resources are being used efficiently and effectively.
◆ Help people to analyse their individual situations and see how their activities may be altered in a beneficial manner, thus setting local priority needs.
◆ Enable people to study their own methods of organization and management.
◆ Provide good information for making decisions about planning and project direction.
◆ Increase the sense of collective responsibility for project development, implementation, monitoring and evaluation.
◆ Identify indicators for monitoring and evaluation purposes later in the project.
◆ Conclude with a community action plan (sometimes called a social contract). This plan can be verbal or written. It is can only be formulated once all sections of the community are in agreement and understand its implications.

The above process can take several months, but it is the most important phase because it is the foundation for all future activities. The complexities – both political and geographical – of reaching the ordinary livestock owners as opposed to their local authority representatives should not be underestimated. It is this phase that poses the biggest financial burden on the project (and a prospective private veterinary practice), and a considerable investment in terms of project facilitation is also required. It does not preclude provision of relatively simple financing schemes to suitably committed private individuals.

Taking a long-term perspective: sustainability issues

Andy Catley, Tim Leyland and Boniface Kaberia

CONTENTS

3.1   Introduction

Experience from around the world has shown how community-based animal health workers (CAHWs) can provide basic veterinary care and improve the health of livestock in rural areas. With proper selection and training, CAHWs can adequately diagnose important diseases and prevent or treat diseases. In some areas, CAHWs are important sources of advice for livestock keepers or they act as reporters of disease outbreaks. Clearly then, CAHWs have useful roles to play in primary-level veterinary service delivery. Despite this situation, the sustainability of CAHW systems is often questioned, and rightly so.

This chapter describes experiences related to the sustainability of CAHW systems and explains how project sustainability can be strengthened. By 'sustainability', we mean that CAHWs can continue to work effectively after an agency such as a non-governmental organization (NGO) or government has withdrawn direct financial assistance. Also, the CAHW system should be able to respond to new opportunities and challenges, and draw on technical support when it is required. To a large extent, sustainability is linked to community participation. When local people have a say in the design and implementation of services, such services are more likely to be used and supported. The important participatory elements of CAHW services during the 'getting started' phase are described in Chapter 2, and in this chapter we develop some of these ideas further by looking at different levels of participation in community-based projects.

In addition to issues of community participation, CAHW services are often constrained by poor financial sustainability. Therefore, in much of this chapter we take a detailed look at the need for CAHWs to acquire veterinary medicines from an efficient and high-quality outlet. Typically, such outlets are operated by the private sector. We also explain how a clear explanation of the roles and responsibilities of the different players in any CAHW project is vital in order to avoid confusion. In the long term, CAHWs require monitoring and supervision by a veterinarian or other qualified worker. As new veterinary products come onto the market and as their experience grows, refresher training of CAHWs is also required. These features of CAHW systems mean that the costs of monitoring, supervision and refresher training have to be built into the system. Training of CAHWs is described in Chapters 4 and 5, and CAHW monitoring is described in Chapter 6.

From a broader perspective, sustainability also requires consideration of environmental issues. These include careful use of veterinary medicines and disposal of unwanted medicines to avoid environmental contamination and human health risks. Also, increased off-take of livestock from areas with limited natural resources may be required. This can mean that marketing systems have to exist in the project area, or evolve as animal health and production improves. Livestock marketing is also related to people's ability to acquire cash to pay for veterinary services, and therefore livestock production, livestock health, marketing and environmental sustainability are closely interrelated.

In addition to financial, environmental and marketing issues, the long-term survival of CAHWs depends on appropriate policies and legislation. This is a crucial and growing feature of CAHW initiatives and assumes that formal recognition or certification of CAHWs will improve the sustainability and quality of service they offer. Numerous experiences on policy and legislative reform are described in Chapter 8, with advice on 'how-to-do-it'.

A livestock market in western Eritrea.

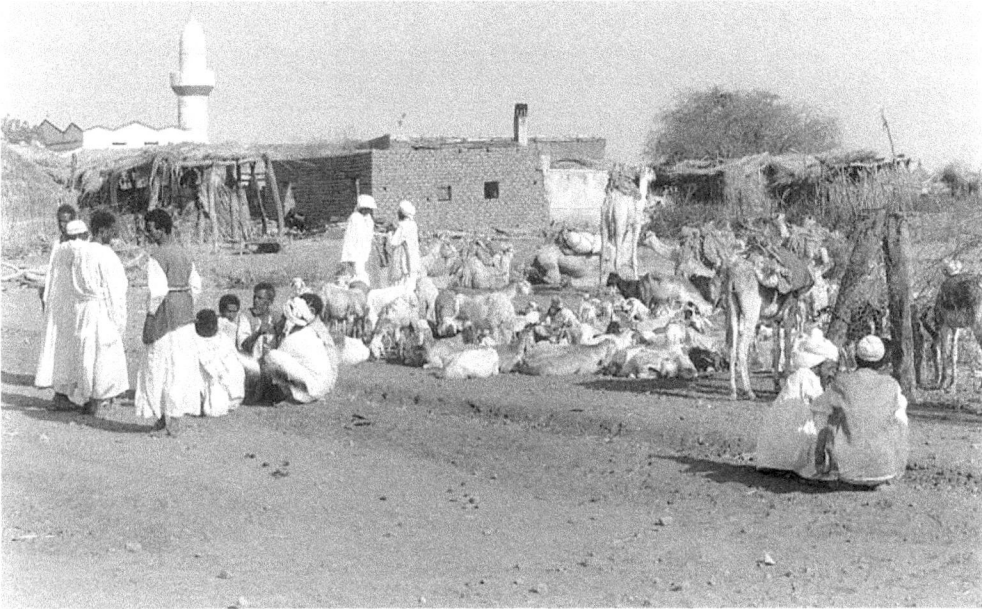

Plate 3.1 Active livestock markets are a major influence on the long-term viability of CAHW services. (*Andy Catley*)

Box 3.1 What do we mean by 'sustainability'? Factors affecting the sustainability of CAHW services

Continuation of CAHW work independent of day-to-day project support

◆ level of stakeholder and community participation when establishing the project;
◆ proper selection of the CAHWs;
◆ CAHWs offering appropriate treatments and services;
◆ good-quality training;
◆ clear understanding within the community about how the finances of the system work, including the incentives for the CAHW to keep working, and pricing of drugs and services;
◆ clear understanding within the community about roles and responsibilities.

Financial sustainability

◆ stakeholder and community involvement in financial discussions from the start;
◆ a clear understanding about who pays the incentive to keep the CAHWs, AHAs, vets etc. working;
◆ an understanding of who pays for different layers of the service (training, support, supervision etc.);

- issues of subsidy, hidden costs, free drugs or services – if these are part of the project they are recognized and discussed;
- small business training to CAHWs, community drugstore owners, village committees etc. as necessary;
- competition – affected by policy and legislation.

Continuation of the system within which the CAHWs are working

- policy and legislation;
- competition from other systems, for example government vets, private vets, other NGOs with different agendas;
- training on community development, participatory training available for vets and others;
- subsidies and cost recovery issues.

Consistency of service

- refresher training;
- training of future CAHWs;
- support and supervision.

Marketing and monetization

- understanding changes within the community such as increasing needs for cash of which the CAHW project is only one part;
- marketing of animals and animal products and whether this can realistically be facilitated;
- small business training.

Environmental considerations

- care in choice and use of drugs;
- care in approach to ethnoveterinary knowledge (EVK), especially if some plant treatments are to be endorsed or encouraged;
- understanding of subliminal effects of the project – the way that external project personnel behave towards the environment in the use of vehicles, fuel and other natural resources.

3.2 Community participation, sustainability and training needs

Community participation in the design and running of CAHW services has very real implications for the sustainability of services. Many of the participatory activities described in Chapter 2 are intended to ensure that local people are involved in defining problems, proposing solutions and implementing projects in partnership with technical staff. While on paper this type of approach seems to be widely accepted, in reality veterinary professionals have different views about the meaning and application of community participation. In some projects, participation is viewed as a process of simple 'involvement'. Here, it is argued that because people are involved in the project they must be participating, even though they do not have any decision-making responsibilities. Such projects tend to have poor sustainability because, ultimately, local people have limited say on key issues such as the most important livestock diseases to be addressed, the criteria for selecting CAHWs or the prices of veterinary drugs. Other projects aim to support 'interactive community participation', as summarized in Box 3.2. With this approach, the project is very much the community's project and the community members have major decision-making and implementing responsibilities. By encouraging a strong sense of local ownership and control, services are more likely to be sustained in the long term.

Box 3.2 Types of community participation and sustainability: which type of participation best describes your project?

1.	Manipulative participation (Co-option)	Community participation is simply a pretence; people's representatives on official boards are not elected and have no power.
2.	Passive participation (Compliance)	Communities participate by being told what has been decided or already happened. Involves unilateral announcements by an administration or project management without listening to people's responses. The information belongs only to external professionals.
3.	Participation by consultation	Communities participate by being consulted or by answering questions. External agents define problems and information-gathering processes, and so control analysis. Such a consultative process does not concede any share in decision making, and professionals are under no obligation to take on board people's views.
4.	Participation for material incentives	Communities participate by contributing resources such as labour, in return for material incentives (e.g. food, cash). It is very common to see this called 'participation', yet people have no stake in prolonging practices when the incentives end.
5.	Functional participation (Cooperation)	Community participation is seen by external agencies as a means to achieve project goals. People participate by forming groups to meet predetermined project objectives; they may be involved in decision making, but only after major decisions have already been made by external agents.

6.	Interactive participation (Co-learning)	People participate in joint analysis, development of action plans and formation or strengthening of local institutions. Participation is seen as a right not just the means to achieve project goals. The process involves interdisciplinary methodologies that seek multiple perspectives and make use of systemic and structured learning processes. As groups take control over local decisions and determine how available resources are used, so they have a stake in maintaining structures or practices.
7.	Self-mobilization (Collective action)	People participate by taking initiatives independently of external institutions to change systems. They develop contacts with external institutions for resources and technical advice they need, but retain control over how resources are used. Self-mobilization can spread if governments and NGOs provide an enabling framework of support. Such self-initiated mobilization may or may not challenge existing distributions of wealth and power.

(source: IIED)

Despite the importance of community participation in CAHW projects, it is common to find projects that were established by veterinarians with limited knowledge of community-based methods of working (Box 3.3). This problem applies to both government and non-goverment organizations, and indicates that investments in staff training are an important step in developing sustainable community-based services. Training in participatory approaches and methods, and study tours are described in Chapter 2.

Typical problems with more 'top-down' styles of implementation include:

◆ failure to address the community's most important livestock health problems. For example, veterinarians alone identify which diseases should be tackled and the other duties of the CAHWs, such as castration or hoof trimming;

◆ failure to select CAHWs using locally defined criteria for selection. Community and professional views can sometimes differ regarding the ideal qualities of a CAHW. Livestock keepers are less likely to support a worker who has not been selected by the community. In some countries it is common for senior policy makers to point towards the many unemployed veterinary technicians as a reason for not training CAHWs. However, when given a choice, communities rarely select such people to provide veterinary services for them;

Box 3.3 The importance of effective communication and of providing field staff with training in community-based approaches

Extract from a review of community-based animal health services in the southern Africa, 1999:

> The Directorate of Veterinary Services and various national livestock development projects have all been active in local level animal health. These activities represent a commendable effort and highlight the interest of the Ministry and its staff to provide animal healthcare solutions to the area in question. However, not all of these activities could be described as participatory or community-based. The communities were not always engaged in meaningful dialogue leading to community agreements based on empowerment, ownership and self-sufficiency. Essentially, some communities were the beneficiaries of training and inputs in the context of a local institutional vacuum.
>
> Judging from the activities of national livestock and rural development projects, it did not appear that the project staff or experts had direct, previous experience in the establishment of community-based animal health programmes.

In east Africa, field staff working on community-based animal healthcare realized the weaknesses in their dialogue with livestock keepers:

> The root causes of the problems have been discussed with the various organizations concerned, and to some extent lie with the skills and knowledge of the field staff. Many of the field staff said that they were unclear about all the issues they should be discussing with the community, and how to actually carry out effective community dialogue. Community dialogue is probably the single most difficult task in developing community-based projects, but without it the programme has little chance of success. The field staff are asked to do a very difficult job … they must be provided with the skills and knowledge they need.

In west Africa, an impact assessment of the Community Livestock Worker programme in 1999 concluded:

> A further limitation to the effectiveness of the CLWs is the confusion surrounding their legitimate role as livestock service providers. This includes the level of education and information available to communities and other service providers about the aims of the CLW programme. Despite initial meetings, many producers remain unclear as to the precise role and training of CLWs … '

(see 'Further reading' section for details of specific reports)

- rushed selection of CAHWs by the community or selection by a single, powerful community member rather than patient, careful and transparent selection via community meetings and discussion. For example, it often takes considerable time and effort to reach pastoral livestock owners. If this effort is not made then inappropriate village-based people may be selected as CAHWs because the real livestock carers and potentially excellent CAHWs were 'away with the herds';
- confusion over the roles and responsibilities of the community, the CAHW and the project staff. For example, who should feed a CAHW who visits a remote herd to treat sick livestock and is forced to stay overnight there?
- confusion over the type of service offered by the CAHW;
- confusion over the prices of veterinary medicines and the financial incentives for the CAHWs (see below). This commonly leads to damaging accusations or rumours that individuals are selling drugs that have been given freely by an NGO or the government;
- inappropriate training approaches and methods. For example, too much emphasis on classroom-based lectures and course content which is too technical (see Chapters 4 and 5).

3.3 Some key constraints to financial sustainability

Limited privatization and hidden subsidies

The last decade has seen major changes in veterinary service delivery in developing countries. Moves towards privatization of veterinary services have led to a gradual withdrawal of free or subsidized services by government and a corresponding increase in private sector activity. In the case of the basic clinical services provided by CAHWs it is increasingly recognized that these services can be provided more efficiently by the private sector, while government and veterinary boards have important monitoring and regulatory roles. However, many veterinary services are still in a state of transition and the private sector has to compete with various forms of subsidized service provided by the state or poorly co-ordinated aid programmes. For example, many countries in east Africa have national policies on veterinary privatization that, in theory, exclude government veterinarians from engaging in private practice. In reality, however, low salaries in government service encourage state veterinarians to engage in informal private activities. Furthermore, because government employees have use of government facilities they can often undercut the prices of the true private sector.

Given this situation, it is perhaps not surprising that a common constraint to effective CAHW services is weak financial sustainability. This means that many projects are dependent on an external source of support, usually in the form of subsidies for veterinary equipment or medicines. When the external support is withdrawn, the subsidies disappear and systems have not been put in place to cope with full cost recovery and project running costs. Therefore, many CAHW projects collapse when NGO or government funding dries up. Alternatively, if government funds are limited, the service can continue to operate but suffers from economic inefficiency and low coverage. In Box 3.4, Mesfin Ayele describes experiences from a project in northern Ethiopia. The veterinary drug supply system operated by this project represents a fairly typical government procurement and administrative set-up. For example, there are several tiers to the system, each with its staff, administration and other costs. This arrangement is expensive and probably too bureaucratic.

Box 3.4 Sustainability lessons from a community-based animal health project in northern Ethiopia

Background

Northern Ethiopia is characterized by high, mountainous terrain and very poor infrastructure. Livestock form an important part of the rural economy and people keep donkeys, horses, sheep, goats and chickens. However, cattle are particularly valued because they enable people to plough their land.

In common with other countries, many government vets in Ethiopia were sceptical of the community-based animal health worker (CAHW) approach. In northern Ethiopia for example, a large-scale Community Veterinary Agent project had collapsed due to poor monitoring and drug supply. Also, some vets believed that livestock keepers could not be trained to provide veterinary care.

In 1996, Save the Children, UK (SCF(UK)) decided to revisit the idea of developing CAHW systems in Region 3, northern Ethiopia. At that time, preventive and curative services were provided by the government veterinary service through veterinary clinics and subclinics. However, coverage was limited to a few kilometres radius of these facilities as government veterinary workers often lacked transport. Another important feature of the government system was limited commitment towards privatization of services.

Because of previous negative experiences of community-based approaches in Region 3, SCF(UK) decided to work closely with local government vets to examine past failings and expose vets to more successful projects and new ways of working. It was hoped that this approach would lead to the design of a CAHW pilot project that would enable the government vets to test the community-based approach.

Some project activities

Work began in mid-1996 with a series of meetings and workshops. A study tour was used to expose ministry staff to community-based approaches and examples of CAHW

---

projects in other countries. An extensive ethnoveterinary survey was conducted and veterinary staff received training in participative training techniques. Based on these activities, a CAHW training course was then designed.

However, an important experience at this stage of the project was a difference in community and government priorities and perceptions. Although ethnoveterinary surveys showed that livestock keepers prioritized anthrax and blackleg, the government insisted in restricting CAHW activities to the treatment of internal and external parasites, treatment of wounds and castration. Therefore, the CAHW training course focused on these activities and CAHWs were not trained to vaccinate livestock.

During more workshops, a system was designed for working at community level to select and monitor CAHWs. The lowest level of public administration in Ethiopia was the Peasant Association and, at this level, Animal Health Steering Committees were formed to act as a link between the project and the community. These Steering Committees were responsible for selecting the CAHWs for training, overseeing the supply of drugs and equipment to the CAHWs and monitoring the CAHWs. The Steering Committees received technical support from staff working in government vet clinics or subclinics, such as Animal Health Technicians (AHTs).

SCF(UK) provided an initial supply of drugs for the CAHWs and these drugs were then sold to livestock keepers. The government veterinary service was responsible for replenishing the drugs. The financial incentive for the CAHWs was a 25 per cent surcharge on the cost price of the drug. This system is summarized in Figure 3.1.

The monitoring system comprised four types of monitoring activity:

◆ monitoring of CAHWs by government AHTs based in vet clinics – every two weeks;
◆ monitoring of CAHWs and AHTs by veterinarians – every month;
◆ meetings of CAHWs, AHTs, SCF(UK) and other players – every two months;
◆ community assessments of project and CAHWs – every six months.

Following the design of the CAHW training course, 40 CAHWs were trained in late 1997. In 1999, monitoring reports for 25 of these CAHWs showed that they had treated 40 000 animals during the previous 20-month period. The most active CAHW treated 4802 animals.

Some key sustainability issues and lessons learnt

Community priorities versus government officials' perceptions

As the project evolved, livestock keepers began to ask the CAHWs to provide a wider range of services. In particular, vaccination of livestock against bacterial diseases was frequently

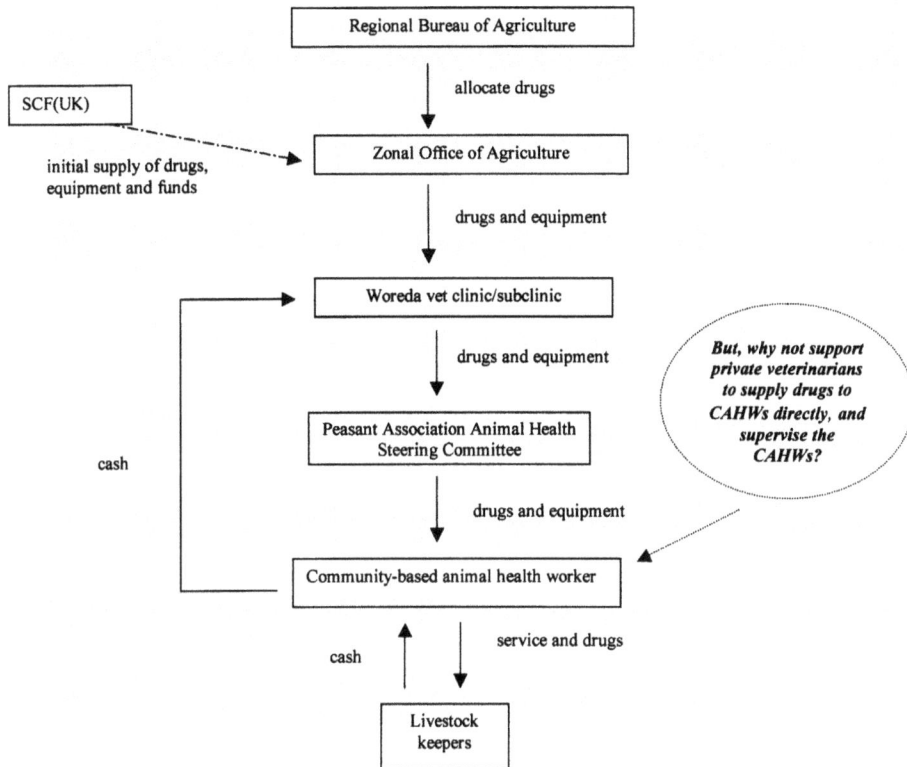

Figure 3.1 The government-operated CAHW system in Region 3, northern Ethiopia

mentioned as an important role for the CAHWs. In September 1999, a zonal-level policy workshop with the theme 'Towards a Co-ordinated Strategy for Improved Animal Health Delivery' was organized in North Wollo that brought CAHWs face-to-face with regional veterinary officers. This interaction was important because these officers were mandated to formulate regional policy on CAHW services. At the time of writing, a draft regional policy was being formulated and it was hoped that a broader range of CAHWs would be officially endorsed.

A government-managed veterinary drug supply system

The diagram above shows that the veterinary drug supply system for the project required drugs to pass through various administrative levels before reaching the CAHWs and livestock keepers. At each level, paper work and people's time was needed and, therefore, costs were involved. Government staff were also responsible for monitoring the CAHWs. These costs were a form of 'hidden' costs to the government within the system and, therefore, the system was subsidized. A key question was: 'Is this system financially sustainable?' Again by reference to the diagram, it can be seen that a private veterinarian could probably have supplied drugs to CAHWs more efficiently than the government system.

A key lesson for the project was, although northern Ethiopia was a very poor region, livestock keepers were willing to pay CAHWs for anthelmintic and acaricide treatments at 25 per cent above the cost price of the medicines. The very large rural population of livestock keepers represents a substantial market for basic veterinary services.

The project demonstrated very promising results and showed that farmers could be trained to provide a service that was very much valued and supported by their communities. The government veterinary service had a very strong and positive stake in the project, and many vets became convinced that CAHWs could be useful service providers. The main challenges for the project were 'sustainability challenges' such as the need for policies that supported a wider range of CAHW activities and private sector development of drug-supply systems.

(contributed by Mesfin Ayele, Save the Children UK, Ethiopia)

While many state veterinary services have tried to improve financial sustainability by introducing 'cost recovery' for veterinary medicines and even adding service fees, in reality these systems often fail to cover core costs. This problem also affects CAHW projects in which veterinary medicines are sold by CAHWs at cost price, with or without an additional service fee for the CAHW. When these systems are operated by NGOs or government, there are usually hidden subsidies in the form of transport costs, storage costs, administration costs and staff costs to manage the drugs. These hidden costs can be substantial and mean that many projects, despite commitment to a cost recovery system, cannot be sustained in the absence of external finance. In another example from Ethiopia, a cost recovery study with a comparison of public and private sector delivery models showed dramatic improvements in financial efficiency for the private sector approach, particularly for private practices linked to CAHW networks (see Box 3.5).

The diminishing revolving fund syndrome

A common feature of cost recovery systems for primary-level veterinary services has been the use of revolving funds. Revolving funds were usually intended to use the revenue from drug sales to finance the purchase of new drug supplies. Although this idea is relatively simple, revolving funds have rarely been sustained and, as the value of the funds declines, drug supply to CAHWs or other workers also declines. Some typical experiences with revolving funds for veterinary drugs are described in Box 3.6 but, in summary, poor management, excessive bureaucracy and use of fund revenue for non-veterinary purposes are common problems. The last problem was often associated with drug revenue entering the government treasury rather than a specific bank account controlled by project staff.

Box 3.5 Financial inefficiencies in government-managed veterinary services: an example from Ethiopia

In 1997, PARC Ethiopia conducted a cost recovery study of veterinary services. The study included a questionnaire survey in 13 districts with 72 government veterinary staff, 21 private practitioners and 217 livestock owners. At the time of the study, government policy aimed to construct more veterinary clinics and staff them with government employees. However, existing clinics suffered from irregular supplies of drugs, and shortages of transport and consumables.

The study findings included:

◆ Each veterinary clinic covered an area of radius approximately 7.5 km. In each district, this meant that only approximately 28 per cent of livestock had regular and relatively easy access to government-provided veterinary clinical service. This finding indicated opportunities for community-based systems and the private sector to service up to 70 per cent of livestock per district.

◆ For an average government veterinary clinic, it was estimated that drug revenues accounted for only 45 per cent of the total costs of providing the service. In other words, the government subsidized the cost of the service by approximately 55 per cent.

◆ By comparison of the existing public sector delivery system with models of private delivery systems, it was calculated that staff costs in a private system per unit volume of drugs delivered would be 30 per cent of those in large, overstaffed public sector clinics.

◆ The retail veterinary drug market was very competitive and private providers had to contend with a highly subsidized public sector (see above), 'unofficial' private practice by public sector employees, and the activities of informal traders.

◆ Study findings indicated that the optimal animal health service delivery model would be a rural practice owned and supervised by a veterinarian, and comprising a practice-owned network of satellite Animal Health Technicians or, preferably, a community-owned network of CAHWs. Economic charges should be levied.

◆ Contracting implementation of compulsory vaccination programmes to the private sector would be feasible and cost-effective if combined with village/community-based private veterinary practices.

(source: Peter Moorhouse and Ayelew Tolossa – see 'Further reading' section)

Box 3.6 The diminishing revolving funds syndrome

Working in north-east Thailand in the early 1980s, the German development agency GTZ established a large-scale CAHW-type system in partnership with the Thai Government. A drug revolving fund (DRF) was established at the Department for Livestock Development Headquarters in Bangkok. Proceeds from drug sales were paid into the DRF and, subsequently, into the treasury. When describing the system some years later, Dr Karl Leidl noted:

> The assumption that the Central Administration was capable of efficiently running the Revolving Fund turned out to be false. Drug replenishment of keymen was initially done through the stock ordered. There was no restocking of drugs via the administrative route. Whenever enquiries were made regarding the proceeds from drug sales paid back to Central Administration we were told that the programme was running smoothly and that most of the keymen, District Livestock Officers and Provincial Livestock Officers were collecting and transferring fees regularly. In fact, the Central Administration failed to order new drugs, and the project had to assist further with supplying drugs to avoid delays in drug replenishment.

> It took us time to discover that there was a misconception between our understanding and the Thai understanding of the word 'revolving'. For us it meant ongoing, under the assumption that all preconditions for value preservation of the fund were ensured. The Thai understanding of a revolving fund, as explained to me by one of my Thai colleagues later, was 'revolving simply means recovering the money once' and this was the official view of administrators at Headquarters.

> Looking back at the problems we encountered, it demonstrates that, without thorough planning, particularly of management and administrative aspects of a DRF, the sustainability of such a programme can be jeopardized – even with a sound technical package that was clearly accepted by farmers. I also believe that the involvement of the Thai Government at a regional level should have been changed into a privatization scheme ... '

Some years later in 1992, the South East Rangelands Project (SERP) in Ethiopia established a revolving fund system for veterinary drugs. The animal health component of this large, African Development Bank-funded project was comparable to a government veterinary service and, in theory, covered an area of around 400 000 km² in eastern Ethiopia. In mid-1997, the following problems with the fund were identified:

◆ At its inception, SERP was organized under the Government's Third Livestock Development Project and, consequently, it inherited well-established but outdated accounting systems. Finance personnel were not accustomed to managing revolving fund systems and some of the new accounting procedures required did not feature in the accepted system of the time. It proved extremely difficult to force a change in the financial bureaucracy.

◆ From 1992 to the present time, the official sale price of most drugs has been below cost price. Inevitably, this approach means that drug assets suffer a reduction in value between the supplier (whether government stocks, NGOs or private) and SERP stores. Therefore, it becomes impossible for the project to collect sufficient revenue to replace drug stocks.

◆ According to government accounting systems at the beginning of the project, all income (regardless of source or future use) was deposited in a single bank account (GOV 50). This system encouraged the use of drug sale revenue for other purposes.

◆ At various times, SERP has suffered cash flow crises due to delays in the release of funds from the African Development Bank. These delays increased the risk of alternative uses of drug sale revenue that was deposited in the GOV 50 account.

◆ Livestock owners were not well-informed about the official sale price of the drugs and some veterinary staff were working in remote areas; staff salaries were low and often payment of salaries and per diems was delayed. In this situation, the temptation to sell drugs at greater than the official selling price must have been considerable.

◆ Infrastructure and communications in the region are extremely weak. Adequate follow-up of veterinary drug distribution and reporting proved to be problematic, if not impossible.

During the last two years, SERP has improved the management of the revolving fund by opening a separate bank account for drug sale revenue and developing a quarterly financial reporting system for drugs supplied. Although it is possible that improvements in the management of the fund will continue, after five years of the revolving fund system the combined capital assets and cash assets of the fund (approximately Birr 1.5 million) fall far below the estimated veterinary drug requirements for the region of value Birr 9.3 million (according to SERP estimate). In addition, almost all of SERP's drugs have been provided by aid agencies.

In common with the situation in Thailand, problems with the sustainability of revolving funds prompted moves towards privatization of veterinary services in this region of Ethiopia.

Free or subsidized veterinary drugs and the problem of dependency

Despite the trend towards privatization and national policies that discourage subsidized or free veterinary services, in many areas veterinary medicines continue to be provided free of charge or at highly subsidized rates. There are various reasons why this practice continues, but typically they relate to institutional or organizational weaknesses within the implementing agency:

Political factors

Within government, livestock issues can have substantial political significance and the provision of free or heavily subsidized services is a useful vote-winner. In addition, more extreme socialist ideologies can support subsidized state services, albeit with limited coverage.

NGO agendas

Unfortunately, a small proportion of NGOs use the promise of free veterinary services to encourage people to participate in religious activities. Other NGOs continue to associate privatization with capitalism and exploitation of communities by multinational pharmaceutical companies.

Technical naivety

Both NGO and government programmes can involve very limited technical input from professionals with experience of community-based approaches. Many programmes lack a clear exit strategy.

In all three cases, the argument that 'people are too poor to pay' is often heard though rarely supported by evidence of discussions with livestock keepers during which the pros and cons of free or subsidized services have been analysed in a participatory manner. This kind of participatory analysis is discussed in more detail in Chapter 2 and in section 3.4 below.

The provision of free or subsidized veterinary care means that programmes almost certainly disintegrate when the implementing agency withdraws or, in the case of government, funds for field operations start to shrink. However, these programmes also hinder future financial sustainability by encouraging livestock keepers to expect cheap veterinary services. Consequently, any new programme aiming to promote more sustainable approaches often has to overcome the behaviour of dependency at community level. Again, this requires patient community-level analysis leading to understanding of the short-term nature of free or subsidized services versus the long-term potential for services that operate without subsidy.

Confusion over drug prices, incentives for CAHWs and other issues

Many reviews of CAHW projects mention confusion among livestock keepers regarding the correct prices for veterinary medicines, incentives for CAHWs, payments for equipment and other important financial issues. Such confusion is an important reason why livestock keepers choose not to use the services of the CAHW and indicates weak community participation during the start-up phase of the project. Ways to overcome this problem are discussed in Chapter 2 and section 3.4.

Box 3.7 Examples of poor communication about financial issues in community-based animal health programmes

In a community livestock worker (CLW) programme in Ghana:

The payments arrangements for CLWs are misunderstood by many livestock producers and other service providers. Literal use of the expressions 'voluntary' and 'community payment' have left confusion in many communities as to whether CLWs are supposed to draw any profit at all from their activities.

In southern Africa:

The participants were not asked to contribute to the cost of the CAHW's kit, but the CAHWs will be asked to sign a contract regarding the kit. After almost nine months from the date of the training, the kits had not been distributed due to reluctance on the part of the Treasury to authorize the distribution. At the community meeting in Ruacana, it was clear that the ownership of the kit and terms of payment had never been discussed with the community or the CAHW. The community members could not be described as participants, as they had never been consulted.

In east Africa:

Some community members and CAHWs interviewed were under the impression that an educated person had to be selected (for training as a CAHW) and that they would be paid a salary and/or employed by the government or an NGO. Clearly, CAHWs are not going to be employed, but the fact that people are unsure about this illustrates that community dialogue has been insufficient.

(see 'Further reading' section for details of specific reports)

In areas previously lacking animal health services, the start of a CAHW project is often met with considerable enthusiasm by the community. In this situation, both the community and the implementing agency can become convinced that CAHWs should work on a voluntary basis and receive no material incentives as payment for their efforts. With this approach, there is an assumption that CAHWs will receive benefits in the form of heightened status in the community or occasional payments of money, livestock or other items. In some projects, there is also an assumption that the authority of community leaders is sufficient to 'encourage' CAHWs to continue to work, again, in the absence of clear incentives. Although this approach can work in the short term, there are very few examples of CAHWs continuing to work as unpaid volunteers. Sooner or later, there will be requests for incentives and, in the absence of incentives, CAHWs will drop out of the system. The lesson here seems to be that people do not work for nothing. Financial incentives should be clearly defined for CAHWs at the start of a project, and documented in agreements between the various players. Furthermore, experience from both government and NGO projects shows that implementing agencies should aim to promote CAHWs and their supervisors or drug suppliers as private operators. This means avoiding salaries because, inevitably, the salaries disappear when the NGO project ends, or government salaries are delayed or insufficient.

The emergency and relief scenario

In emergency and relief situations such as drought, conflict or livestock disease epidemics, a common response of aid agencies is to provide free or subsidized veterinary drugs. However, without careful planning with communities, CAHWs, government and private suppliers of veterinary products, these programmes can seriously undermine the financial sustainability of existing services. For example, private veterinarians who have been working hard to establish new businesses can find themselves in a situation where cheap drugs are being supplied directly to livestock keepers by an aid agency or government veterinarians. These programmes also create much confusion among livestock keepers, particularly if another programme has been working with them to develop a privatized system based on real market costs.

Privatization efforts in the risk-prone regions such as the pastoral areas of the Horn of Africa will inevitably have to take into account the regular cycle of drought. What does a private business do when people's livelihoods are severely threatened by environmental disaster? Some vets who have experienced several cycles of drought are now realizing that there are in fact increased opportunities to supply veterinary services to livestock owners during such times. For example, deworming small ruminants and camels that are nutritionally stressed can increase their chances of survival; vaccinating against diseases such as anthrax that tend to be more prevalent as animals crowd or die around scarce water sources can save large numbers of stock. Likewise, livestock owners will invest in keeping their best breeding stock healthy during the hardship period.

Privatization of services in these harsh environments presents special challenges. It is important that local authorities, NGOs and donors start to respect private sector initiatives when developing drought contingency plans. This could allow relief efforts, with appropriate monitoring, to be channelled through the private sector. In the 2000/01 drought in northern Kenya, CAHWs were paid to administer and distribute subsidized veterinary medicines and vaccines as part of the drought relief effort. A concerted effort to help pastoralists market their excess stock as range resources diminish can allow them to cope with drought, invest in improved health for remaining stock and purchase food.

In situations such as post-conflict recovery, lack of civil society and strong local expectations may justify free or subsidized services. However, the overall strategy should be to move towards full cost recovery as soon as possible. Again, the strategy can include support to the private sector so that activities such as veterinary drug supply become 'privatized' as soon as possible.

The effect of poor drug supply on CAHW systems

The preceding sections all show how the supply of veterinary drugs to CAHWs can be insufficient or irregular. These weaknesses in veterinary drug supply have important consequences for the sustainability of CAHWs. For example:

No drugs means no incentives

In many projects, the cash incentives for CAHWs are derived from drug sales and treatments. As drug supplies fail, so do the rewards for the CAHWs.

No drugs means no credibility

Livestock keepers become frustrated when CAHWs are unable to provide the services that were agreed during the initial stages of the project. Trust in the system wanes as people realize: 'Yes we have a CAHW, but still our animals are sick'.

Limited drugs means pressure from the powerful

In some communities, when drug supplies are limited the CAHWs face pressure from powerful members of the community to either 'Treat our animals first' or 'Keep the drugs in case our animals become sick'. When CAHWs succumb to this pressure, other people feel resentment and lose trust in the system.

Limited drugs mean limited monitoring and refresher training

Drug distribution to CAHWs from a project or government store is often an opportunity to collect monitoring reports from the CAHWs or provide updates about new drugs. If CAHWs suspect that drugs may not be available, they visit the store less frequently and contact is weakened or lost.

Drugs from alternative sources

If drug supply via a project or government fails, some CAHWs will seek drugs elsewhere. This behaviour is not always a problem if good-quality drugs are available from other sources but is a problem if CAHWs obtain poor-quality drugs from markets or illegal traders. It is this latter scenario that commonly occurs after NGOs 'train and release' large numbers of CAHWs. Veterinarians rightly criticize such projects because the CAHWs purchase all drugs unsupervised and commonly call themselves 'doctor'.

These concerns show why the development of a sustainable veterinary drug supply system is central to the sustainability of the whole system.

3.4 How to improve financial sustainability in CAHW services

As indicated previously, increasing privatization of veterinary services assumes that the private sector should be handling important components of the service, such as disease preventive and curative activities. Considering the strong economic logic of this approach and the poor sustainability of many CAHW projects, this section focuses on ways to encourage private sector involvement in sustaining CAHW networks. In order to do this, we use three different policy contexts that can exist at the start of a project and suggest how project approaches and activities should vary accordingly. The three policy contexts range from clear government policy on veterinary privatization and strong commitment to the policy, to absence of government and, therefore, absence of policy.

When using this approach, it should be recognized that veterinary privatization is only one part of national, macro-economic policy and so a wide range of political and economic factors will influence the outcome of privatization programmes. For example, although state veterinary services may be committed to restructuring themselves and promoting privatization, macro-economic conditions may limit the capacity of veterinarians to access credit and the capacity of livestock keepers to pay for services. In other countries, privatization polices are well-defined on paper but not fully supported by the state for political or other reasons. Whatever the case, efforts to support private sector activities locally will be influenced by trends that are outside the control of your project. In project proposals, these trends are usually detailed as 'Risks and Assumptions'.

Where there is clear policy and strong commitment to veterinary privatization

In some countries, governments show strong commitment to veterinary privatization. Such commitment might be demonstrated in clear and well-publicized policies, or in meaningful support to national veterinary privatization programmes. In these areas, new private veterinary businesses will be appearing although they may be restricted to towns or 'high-potential' farming areas with relatively intensive livestock production systems. Experience from many developing countries indicates that, apart from small animal clinics in capital cities, private veterinary practice is based on the sale of veterinary pharmaceuticals with relatively little hands-on clinical work for veterinarians. Furthermore, many veterinary practices or pharmacies perform well but are unable to generate sufficient profit to support vehicles and provide an on-farm service. In other areas, difficult terrain and poor roads are also limitations to reaching livestock-rearing communities.

An important principle behind privatized CAHW networks is that the profitability, and therefore the sustainability of a private veterinary business, is heavily dependent on drug turnover. For a veterinarian running a pharmacy, CAHWs provide an opportunity to reach new clients and expand a business into areas that might otherwise be inaccessible (see Box 3.8). While veterinarians are usually unwilling to walk up steep mountainsides, wade through swamps or trek across deserts, CAHWs are accustomed to these discomforts and will move long distances on foot or use donkeys, mules, camels, canoes or bicycles.

Box 3.8 A model for a privatized CAHW network

This model is based around a town. The veterinary pharmacy in town is managed by a veterinarian who supports 16 CAHWs by supplying drugs and providing technical supervision, as required by the national veterinary board.

The direct service from the veterinary pharmacy covers an area of radius 10 km. This is the distance that the vet can cover on foot, although such journeys are not worthwhile unless, at the end of the journey, a substantial number of livestock require treatment.

The CAHWs provide a service to communities up to 60 km away from the main town. The CAHWs travel on foot or sometimes get a ride on a truck or bus travelling to or from the villages. The journey to town usually takes around two days.

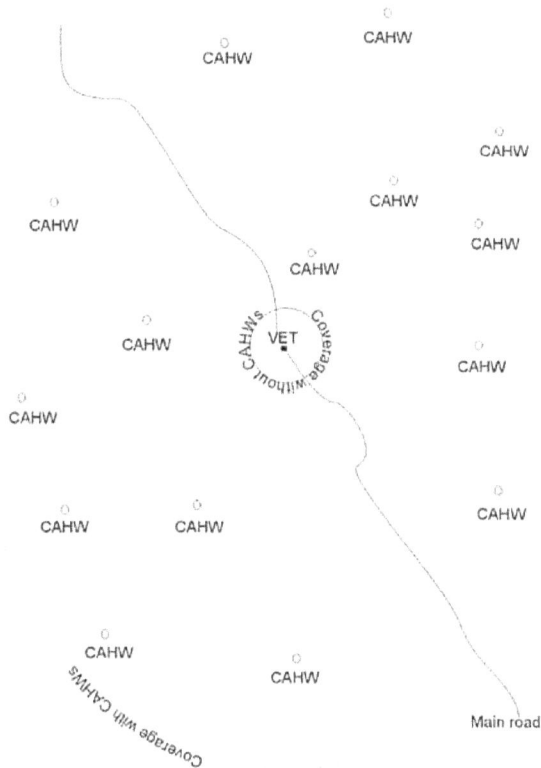

Another important opportunity for new, private veterinary businesses is the contracting out of compulsory vaccination programmes. Private, veterinary supervised CAHWs can easily match the vaccination efficiency achieved by government implemented vaccination programmes, and have the advantage of substantial cost

71

savings. In marginal pastoral areas, revenue for private practices generated by vaccination or surveillance programmes can have a significant positive impact on the sustainability of the practice (see Box 3.9).

Box 3.9 Linking private veterinary practice to CAHWs: an example from Chad

In considering CAHW projects in different communities established through various projects, NGOs or veterinary services, it appeared that the resupply and monitoring of CAHWs were the most significant constraints to the sustainability of the programmes. Inevitably, the sponsoring organization withdrew or found other priorities. The CAHWs and communities were left to their own resources and, if dependency had been designed into the programme, it collapsed. This led one to hypothesize that, if both the resupply of medicines and the monitoring were established on market-based incentives, the programmes would be truly self-sustaining.

In order to test this, a CAHW network was established in Salamat, a remote region of eastern Chad on the border with the Central Africa Republic, as part of a private veterinary practice – 'a community-based veterinary practice'. The practice delivered curative treatment and vaccination through CAHWs. The practice benefited from a sanitary mandate and vaccination contract for rinderpest vaccination, which was executed by the CAHWs under the supervision of the veterinarian using thermostable rinderpest vaccine.

Establishment of the community-based practice was facilitated by a loan to the veterinarian for the purchase of initial drugs and equipment and technical assistance from the extension department and veterinary services on the set-up of a CAH network and training of CAHWs. The veterinarian took the lead in contacting the communities, conducting initial participatory assessment, community dialogue and training, with the 'experts' mainly providing back-up and guidance. Training of the veterinarian in community development approaches was very much conducted 'on-the-job'. In this manner, the community perceived the veterinarian as a catalyst for community development and developed a sense of loyalty and confidence in the community-based veterinary practice.

The veterinarian employed two veterinary assistants and eventually established a network of 40 CAHWs. The veterinary practice earned its income through the reselling of medicines and vaccines through the CAHWs and by retaining a percentage of the rinderpest vaccination fees. At that time, livestock owners covered about 50 per cent of the cost of rinderpest vaccination and the government contributed the remainder. The CAHWs collected this fee from the cattle owners when they vaccinated, retained a fixed amount per head for their own incentive and returned the remainder over to the practice. The veterinary assistants also received a fixed amount per head vaccinated in their respective areas and a percentage of all sales receipts. In this way each level of the system received an incentive based on the quantity of work performed.

During the first year of operation, about 40 000 head of cattle were vaccinated against rinderpest and the practice was well-established. Livestock owner and CAHW satisfaction was high. Due to an unfortunate accident, the veterinarian passed away and the trial was interrupted. The government of Chad, which was originally reluctant, expressed strong interest in replacing the veterinarian and continuing to develop such delivery systems.

(contributed by Dr Jeffrey Mariner)

These opportunities can enable sustainable, private CAHW networks to be established using an approach such as that outlined in Box 3.10. The idea is to link a professional veterinary worker with a clinic or pharmacy to a group of CAHWs. The veterinarian (or other worker) provides technical supervision and, according to national regulations, assumes legal responsibility for the actions of the CAHWs under his or her direction. The statutory bodies responsible for the provision of veterinary services in the country should determine training standards for CAHWs and define what constitutes 'supervision' of CAHWs. The private nature of the system ensures sustainability, or at least better sustainability than government- or NGO-managed projects.

When producing business plans for private community-based veterinary practices it may be vital to think 'out of the box'. For example, when establishing a network of CAHWs in an area, what are the other work opportunities beyond clinical animal health service delivery? It is feasible for the CAHW networks to trade hides and skins, link milk supplies to village areas, become paid extension agents for other sectoral initiatives such as human health or collect information for those looking for specific information in their area e.g. wildlife disease outbreaks. Some examples and ideas of how this could work are provided in Box 3.11.

a. Participatory analysis with communities and potential private veterinarians

For projects aiming to develop privatized CAHW networks, an important step is to identify either an existing private veterinary pharmacy or clinic that is suitable for expansion (to cover more remote areas) or veterinarians who wish to open new businesses in the project area. In some areas, it will be difficult to find suitable veterinarians but privatization policy might allow an animal health assistant or other worker to run a small business. In other situations, restructuring of government veterinary services can lead to government vets looking for new opportunities and these vets could be candidates for running privatized CAHW systems.

The next step involves working with candidates for privatization to conduct participatory surveys in target communities. Typically, this will involve training in participatory approaches and methods (as described in Chapter 2) and analysing a wide range of issues with livestock keepers in order to determine the most appropriate

Box 3.10 Pathways for improving financial sustainability in CAHW sevices: countries where there is enabling government policy on veterinary privatization

Policy context

- ◆ clear government policy on veterinary privatization;
- ◆ strong government commitment to policy.

⬇

Approach

Establish and test an integrated system with:
- ◆ private veterinarian(s) supporting a CAHW network by supplying medicines and providing technical supervision;
- ◆ state veterinary service providing regulatory support.

⬇

Key activities

1. Identify existing or potential private veterinarian(s) or other suitably qualified workers.
2. Training:
   - ◆ participatory approaches and methods;
   - ◆ small business planning;
   - ◆ participative training techniques.
3. Participatory analysis:
   - ◆ with community to identify key needs and solutions;
   - ◆ leading to information to develop a business plan;
   - ◆ identify source and clarify prices of drugs and incentives for CAHWs.
4. Develop business plan.
5. Identify sources of credit (if required) and use business plan to secure credit.
6. Work with communities to select and train CAHWs.
7. Close monitoring of CAHWs activities and business performance.

Box 3.11 Alternative sources of income for community-based animal health delivery systems

Contracting CAHWs as extension agents: a missed opportunity

In the mid-1990s in southern Sudan, a major human Guinea worm eradication programme organized by a consortium of well-funded NGOs and international agencies requested CAHWs and their supervisors in remote areas to provide water filtration cloths and Guinea worm prevention extension messages to remote livestock owners. These owners were not easily contactable by any other means and were at serious risk of both contracting and spreading the disease. The CAHWs did this work voluntarily for a time but, because no incentives or follow-up were provided, apathy soon developed.

Milk marketing networks: an opportunity waiting to happen?

In Somali areas of north-east Kenya, there are well-developed networks of women milk-sellers. Women send small containers of milk, by vehicle, to intermediaries in towns on a daily basis. Strapped to each container is a note with coded instructions on what to do with the revenue – e.g. purchase tea – that is sent back with the container. Such sophisticated delivery and return mechanisms that are already functioning and rely on a high level of trust could be used for the regular provision of veterinary drugs to women CAHWs and disease information to supervisors.

Payment for public good services

As disease surveillance becomes increasingly important to national governments promoting international trade in livestock and livestock products, the possibilities and incentives for contracting these services to CAHW networks becomes more likely. CAHWs provide an excellent 'front line' source of both disease information and simple sample collection (see Chapter 7).

In many pastoral areas of Africa there are networks of community monitors collecting information on the food security situation for famine early-warning systems. Could these networks provide supplementary training and contract some of the CAHWs to provide such monitoring information?

way to establish the community-based system. At this stage, those vets who wish to establish private businesses should also be thinking about developing business plans and, in particular, can use the participatory assessment to help develop the 'market research' component of the business plan (see below). Community-level analysis should also provide insights into the appropriate number of CAHWs required to cover each community, local priorities for different vaccines or treatments, local perceptions about fair prices for vaccination and treatment, and how to remunerate CAHWs for their services. All this information is useful when drawing up a business plan.

While examining the needs for and roles of CAHWs it is important that female CAHWs are not overlooked. There is an increasing amount of evidence to suggest that women make excellent CAHWs. Not only do they interact well with that section of the population – women – who commonly care for the young, lactating and sick livestock, but they also take extra care not to provide credit and manage their financial resources wisely. It should be noted that in some cultures the working patterns and roles of female CAHWs may differ from male CAHWs. These roles can be determined through dialogue.

As described in section 3.3, confusion over prices of drugs, service fees for CAHWs and other financial issues are crucial topics for discussion at this stage. In addition, local expectations regarding free or cheap veterinary drugs may also arise and will need to be addressed. There is no standard methodology for facilitating discussion on financial matters, but some of the methods below can enable local analysis of costs, benefits and sustainability of services.

One approach is to use the market value of different livestock species as the basis for prompting discussion on the benefits of treating sick livestock (see Box 3.12). The idea is to encourage people to compare the economic value of livestock with the price of veterinary medicines. The basic structure of the key question is: 'If you have an animal of market value x and that animal is suffering from disease y, what is the value of the medicine that can cure the animal?' Discussions can be repeated with different wealth groups in a community using different types of livestock suffering from different diseases. This helps the project to determine if and how wealth affects people's perceptions of the value of veterinary medicines and, indirectly, their willingness to pay.

Box 3.12 Discussions on the cost–benefit of treating livestock and the value of veterinary treatments

For people who have been accustomed to free or subsidized veterinary medicines, careful and patient discussion is often required to 'discover' the real value of drugs.

Karamoja, Uganda

In Karamoja, Uganda, discussions were developed on the value of veterinary drugs for some common diseases. The types of questions asked were: 'If you have a bull and that bull is worth Uganda shilling (UgSh) 300 000, how much is the medicine worth which can prevent the bull suffering from CBPP?' Examples of responses were:

Different things can be sold to buy the medicine such as a large cockerel (value UgSh 3000), a goat (value UgSh 25 000) or some grain. Alternatively, a drum of beer can be brewed and sold (value UgSh 10 000).

(women's group in Karenga)

Regardless of whether a man owns ten cows or 100 cows, he should sell one cow to buy the medicine.

(male informants, Sidok)

With a group of men in Karenga a cost–benefit discussion was developed using an example of a farmer whose four young adult goats (three does and a buck, valued at UgSh 160 000) died from a disease. If these goats had survived then they might have produced up to 30 kids during their lifetime; assuming these kids were 15 males and 15 females, their sale value would be around UgSh 1 050 000. The cost of the CAHW service to treat the four sick goats would have been around UgSh 2000 and this money could have been obtained by selling only one chicken worth UgSh 3000. The early treatment of the goats would have resulted in a huge benefit that was recognized and discussed by the group. This discussion was aided by the use of piles of stones to show the different costs and benefits.

Sanaag region, Somaliland

In the ActionAid, Somaliland Animal Health Programme, a subsidized veterinary drug supply system for CAHWs was set up soon after the end of the civil war in 1992. This system proved to be very useful for establishing the CAHW network, but depended heavily on ActionAid for procurement of drugs and transport to the project area. During a review of the programme, numerous groups of livestock herders were asked to consider two scenarios.

◆ In the first scenario, they had 100 sheep suffering from *caal* (worms) and were asked to calculate a fair price for a medicine to treat the sheep, assuming that one sheep was worth Somali shilling (SomSh) 200 000.
◆ In the second scenario, they had a sick camel suffering from *dhukaan* (trypanosomiasis) and were asked to calculate the value of the medicine that would cure the camel. A healthy camel was valued at SomSh 1 million.

The most common response to both questions was that a single sheep should be sold to cover the cost of the medicine. In the case of the sick camel, one man explained how this was similar to a traditional remedy for the treatment of *dhukaan*, involving the slaughter of a sheep or goat to make a broth for the camel.

Jijiga, Ethiopia

During a stakeholder analysis of veterinary services in Jijiga, Ethiopia, groups of livestock traders were asked to describe reductions in the market value of livestock due to different diseases. The discussion was assisted by a simple proportional piling method and results were used as an indirect measure of the value of disease prevention or treatment. An example of results is provided below.

Table 3.1 Trader's perceptions of reductions in livestock value as a result of disease

Livestock type	Value (Birr)	Main diseases affecting value	Reduction in value (Birr)	Reduction in value as percentage
Cattle	1000	Bovine ephemeral fever	400	40
	1000	Foot-rot/foot injury	300	30
	1000	Foot and mouth disease	150	15
Camels	1200	Respiratory disease	700	58
	1400	Trypanosomosis	600	43
	800	Helminthosis	300	37
	1200	Abscesses	300	25
	1200	Mange	120	10
Sheep and goats	200	Tick-associated disease	160	80
	150	Helminthosis	75	50
	200	Foot-rot/foot injury	60	30
	200	Pox diseases	20	10

b. Developing a business plan

The formulation of a good business plan is a crucial stage in the development of a new or expanding veterinary pharmacy or clinic. It is comparable to a project proposal, but includes detailed financial information and predictions of economic performance of the business. Essentially, the business plan also allows potential investors to assess the feasibility of the business and the returns on investment. Many veterinary

---

Box 3.13 Improving awareness about usage of veterinary medicines

Livestock owners, particularly pastoralists, are often accustomed to using certain brands of drug for certain treatments. Even if the dose rate used is wrong or newer more appropriate drugs are available, they insist this product is best. It is common for extremely low doses to be used as one-off treatments. Sometimes the livestock owners have been practising this for so long they have no experience of what might be achieved with proper dosing and newer drugs.

While recognizing that even small doses of certain drugs may give transient improvements in health, private veterinary technicians should encourage proper use of efficacious and cost-effective products for their clients. Changing the habits of livestock owners and persuading them to pay more for a better product and using it at proper dose rates, let alone preventative treatments, is not easy. As with any attitude change it requires trust and confidence in the technician and experience of an improved result.

The following methods can be used to both highlight the problems of underdosing or use of inferior drugs and to persuade clients to pay more for better products.

◆ problem plays on the results of inadequate versus adequate treatment or prevention;
◆ using easily understandable community dialogue sessions to allow exchange of experiences;
◆ drug use demonstrations plus physical displays of various types of drug with appropriate discussion;
◆ display or leaflets describing fake or non-efficacious products;
◆ in collaboration with drug manufacturers or wholesalers, initial subsidies to encourage use and therefore experience of better, but more expensive drugs;
◆ training on proper storage of drugs and vaccines.

Using problems plays in Turkana to reveal sustainability issues

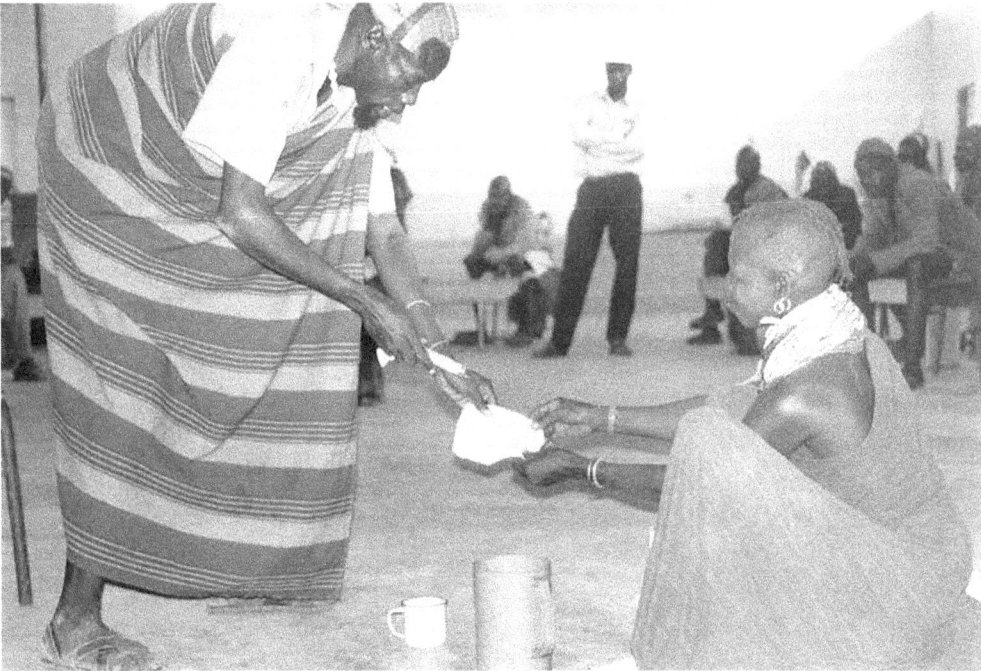

Plate 3.2 Problem plays about the value of veterinary medicines or provision of subsidized services can help people consider the long-term implications of cheap drugs. (*PARC Communications Unit*)

privatization programmes provide training in business planning and proposal writing. An outline of a training programme is provided in Box 3.14 and the key elements of a business plan are summarized in Box 3.15.

As the development of business plans is such an important aspect of developing the skills and knowledge of veterinarians who will manage CAHW

Box 3.14 Outline of a training course for veterinarians on business planning and proposal writing

This example (and the business plan format in Box 3.15) is drawn from the Veterinary Services Support Project run by Save the Children, UK and the Regional Bureau of Agriculture, Somali National Regional State, Ethiopia. This course was organized for government veterinarians who were interested in developing private clinics or pharmacies.

Training objectives and learning needs

Objective 1

At the end of the training the trainees will be able to describe current economic and structural reform of veterinary services in Africa and ongoing veterinary privatization programmes in Ethiopia and Somalia.

Learning needs

◆ historical aspects of veterinary service development in Africa; the colonial period and post-colonial period; the funding crisis in African veterinary services; structural adjustment; the failures of cost recovery and government-managed revolving funds in veterinary services;
◆ economic theory and veterinary privatization; definitions of public goods and private goods; defining 'who does what' using economic theory; asymmetries of information, externalities and economies of scale;
◆ updates on progress and lessons learned from veterinary privatization programmes in Ethiopia and Somalia; special challenges facing pastoral areas.

Objective 2

At the end of the training the trainees will be able to describe the importance of business planning and understand financial terminology used in planning and basic accounting.

Learning needs

◆ the principles of planning small businesses; why do we need a business plan?
◆ new terminology – capital, working capital, fixed assets, depreciation, cash flow, profit and loss, collateral, equity, net present value, internal rate of return.

Objective 3

At the end of the training the trainees will be able to prepare a detailed business plan for a private veterinary pharmacy or clinic.

Learning needs

◆ the format of the business plan (see Box 3.15);
◆ how to acquire and present information for the business plan;
◆ how to calculate cash flow, depreciation, profit and loss charts and internal rate of return;
◆ how to bring all the information together and produce the final business plan.

Box 3.15 Format for a business plan

1. Statement on the purpose of the loan

The statement should detail the services that will be offered by the business in terms of clinical services; vaccination; prophylaxis (e.g. for tick control or trypanosomiasis); diagnosis; certification of livestock (e.g. for export); training of CAHWs; drug supply to CAHWs.

2. Details of capital costs
Fixed assets

◆ surgical equipment;
◆ medical equipment;
◆ laboratory equipment;
◆ office equipment;
◆ replaceable equipment (syringes, needles, etc.);
◆ transport equipment;
◆ spraying equipment.

Working capital

◆ essential drugs;
◆ rental of premises;
◆ salaries and wages;
◆ utilities;
◆ supplies;
◆ transport expenses.

Statement on sources of finance for fixed assets and working capital

3. Sources of finance

◆ own savings;
◆ loan from relatives/friends;

- ◆ bank loan;
- ◆ bank overdraft;
- ◆ veterinary pharmaceutical companies;
- ◆ other;
- ◆ total.

4. Market survey

- ◆ estimated livestock population in the area that will be serviced by the business. The livestock population should be broken down into species (camel, sheep, goat, etc.);
- ◆ details of any important competition to your business e.g. from other private businesses or from government veterinary facilities. What proportion (percentage) of the market does your business expect to cover?
- ◆ monthly statistics of the most important clinical cases for the last two years in the project areas;
- ◆ estimated number of cases by species and diseases that your business expects to handle on a monthly basis;
- ◆ prospects for developing new business activities e.g. linking with CAHWs in order to improve the distribution of drugs, or undertaking contract vaccination work for the government;
- ◆ details of infrastructure in the area covered by the business e.g. telephones, roads, electricity and so on.

5. Cash flow forecasts

a. cash flow forecasts for 12 months;
b. cash flow forecasts for six years

6. Profit and loss budgets

a. profit and loss budget for 12 months;
b. profit and loss budget for six years.

networks, it is worthwhile taking time to identify a suitable trainer for the business planning courses. A good trainer knows about participative training techniques (see Chapter 4), has the right technical knowledge on small business management and, ideally, understands the culture, economy and practicalities of establishing a business in the project area. Therefore, a balance of business theory and hands-on experience is required.

An important part of a business plan and training in business planning is market research. Market research shows that the business proposer (i.e. a vet or group of vets) has a good understanding of the needs of the clients and the volume of work that these clients are likely to support. In a veterinary business, market research includes estimates of livestock populations by species, community views on priority livestock diseases, estimates of disease prevalence, estimates of numbers of animals requiring different vaccinations or treatments and understanding of local capacity and willingness to pay. A business proposer should also be able to describe existing and potentially competing businesses and estimate the proportion of the market that the new business will acquire. The proposer must also be able to assess the risks posed to the business –for example, regular cycles of drought – and to take them into account.

At this point, many readers will have realized that much of this information can be derived from the participatory assessment (see Chapter 2) supported by government reports on livestock populations and records of livestock vaccinations and treatments (see Box 3.16).

During the formulation of a business plan, it will become apparent that drug turnover (i.e. the volume of drugs sold in a given time period) strongly influences cash flow and profitability. In order to increase drug sales, a small veterinary pharmacy can use a network of CAHWs to reach livestock keepers located outside the direct coverage of the pharmacy. There are no golden rules concerning how many CAHWs are required, but each business can estimate an appropriate number based on the market research, required mark-ups on veterinary drugs and the expectations of the CAHWs in terms of financial incentives. At this stage, it should be noted that CAHWs are commonly part-time workers who use incentives from animal health activities to

Training in business planning for veterinarians in Ethiopia

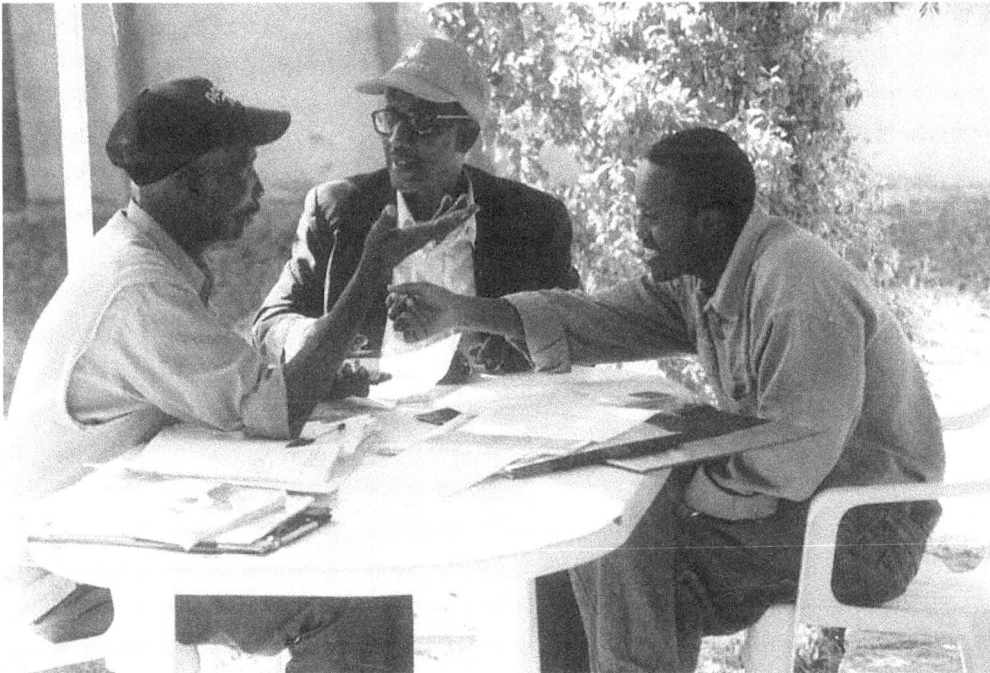

Plate 3.3 Training courses in business planning and proposal writing are an important stage in the privatization process. (*Andy Catley*)

Box 3.16 Combining participatory assessment and market research during the formulation of business plans

Information required for market research section of a business plan	Participatory method	Secondary data sources
Definition of area(s) to be covered, including estimates of human and livestock populations, and infrastructure	Participatory mapping, key informant interviews	Official maps, human census, livestock census
Proportion (and number) of households owning livestock by livestock type	Proportional piling	
Relative importance of different livestock types, with reasons	Livestock species scoring	
Relative importance of different livestock diseases, with reasons	Livestock disease scoring	Government veterinary clinic reports
Prevalence estimates for important livestock diseases	Proportional piling	Laboratory reports, disease survey reports
Seasonal variations in important livestock diseases and disease vectors	Seasonal calendars	Government veterinary clinic reports analysed by month or season
Geographical variations in important livestock diseases and disease vectors; seasonal movement of herds	Participatory mapping	Disease or vector survey reports
Existing veterinary services (public, private, informal, indigenous)	Service maps	
Number of CAHWs required per target area	Participatory mapping	
'Demand' for veterinary services and capacity and willingness to pay	Individual interviews, group interviews, problem plays, proportional piling	Government veterinary clinic reports

supplement their usual farming, livestock herding or other sources of income. The implications of training part-time CAHWs on business plans have yet to be assessed. Inevitably, some CAHWs will work very hard and derive almost all their income from animal health work and perhaps quickly invest in a bicycle to improve coverage. Such CAHWs are a good investment in terms of the time and money taken to carry out community dialogue, training and refresher training. As private CAHW networks become established, will private vets demand selection of people who want to work as full-time CAHWs? If communities prefer part-time workers, how will such a difference be resolved? These are outstanding learning issues for privatized CAHW networks.

The final stages of a business planning training course should involve practical sessions during which groups of participants prepare mock business plans using criteria provided by the trainer. The participants then present their business plans to the rest of the group, who act as potential investors and ask questions to test the understanding of the presenters. This can make a lively final session and enables the participants to see their learning efforts being turned into actual business proposals. It also enables the trainer to check that the training objectives have been met and, if not, provide further guidance on topics that were not properly understood.

c. Using sources of credit: formal and informal

A common constraint to veterinary privatization has been poor access to credit for veterinarians wishing to establish private businesses. For those veterinarians who have been working for government, poor salaries can mean that personal savings are low and equity in the form of insurable property or other assets is minimal. This situation limits their capacity to acquire bank loans under conventional lending arrangements. Other common constraints include high interest rates for loan repayments and assumptions on the part of lenders that remote rural areas cannot support veterinary businesses. For example, pastoral areas of Africa are usually termed 'low potential' with respect to livestock production although livestock numbers are substantial.

In some countries, there will be opportunities to support linkages between projects aiming to develop private CAHW networks and national veterinary privatization programmes. The latter can include business management training for veterinarians, assistance with writing a business plan and access to credit at favourable interest rates. Such programmes often establish a loan scheme with a national bank and use programme funds to guarantee some of the loans. Programme staff may monitor the performance of businesses under the scheme and provide financial advice if problems arise. Therefore, partnerships between these programmes and CAHW programmes can be extremely useful, with one side providing the business management support and credit facilities, and the other side providing the community-based support.

Another option for credit includes encouraging veterinarians to seek business partners who possess sufficient equity to source loans for the business. This is probably one of the strongest loan arrangements because it combines technical veterinary know-how with the business savvy of an existing, successful businessperson. The arrangement is not dependent on aid inputs in the form of finance, but only by way of technical support, training and monitoring. In different cultures, different lending systems exist and, where possible, projects should try to use these existing loan arrangements. A further option is to approach the pharmaceutical manufacturers and their agents. These companies are constantly looking for new markets and they may be interested in investing in a private practice if that means opening up new market areas for their products.

In the absence of a national privatization programme, a CAHW project can offer to guarantee a bank loan for private veterinarians. This form of assistance requires very careful design and, ideally, a substantial personal investment from the veterinarian (or group of veterinarians) in order to demonstrate commitment to the project. In the absence of such investment, an aid-funded project should probably avoid the guarantee arrangement because the guarantee can easily be regarded as 'soft' by the veterinarian, because it is based on aid funds rather than being a genuine commercial enterprise. Consequently, there is less pressure on the loan recipient to keep up loan repayment because the project, not the veterinarian, will be held financially responsible.

d. Selection and training of CAHWs

In a privatized CAHW network, the private veterinarian will be responsible for supervising the CAHWs in addition to supplying them with veterinary medicines. Consequently, a project can assist a private veterinarian to work with communities to select and train CAHWs. The overall approaches and methods to be followed for CAHW selection are described in Chapter 2, and training issues are described in Chapters 4 and 5.

The project and the private veterinarian will have to decide if and how to incorporate CAHW selection and training costs into the business plan. Although initially, these costs might be met by the project, future training events (e.g. refresher training) should be funded by the private business as part of the business running costs.

e. Monitoring performance

An important feature of establishing new CAHW networks is proper monitoring. This includes early 'post-training' monitoring in the first few weeks after training (see Chapter 5) and establishing a regular monitoring system (see Chapter 6). In a privatized CAHW network, monitoring of financial indicators is particularly important and can form part of the loan agreement, particularly if the agreement is with a privatization programme or NGO.

Where is there is weak commitment to veterinary privatization

In some countries, governments have not yet fully committed themselves to veterinary privatization. In these countries, privatization policy may not exist or it remains suspended in 'draft' form. Even when clear policies are evident, they may not receive the required political support to ensure enactment. In these situations, the aim of sustainability in CAHW systems is a major challenge because the real policy environment does not support private sector development and yet governments and NGOs have a poor record in sustaining community-based projects. One approach in these areas is to work with government to design and test CAHW networks or 'pilot projects' based on full cost recovery. With this approach, the project provides the bulk of the start-up costs for the network but runs the CAHW system using the principles of small business management.

Box 3.17 Pathways for improving financial sustainability in CAHW services: countries where there is weak commitment to veterinary privatization

Policy context

- ◆ no government policy on veterinary privatization; or
- ◆ policy exists but weak government commitment to support policy

⇩

Approach

Establish and test a system with:
- ◆ 'the project' supporting a CAHW network by supplying medicines and providing technical supervision;
- ◆ 'the project' based on sound, small business development principles;
- ◆ 'the project' acting as a pilot system to inform policy on veterinary privatization.

⇩

Key activities

1. Identify government partners for developing and testing the pilot system.
2. Training:
   - ◆ participatory approaches and methods;
   - ◆ small business planning;
   - ◆ participative training techniques.
3. Participatory analysis:
   - ◆ with community to identify key needs and solutions;
   - ◆ leading to information to develop a project business plan;
   - ◆ clarify prices of drugs and incentives for CAHWs.
4. Develop the project business plan.
5. Use project resources to begin implementation.
6. Work with communities to select and train CAHWs.
7. Close monitoring of CAHWs activities and business performance.
8. Regular reporting to government.
9. Relay experiences to policy makers; facilitate stakeholder analysis of experiences and opportunities e.g. handing over the CAHW network to the private sector.

When using this approach, government veterinarians are exposed to alternative ways of working, including both community-based approaches and the management of cost recovery for services. Ultimately, a model CAHW network can emerge that not only informs government policy reform, but that can also be handed over to the private sector when the opportunity arises. Well-designed cost recovery studies, such as that outlined in Box 3.5, can be useful for comparing public sector and private sector delivery models, and improving understanding of financial sustainability among government players.

When designing this type of project, it is important to include specific policy-related outputs and activities in the project proposal and ensure government support at an early stage. An optimistic output might be 'Revised government policy in place to support privatized CAHW networks' whereas a more cautious output could be 'Increased awareness of CAHW systems among policy makers'. These types of project outputs need to be supported by activities that bring together stakeholders at various stages of the project. These events can be used to involve government players in the design of the project and conduct frequent reviews to check progress and revise activities as necessary. Information dissemination can also be very important in this type of project and so, again, this activity has to be planned and budgeted. More detail on ways to influence policy is provided in Chapter 8.

Other important components of the project are similar to those already mentioned in the previous section and in other chapters of the book. These include training of project staff in participatory approaches and methods, and participative training techniques, exposure to experiences in other countries through study tours, and close day-to-day support to ensure meaningful community participation in the project.

Where there is no government

Community-based animal health approaches have often been used in areas suffering from conflict and where no recognizable government is present. In acute situations, sustainability issues can be very difficult to address because communities can be facing extreme food security or other problems, and the immediate need is to keep people alive and protect their livestock. Therefore, in emergencies the provision of free veterinary care is sometimes a necessity. However, pre-existing veterinary services should be considered as a means to deliver assistance and, in the case of the private sector, efforts should be made to limit negative impact on small businesses in the area in question. For example, an emergency project might buy veterinary medicines from local suppliers at normal market rates and contract CAHW networks to disseminate the drugs and provide the treatments.

In more long-term or chronic conflict-affected areas, the establishment of sustainable CAHW networks is largely dependent on at least four important factors:

◆ the presence of sufficient numbers of veterinary professionals to work with projects to establish and manage CAHWs, ideally on a private basis. During conflict, many people can be forced to flee from an area and sometimes become residents of neighbouring countries or move overseas;

◆ the presence of active livestock markets which enable communities to turn animals into cash to pay for basic veterinary services. Conflict can sometimes destroy market infrastucture and holding grounds, or prevent movement of livestock. Banking systems can also collapse and there may be no formal facilities for foreign currency exchange;

Box 3.18 Pathways for improving financial sustainability in CAHW services: countries where there is no government

Policy context

◆ no effective government in place
◆ no official policy on veterinary service delivery

⇩

Approach

◆ Establish a CAHW network.
◆ Supply medicines according to local capacity to pay.
◆ Co-ordinate aid agencies; develop best practice guidelines and common strategy for CAHW services.
◆ Seek private sector involvement as soon as possible.
◆ Promote policy debate among potential future administrations.

⇩

Key activities

1. Training:
   ◆ participatory approaches and methods;
   ◆ participative training techniques.
2. Participatory analysis:
   ◆ with community to identify key needs and solutions;
   ◆ clarify prices of drugs and incentives for CAHWs.
3. Use project resources to begin implementation.
4. Work with communities to select and train CAHWs.
5. Close monitoring of CAHWs activities and performance.
6. Hand over veterinary drug supply to private sector as soon as feasible.
7. Relay experiences to potential policy makers; facilitate stakeholder analysis of experiences and opportunities.

- the presence of reasonably strong local administrations to ensure security in the area and safe working conditions for CAHWs and other workers. Local administrations can vary from those established by independence movements to self-declared independent states;
- co-ordination of animal health projects to ensure common approaches in adjacent areas. For example, varying approaches to cost recovery by different agencies causes confusion among communities.

Considering these factors, it is likely that sustainability is not a realistic objective in many conflict situations or where government is absent. Despite this, it is often possible to establish CAHW networks with a strong element of cost recovery built into the system. For example, veterinary medicines can be provided through CAHWs at

---

Box 3.19 Towards sustainability in the CAHW programme in southern Sudan

The current cost recovery system aims to prepare for a future privatized animal health service, where livestock owners pay full cost for vaccinations and treatments to CAHWs. The CAHWs would make a profit from their services and would be supervised by Animal Health Auxiliaries or equivalent who in turn would be supervised by private veterinarians. The veterinarians would carry out community dialogue to identify needs and involve the community in the development of animal health services, provide training, ongoing follow up to CAHWs and run pharmacies to supply medicines to the CAHWs. The more active the CAHWs the better the availability of services to the livestock owners and the greater the profit for the CAHW, supervisors and veterinarians.

The role of the government would be policy development and regulation of the private system to ensure that training of CAHWs is standardized and of good quality, and that animal health services and pharmaceutical suppliers meet technical standards. In southern Sudan, for such a system to be in place the infrastructure and economy need to be sufficiently developed to allow importation of medicines and equipment through established trade routes. At present, export trade in southern Sudanese livestock and teak is just being re-established to Uganda and Kenya. The programme is currently working to facilitate trade in livestock to improve the trading situation and by influencing Sudanese professionals who may be interested to invest in medicine supply to southern Sudan. However, for the system to be sustainable, there needs to be peace.

(source: Jones et al., 1998 – see 'Further reading' section)

---

commercial rates rather than being given free of charge or subsidized. Although implementing agencies will bear procurement, administration and transport costs, at least a cost recovery approach helps to reduce expectations about free or cheap services. Consequently, when conflict ends people are accustomed to paying for services and this helps the private sector to develop.

Similarly, engagement with local administrations, whatever their form and legitimacy, often encourages them to develop their policies. Unless the local authorities understand the approach, see it working and appreciate it, there is a risk that unsupportive policies may be put in place as circumstances change, displaced policy makers return and the administration consolidates.

3.5 Can privatized CAHW networks really work? A case study from Kenya

This section is a short case study of FARM Africa's privatized CAHW service in Meru and Tharaka-Nithi Districts, Kenya. This project was the winner of the News International Not-for-Profit Award 2000 for 'promotion of sustainable economic development in poor communities in the developing world through the use of commercial best practice'.

Background

In Kenya, both large- and small-scale farmers practise livestock farming throughout Meru Central and South Districts. However, livestock farming is predominantly undertaken by the small-scale farmers. Clinical veterinary service delivery in the country has experienced problems, particularly in the wake of privatization of veterinary services. In the past, the Government of Kenya provided veterinary services at subsidized rates. However, these services stopped in 1985 because the Government was unable to sustain the heavy investments and subsidies involved.

By 1998, a few vets had taken up the challenge and opened private practices in the country. However, most of them located their practices in the high-potential areas where dairy activities were predominant. In these areas, the practices were found in markets or operated from the homes of the veterinarians. Therefore, the rural people had to travel long distances to look for services, which was time-consuming and costly.

Project approach and activities

FARM Africa's approach in Meru and Tharaka-Nithi Districts was to develop a veterinary-supervised, private and community-based animal healthcare system. Through the process of identifying potential candidates and preparing business proposals, it became clear that there were a number of trained Animal Health

Box 3.20 FARM Africa's veterinarian-supervised private animal healthcare system in Meru and Tharaka-Nithi Districts, Kenya

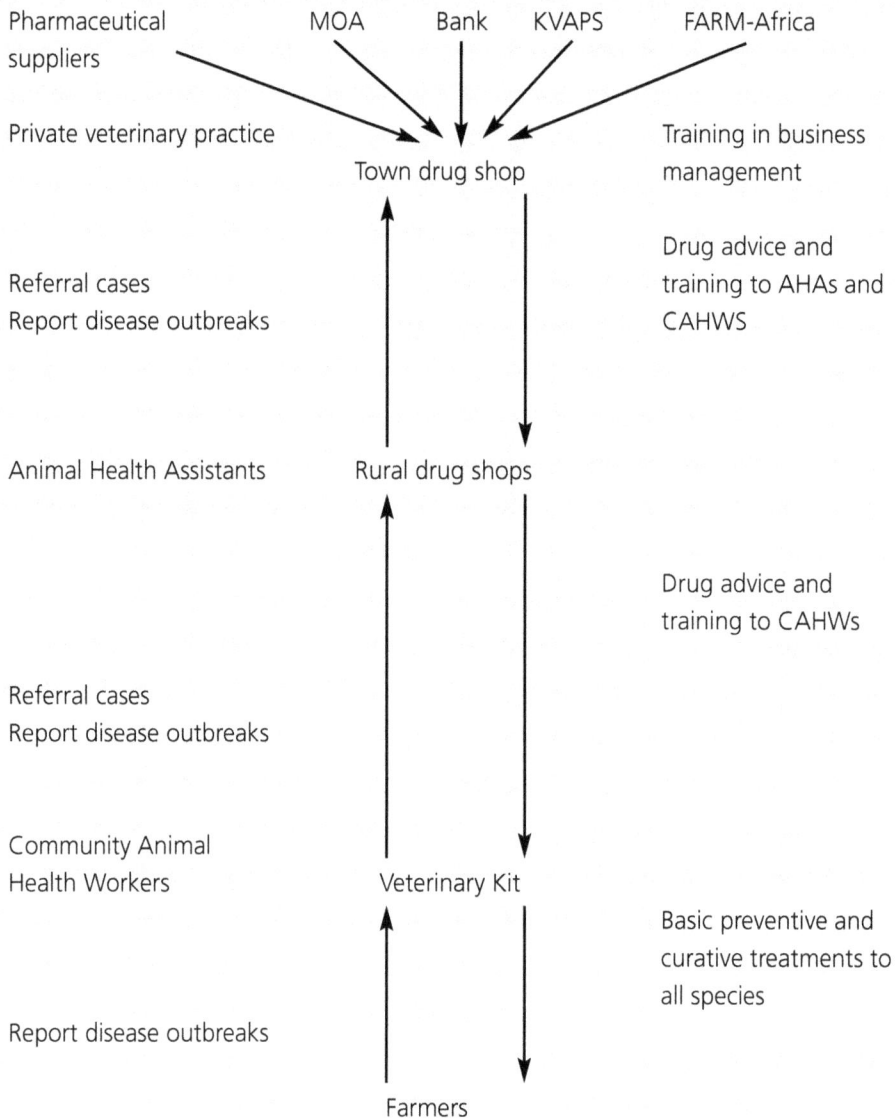

Pharmaceutical suppliers   MOA   Bank   KVAPS   FARM-Africa

Private veterinary practice

Town drug shop   Training in business management

Referral cases
Report disease outbreaks   Drug advice and training to AHAs and CAHWS

Animal Health Assistants   **Rural drug shops**

Drug advice and training to CAHWs

Referral cases
Report disease outbreaks

Community Animal Health Workers   **Veterinary Kit**

Basic preventive and curative treatments to all species

Report disease outbreaks

Farmers

Note:
KVAPS = Kenya Veterinary Association Privatization Scheme
MOA = Ministry of Agriculture

Assistants (AHAs) in the field who were unemployed. The communities suggested that these AHAs could become part of a private system, and so a model was developed in which the AHAs occupied an intermediary position between the vets and the CAHWs (see Box 3.20).

The AHAs were advanced credit to establish rural drug shops, which sold drugs and provided clinical services to farmers. The AHAs also supervised and supplied the CAHWS with drugs. Farmers went directly to their nearest supplier to obtain veterinary services (this includes the CAHWs). By so doing, the project hoped to increase accessibility to animal healthcare services and drug supplies to smallholder farmers in the lower potential areas. This also reduced the cost of services tremendously by eliminating or reducing transport costs. The project linked up with the Kenya Veterinary Privatization Scheme (KVAPS) which was developing private services in high-potential areas (see Box 3.21).

The FARM Africa system operated with two vets (one female, one male), six AHAs (two female, four male) and 44 CAHWs (17 female, 27 male) working in five divisions. Each vet was in charge of two divisions and operated from a practice office within an agrovet shop. The office had a telephone and was located in a main town. AHAs were located in the rural markets and operated a rural drug shop, which supplies drugs and agrochemicals to the farmers as well as the CAHWS.

Box 3.21 Achievements and problems facing national veterinary privatization programmes: the case of Kenya

In November 1994, the Kenya Veterinary Association Privatization Scheme (KVAPS) began as a collaboration between:

◆ the Government of Kenya through the Ministry of Agriculture (MOA) as the implementing line Ministry (though implemented by the MOA the project management is autonomous and free from ministerial interference and control);
◆ the Kenya Veterinary Association as the executing agency through a privatization trust;
◆ the Barclays Bank of Kenya Ltd as the credit intermediary bank;
◆ the European Commission (EC) as the funding institution;
◆ the Organization of African Unity under the Pan African Rinderpest Campaign (PARC). Privatization of veterinary services is a component of the PARC project in Africa.

When reviewing experiences in 1998, KVAPS Assistant Project Manager Mary Kariuki noted the following achievements:

To date, the Scheme has funded a total of 42 practices, 16 of which were pure start-ups. Both pre- and post-loan training has been held for all the participating veterinarians. At least 90 per cent of the funded veterinarians are doing well while the remaining 10 per cent are putting a lot of effort to repay their loans and expand their practices. It is worth noting that the high-potential intensive farming areas hold most of the supported practices.

However, the following problems were also encountered:

> *For the last six months, the Scheme has registered a drop in the number of veterinary surgeons applying for loans under the Scheme. The following factors have been identified as contributing to this scenario:*

> ◆ *Realization that KVAPS is self-sustaining and therefore vigilant in ensuring loan repayment. When the Scheme started, there was an attitude of 'It's another donor-funded project that will soon be terminated'. Those who understand the dire consequences of default are hesitant to borrow as they now realize that they cannot get away with it.*

> ◆ *The prevailing poor economic situation in the country has reduced the purchasing power of the farmers hence reducing demand for artifical insemination and clinical services. Private practice, therefore, has become less lucrative due to the reduced profitability. Veterinarians carrying out a market study realize these facts hence the reduced demand on KVAPS loans.*

> ◆ *Unfair competition in the delivery of animal health services by Animal Health Assistants and government veterinarians.*

> ◆ *When the Scheme started its operations in 1995, the bank base rate was 16 per cent and thus the initial loanees borrowed at 19 per cent. In 1997 and the first half of 1998, the base rate has increased to 26 per cent. The veterinarians in the Government of Kenya service found this rather high as they can borrow from their Co-operative society at lower interest rates. This also adversely affects the veterinarians in the Scheme, as they have to cope with fluctuating interest rates.*

a. Loan arrangements

Both the vets and AHAs conducted feasibility studies with the help of FARM Africa and drew up business plans. Participatory methods such as service and opportunity maps, pair-wise ranking of diseases and seasonal disease incidences were used to predict the expected caseloads per month. Other sources of data were the Divisional Veterinary Officer's files and the District Veterinary Officer's records.

Each vet in the project was given a bank loan through a national bank, with the size of the loan depending on the vet's business proposal. FARM Africa guaranteed about a third of the loan, KVAPS also a third and the vet had to provide collateral for the other third. The vet's portion was a third-party guarantee or a mortgage on equipment e.g. a motorbike. All the AHAs were also given a loan through a national bank. As a show of commitment they had to provide security, be it their own equity or a third-party guarantee. FARM Africa opened fixed-deposit accounts of a similar amount and used the certificate of deposit as collateral in the bank. The interest earned from the fixed-deposit account was used to lower the commercial interest for the AHAs, for example at the start the commercial interest rate was 34 per cent but the AHAs were paying only 20 per cent interest.

b. Duties of the different workers

In the FARM Africa system, the duties of the different veterinary workers were as follows:

Duties of a private vet

- Provide veterinary drugs and agrochemicals to AHAs, CAHWs and farmers. Apart from stocking drug shops for the AHAs, the vet also supplied the CAHWs surrounding the practice but at supply prices offered by the AHAs in the field.
- Provide clinical services.
- Attend to referral cases.
- Practise and run the shop.
- Provide artificial insemination and disease control services.
- Train the CAHWs (frequent refresher courses).
- Compile a monthly report and send it to the District Veterinary Officer, FARM Africa and KVAPS.
- Supervise the activities of the AHAs and CAHWs and organize regular meetings with them.

Duties of the AHA

- Supply the CAHWS and the farmers with drugs.
- Provide clinical services.
- Attend to referral cases and refer those unable to attend to the vet.
- Manage the rural drug shop.
- Report outbreaks to the vet.
- Write monthly reports and send to the vet.
- Supervise the CAHWs and provide them with refresher courses where they found weakness and also organize regular meetings with them.
- Provide extension services and training for farmers in areas identified by the community.
- Carry out monitoring exercises.

Duties of the CAHW

- Treat minor problems such as wounds and carry out routine tasks such as deworming, spraying and castration.
- Monitor and report outbreaks and deaths to the rural drug shops.
- Train fellow farmers on good husbandry techniques.
- Organize training for the community with the vet or the AHA.
- Report on activities in the field.

Impact of the animal health services

a. Information on the animal health service provided

One way of assessing the impact of the services was through the use of participatory methods. For example, a ladder diagram (constructed on the ground from maize stovers with leaves for markers) was used by farmers to show the level of the health of their animals at different time periods: five years ago, at the start of the project and presently. Although the standard of health started and finished at different levels, the trend for every group or individual farmer interviewed (project and non-project) showed an increase since the start of the project.

Reasons given for the improvement in animal health from the start of the project to the present time were as follows:

- availability of project-trained CAHWs or AHAs (73 per cent of the replies);
- non-project-trained CAHWs, AHAs or vets (27 per cent of the replies);
- goat houses ensured that goats were clean and had fewer worms;
- farmers have been implementing what they were taught at seminars;
- farmers have learnt about general hygiene, therefore animals have fewer worms;
- improved feeding.

Between December 1997 and September 1998, project records showed that the CAHWs provided a service to 4180 farmers and treated 6998 animals. The CAHWs referred a total of 248 cases to either an AHA or a vet.

b. Economic indicators

The total value of the drugs sold by CAHWs was KSh222 285.80 (approximately GB£2020). They only treated animals as a part-time activity to complement their usual day-to-day activities. The drug kits were provided in the form of a loan. They were to repay 60 per cent of the drugs cost back to the project. Within a year the CAHWs were able to repay 53 per cent back to the project.

Table 3.2 shows a breakdown of revenue and expenditure for vets, AHAs and CAHWs as a proportion of total annual figures. This shows that, compared with vets, AHAs and CAHWs earned relatively more income from hands-on treatment of livestock. Table 3.3 summarizes some of the results of financial and economic analyses. Each of the listed components is clearly financially viable. All the benefit–cost ratios (BCR) are greater than unity. The break-even sensitivity analysis results indicate that the components are very stable. Total costs could increase or total benefits could fall by large percentages from those used in the base model analysis and the components would still be financially viable. The high BCRs for veterinarian, AHA and CAHW enterprises were a good indication of the potential financial viability of the private animal healthcare delivery system in a dairy cattle system. This demonstrated the potential for extending private veterinary services to other, similar farming systems in Kenya and elsewhere in the eastern Africa region.

Table 3.2 Revenue and expenditure for veterinarians and CAHWs in the FARM Africa privatized CAHW network

	Proportion of total annual revenue and expenditure (%)	
	For private veterinarians	For private AHAs and CAHWs
Revenue		
◆ drug sales	71	71
◆ clinical service fees	21	48
◆ consultation fees	6	3
Expenditure		
◆ drug purchases	74	57
◆ salaries	14	27
◆ rent	3	8
◆ transport	2	5

Table 3.3 Benefit–cost ratios and break-even sensitivity analysis

Indicator of viability	Private veterinarians	AHAs and CAHWs	Overall project
Benefit–cost ratio	2.5	4.2	1.4
Break-even sensitivity analysis:			
- total costs	149	318	80
- total benefits	60	76	25

The break-even sensitivity analysis shows the percentage change required to reduce the benefit–cost ratio to 1.00; total costs need to increase and/or benefits to decrease by the percentages shown above.

3.6 Broader issues affecting sustainability

Animal health services do not exist in a vacuum and are influenced by many economic, political and cultural factors. As mentioned previously, the overall economic conditions prevailing in an area and market activity will affect sustainability. During participatory analysis it is usually possible to identify some of the fundamental problems that limit the sustainability of any private business or community-based animal health delivery system. These vary with country and region but some of the more common ones consist of the following:

- ◆ conflict or insecurity in the work area that prevents overall development or makes private business prohibitively risky;
- ◆ lack of infrastructure (roads, market facilities such as holding grounds or loading ramps, telecommunications);
- ◆ lack of markets for livestock and livestock products;
- ◆ poor use of pasture or range due to lack of water sources, over-grazing, land tenure disputes;

- ◆ weak local representation or poor capacity for communities to organize themselves;
- ◆ marginalization of communities in terms of service provision (education, health services, technical training, water resources, local government);
- ◆ lack of credit.

All of these factors will negatively affect sustainability and may have to be addressed before or during the development of an animal health project. Where communities rate animal health as a high priority, it is possible to use animal health as a vehicle for addressing some of these problems, as described in Box 3.22.

Box 3.22 Animal health services as an entry point to brokering peace among warring pastoralist groups and encouraging integrated development

'Use one stone to kill two birds', so goes the adage.

The Organization of African Unity/Interafrican Bureau for Animal Resources (OAU/IBAR) core mandate is to promote the development of animal resources in the African continent. To this end, OAU/IBAR undertook to eradicate rinderpest from the continent in the 1990s. One of the target areas was the Karamojong cluster, a semi-arid area straddling four countries north-west Kenya, south-west Ethiopia, south-east Sudan and north-east Uganda. The inhabitants of the cluster, consisting of 14 ethnic groups, depend on livestock for their livelihood. Livestock rustling tradition has been practised in the cluster since time immemorial. However, this practice has assumed disturbing proportions in recent times. The factors contributing to this trend include war in the Sudan, easy availability of guns, breakdown of the traditional social control mechanisms, shrinkage of grazing land and lack of water resources and increasing general poverty.

After several years of working with local communities to introduce sustainable animal health delivery systems in the cluster, OAU/IBAR and the partner communities identified insecurity and livestock raiding as one of the key constraints. In 1998, the communities requested IBAR to facilitate intercommunal dialogue to explore avenues for containing the insecurity and bring about reconciliation so that animal health services could be continued effectively. What started out as a relatively informal activity that used concern over animal health to discuss broader development problems soon started to show results and attract a lot of attention from other development actors, including government agencies.

Meetings of elders and community leaders continued throughout the year 1999. Initially, representatives of two neighbouring communities were brought together. The climax of the year was the meeting of all the communities. A total of 100 elders attended this meeting and discussed the problems of raiding and insecurity, identified the root causes, and proposed activities to address the problems. Pervasive poverty was identified as being at the heart of the problem. Among other causes identified were the following:

◆ shortages of grazing lands and water;
◆ the apparent inability of governments to address insecurity;
◆ war in southern Sudan;
◆ easy availability of arms;
◆ breakdown of traditional elders' authority over the youth;
◆ lack of education facilities to engage the youth and offer them alternative ways of earning their livelihoods;
◆ a general lack of development.

The elders then went on to make proposals relating to what should be done to prevent, contain and manage conflict. Governments were requested to collaborate with each other in carrying out the following:

◆ stamping out raiding;
◆ facilitating branding of animals for identification;
◆ intensifying education and training for the youth;
◆ working with communities to make water widely available;
◆ facilitating cross-border trade;
◆ improving communications infrastructure;
◆ generally creating a climate conducive to peace and development

The meeting also made recommendations to development agencies and donors. The following key activities were recommended for action by those agencies:

◆ working with communities to improve animal health provision;
◆ collaborating with governments to initiate and catalyse development;
◆ assisting in the empowerment of youth and women;
◆ generally intensifying and expanding the development initiatives currently being undertaken.

The following key roles, among others, for the communities were also identified by the elders:

◆ intensifying the people-to-people dialogue;
◆ participating in the promotion of education provision for their children;
◆ taking part in the disease control and eradication activities;

- ◆ restoring useful traditions of social organization and control;
- ◆ adopting, where possible, alternative means of earning livelihoods;
- ◆ participating in their development creation;
- ◆ raising high-standard livestock for market.

The community representatives' meetings continue to be held under the facilitation of the OAU/IBAR. Youth and women forums have been organized in the fashion of the elders' meetings. Raiding has been curbed in a few cases, as a result of those meetings. For example, the raids that were prevalent between the Turkana and the Toposa groups have almost ceased and, in a few cases where these have taken place, the elders, working closely with the local authorities, have managed to get the stolen livestock returned.

While all this is happening, community-based animal health delivery systems continue to be developed in the region in a collaborative effort between government vet services, communities, NGOs and the private sector.

(contributed by Dr Darlington Akabwai)

Many of fundamental problems affecting sustainability relate to policy and strategy, but these areas are not normally the direct mandate of NGOs or private individuals. However, co-ordination with mandated organizations (government or international agencies), information sharing and dissemination, and integration of development efforts can all promote improvement in the situation. Therefore, it is in the interests of animal health practitioners and NGOs to find out who is doing what to alleviate fundamental problems and then become directly or indirectly involved.

One long-term approach to overcoming the basic problems of an under-served area is to invest in community development. Successful development projects around the world all have a common theme of local organization-building leading to empowerment of local groups. Once empowered, local groups are much better able to address fundamental problems themselves. One example of groups doing this is given in Box 3.23.

3.7 Summary

This chapter provides guidelines for helping to improve the sustainability of CAHW services. It highlights the importance of community participation for ensuring that local people have a major say in the design and implementation of services. Such services are more likely to be used, supported and sustained. Related to community participation is the need for careful and patient dialogue to ensure that communities agree to the pricing systems that are established, the incentives for CAHWs and the roles and responsibilities of the different players.

Box 3.23 Developing pastoral associations to strengthen local community problem-solving abilities

In Wajir District of north-east Kenya, the NGO Oxfam–GB and the Government of Kenya through the Arid Lands Resource Management Project (ALRMP) have with the local communities invested in the development of pastoral associations (PA). They see these pastoral associations as the core engine by which improvements to people's lives will be delivered. The PAs are responsible for providing and managing services to their pastoralist members in the fields of education, livestock and human health and water, either directly or through subcommittees (e.g. water users' associations). PAs may also play a role in areas such as conflict management and natural resource management, drought early-warning and response, and livestock marketing. The work of PAs is facilitated by a district pastoral association (DPA) whose capacity continues to be strengthened. In Wajir, the DPA has a drug store that stocks drugs for the distribution to the PAs who in turn sell drugs to *Daryelles*, community health workers for both livestock and human health (*Daryelle* means carer or the concerned in Somali). The DPA currently has a full-time animal health technician attached to it from the Department of Veterinary Services and it is hoped that in time the DPA's drug turnover will allow it to employ a full-time veterinarian.

The establishment of associations is a long-term development strategy and is based on strategies different from those to establish private veterinary practices. The list below illustrates some of the key lessons in forming such associations and those organizations interested in developing similar associations should refer to the Oxfam manual in the 'Further reading' section:

◆ long, repeated and frequent visits by the agency are necessary during the PA formation period. The same staff should be involved each time;
◆ the start-up phase of PAs is resource-intensive: initial assessment, continually explaining new concepts, prompt response to the most immediate needs to gain the community's confidence, repeated visits, training and close monitoring. This is all costly but the extent to which it is done and the resources invested in this respect (opposed to emphasis on physical structures) have been shown to be key factors in the success of PA organization;
◆ start funding of some activities during community planning phase: improved animal health builds the community's confidence in the PA's ability to implement and also convinces the community that the agency is serious in its commitment;
◆ do not start too many activities until sufficient groundwork has been laid and the association formed and understood. There is a need to go at pace of the community, not the external agency (for example, large amounts of drugs provided before the PA is well-established have been a mistake);
◆ the importance of community contribution in all aspects of the programme. From

the beginning, communities realized they would have to play the lead in all future activities;

♦ communities must be allowed to go at their own pace – even if slow: take the time necessary to discuss internally and understand the concepts;

♦ many in the community have misunderstood the concept of the PA as a profit-making venture in which they invest shares. This may partly derive from the word – *sherqed* – used for PA in Somali.

♦ part of the challenge is changing attitudes and the accepted way of doing things: this will take a long time – for example, for Oxfam's work in the east of the District, it took three years of the first phase for the idea to be widely understood;

♦ lower community expectations from the beginning; make it clear that the stress will be on the community itself; direct external inputs will be limited in scale and time frame;

♦ develop a thorough understanding of the local context: in particular local elites and social dynamics. Avoid the association relying on a few main elites in the centre;

♦ recognizing but not ingraining clan divisions: raise it as an issue if it appears one clan is being marginalized by the PA;

♦ points for agency capacity: do not try and work with too many PAs at once – it will stretch the agency too far;

♦ avoid PA moving away from focus on pastoralist issues to settlement issues – approach sprouted out of need for pastoral development;

♦ the approach to working with PAs needs to be adapted for PAs at larger settlements: high urban populations with many gatekeepers increases the difficulty of involving *badia* people; the agency may need to devise a separate 'urban programme';

♦ maintain a fine balance between local ownership and external control: the community must direct the process but note the importance of agency being prepared to intervene at some points, for example ensuring representativeness;

♦ agencies supporting PAs should be consistent in their approach, transparent and accountable in their dealings, and maintain commitments made to communities.

The chapter pays particular attention to issues of financial sustainability and explains how private CAHW networks, with veterinarians supervising and supplying CAHWs, can overcome some of the common problems associated with government or NGO projects. Strategies for building financial sustainability into CAHW systems are described in relation to different privatization policy contexts, varying from clear and strong support for privatization, to lack of government and no policy.

Taking a long-term perspective involves taking a broad overview of the situation and looking beyond purely animal health issues. Environmental sustainability means proper use of veterinary medicines and agrochemicals, and looking at the effect of improved animal health on natural resources. For both environmental and economic sustainability, CAHW services need to be aware of the importance of marketing opportunities for livestock and livestock products.

In many countries, policy and legislation does not fully support community-based approaches to animal healthcare. This is a crucial issue for the sustainability of CAHW services, and ways to influence policy are described in Chapter 8.

Ultimately, sustainability is difficult to define. Even in industrialized countries, farming practices can change and private veterinary services that were once thought to be 'sustainable' suddenly find themselves no longer viable (see Box 3.24). With the removal of subsidies for either farming systems or veterinary services, livestock keepers will take more responsibility for the basic veterinary care of their animals.

Box 3.24 The changing face of farm animal practice

Below is an abstract from an editorial in the Veterinary Record, the official journal of the British Veterinary Association, dated October 1998. It discusses the challenges facing private veterinary practices in livestock-farming areas. Although these farm animal practices were once the backbone of the veterinary profession, times change and the removal of farm subsidies by the European Commission prompted debate on farming trends and the viability of private veterinary practice. Some would argue that farm animal veterinary practice in the United Kingdom was indirectly subsidized by the EC, because farming itself was subsidized. Also, little did we know that foot and mouth disease would break out in 2001.

Brave new agriculture

This year's British Veterinary Association Congress featured some excellent debates, but none was quite so thought-provoking as that on the future of farm animal practice. The debate was, of course, prompted by the current crisis in agriculture: if, as some have suggested, British livestock farming is seriously endangered, what of the veterinary practices that serve its needs? Reports of the death of livestock farming may be exaggerated (just) – but there can be no doubt that it is set to change significantly over the next few years. How will this affect the veterinary profession, and how should the profession react to the changes taking place?

Whatever the outcome of the Common Agricultural Policy reforms (i.e. fewer subsidies), the tendency towards fewer, larger livestock units in itself provides challenges for the veterinary profession and it is clear that large animal practices will have to adapt. With fewer farms and fewer practices, veterinarians would have to provide services over a wider area and this might create logistical problems. **Meanwhile, there would be a decline in the amount of routine work of the kind traditionally undertaken by farm animal practitioners, as farmers took on more of these tasks themselves.**

Participative training approaches and methods

Karen Iles

CONTENTS

4.1 Introduction

Overview

Training of community-based animal health workers (CAHWs) is often seen as the high point when setting up a community-based animal health (CAH) system and is received with much anticipation by the community. The training represents the culmination of months of work and preparation, from numerous meetings with the community, government staff and other stakeholders, to surveys, designing the project and selecting the CAHWs. Experience from different parts of the world has shown that the effectiveness of CAHW systems partly depends on the abilities of the CAHWs and, therefore, the quality of the training they have received. Livestock owners need to feel confident about the skills and knowledge of the CAHWs.

Training provided for CAHWs will not necessarily be the same for all projects because the role of CAHWs varies between areas. Effective, good-quality training for CAHWs, specifically designed for the project area, is therefore pivotal to the success of a project and requires careful planning. Teaching directly from textbooks on animal health and husbandry is rarely appropriate. These books are usually too technical for training primary-level workers and tend to focus on high-input farming systems rather than the production systems used in many rural areas. The challenge facing the trainers is to design courses that give trainees the knowledge, skills and attitudes required to address the specific livestock problems in the area that have been identified through surveys and discussions with the community. The advice offered to livestock owners has to be appropriate to the area, make use of local resources and be affordable.

Chapters 4 and 5 describe how to provide effective training for CAHWs. To emphasize the importance of the training approach, Chapter 4 concentrates on participative training approaches and methods. Usually, the trainers themselves need to be trained in participative training techniques and how to design training courses. Trainers also need to receive guidance on how to plan and evaluate training sessions. Chapter 5 concentrates on the detailed design of an actual CAHW training course based on participatory survey data and the needs of the community. Chapter 5 also includes the logistics of organizing training events, and issues such as who pays for the training and how to evaluate the effectiveness of training.

Being flexible and adapting to local situations and resources

The principles and tools set out in this chapter are based on ideal situations and on best-practice recommendations for training. However, while it may be possible and desirable for larger, well-funded projects to commit considerable resources to the training component of a CAHW project, smaller projects or individual veterinarians may not have these resources. This should not prevent people from proceeding with their CAHW training. The basic principles still apply – in particular, the use of participative training approaches and techniques.

4.2   Principles of participative learning and training

Lectures and formal approaches to training

During their formal education at school, college or university, most veterinarians and livestock professionals will have experienced formal training methods such as lectures. Typically, the teacher stands in front of the class and attempts to teach the students by telling them the information they need to know. With the formal lecture, the students take a passive role in the learning process. There is usually little interaction between teacher and students, and limited scope for discussion or asking questions. The flow of information tends to be one way, from the teacher to the students. Opportunities for students to share their experiences either with each other or with the teacher are few. This type of training is said to be 'teacher-centred' where the emphasis is on the teacher attempting to cover the subject matter in the lesson, with rather less concern for whether or not the students really understand what is being taught. Because this approach is not very interactive, it is often difficult for the teacher to know whether or not students have grasped the content of the lesson, other than perhaps to ask at the end of the lesson 'Does anyone have any questions?'

The formal teaching approach may be appropriate for university courses where a large amount of subject matter is covered and students are expected to carry out self-learning in their free time. However, experience in CAH and other rural development projects has shown that this approach is rarely effective for training livestock keepers.

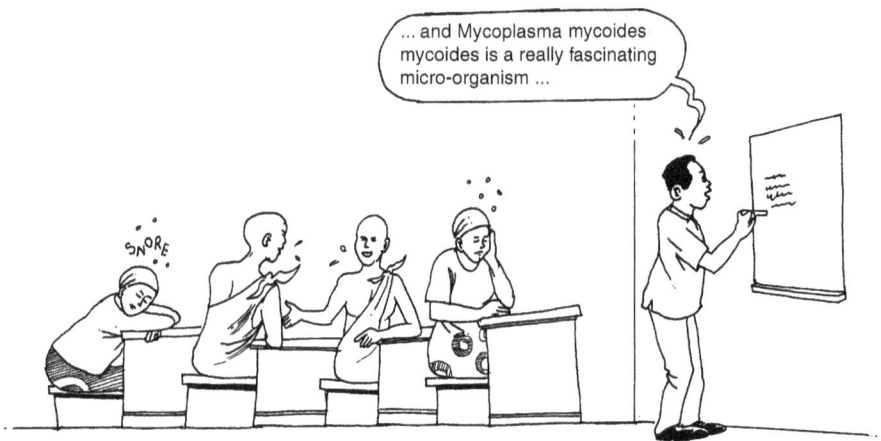

Feeling sleepy? Formal classroom lecturing is never a good way a train CAHWs

Principles of adult learning

The basic premise of adult training is to build on the experience and knowledge that people already have. Participants should be encouraged to take responsibility for their own learning.

Box 4.1 How adults learn

Adults learn best when:

◆ the training is relevant to their daily lives;
◆ they come to learn voluntarily;
◆ they can share their own experiences through discussion;
◆ they are encouraged to present their problems freely;
◆ they are encouraged to analyse problems and find their own solutions;
◆ they learn skills practically;
◆ the training fits with their culture;
◆ the trainer uses discussion, pictures, plays, song, drama, exercises and visual aids (pictures, models, films, photographs, slides);
◆ they understand the objectives of the training.

People with busy lives and many responsibilities have little time to deal with information that they do not think is useful. Effective learning takes place when people see the relevance of what they are learning. Short-term memory can become less reliable as people get older, and so lecture-based learning becomes less effective. People also learn more effectively when they can learn at their own pace, and have the opportunity to analyse, reflect and draw their own conclusions based on their life experience. If they are learning new skills, they need plenty of time and equipment to practise, so that the lesson is reinforced. Adults are rarely satisfied with an explanation from the trainer – they want to do it themselves until they are satisfied they have understood everything.

Many livestock keepers have not had the opportunity to attend formal schooling and some may not be literate. However, they do have a great deal of experience, skills and knowledge of managing farms and livestock systems in complex and unpredictable environments. Experience has shown that farmers and pastoralists usually want to learn more about looking after their animals and want to take an active role in the learning process. They want to learn from each other, share ideas and experiences, be challenged, analyse problems and draw their own conclusions. The learning needs to be a process of discovery and, therefore, training courses need to encourage the active participation of trainees.

4.3   Participative training

Building on local knowledge

Participative training is based on the principles of adult learning. As mentioned above, people already have a wealth of experience. Livestock keepers live and work in complex, sometimes fragile environments. In order to sustain their livelihoods they have learnt over time to manage and respond to these environments, constantly making decisions, weighing up different courses of action and assessing the outcomes of their efforts. Their knowledge and skills include marketing, farm management, crop production, animal health, government policy and the social issues affecting livestock keeping.

Training courses for CAHWs aim to draw out and build on people's existing livestock knowledge and skills. Much of this existing know-how will have been discussed and documented during the initial participatory surveys (see Chapter 2) and, therefore, the trainer will already have some understanding of how people care for their animals. These insights can help to determine the content of the training by identifying strengths and weaknesses in knowledge, and practices that seem harmful to animals. These practices can be discussed and, if necessary, corrected.

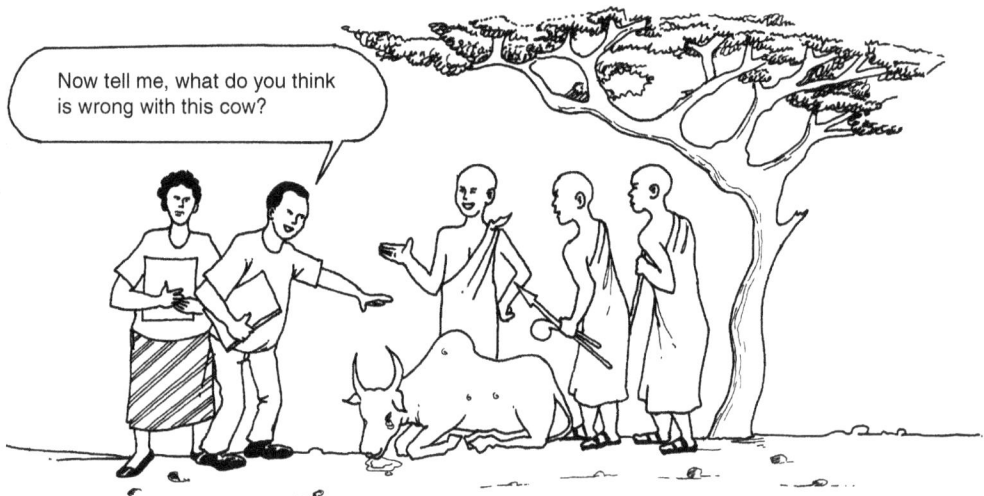

Participatory training methods aim to find out what people know and then build on this knowledge.

Practical methods and problem solving

The aim of participative training methods is to encourage the active participation of the trainees by posing problems and providing a forum for analysing the problems and discovering solutions. These processes take time and can be complex to organize compared with conventional methods like lecturing. However, experience has shown that, using these methods, farmers and CAHWs are far more likely to acquire skills and remember what they have learnt.

Experience from the field

Trainees in southern Sudan were far more confident and competent in handling and using automatic syringes when each one of them had practised dismantling, cleaning and assembling the equipment themselves, rather than just observing the trainer. The trainer was able to assist trainees with any problems, and check that each individual had acquired the relevant skills by the end of the training session. When trainees understood the role of each component of the syringe they were more motivated to maintain the equipment properly. Their increased confidence also showed itself in improved vaccination technique, and in the way they worked with cattle owners to manage vaccination campaigns.

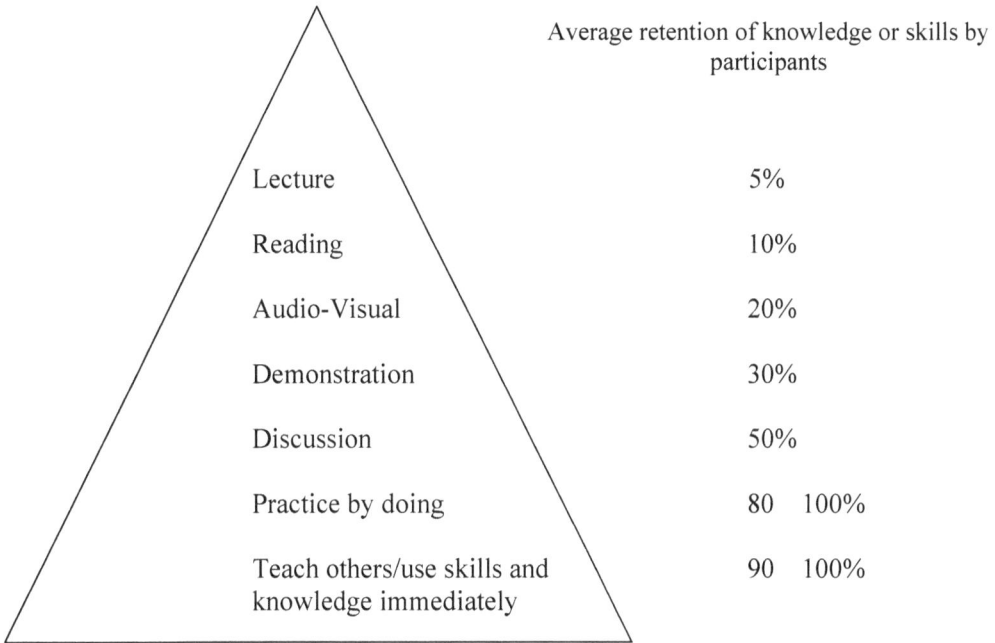

Average retention of knowledge or skills by participants

Lecture	5%
Reading	10%
Audio-Visual	20%
Demonstration	30%
Discussion	50%
Practice by doing	80 100%
Teach others/use skills and knowledge immediately	90 100%

(Source: adapted from Voluntary Service Overseas)

Figure 4.1 The pyramid of learning

Training techniques for illiterate people

It is possible that some or all of the CAHWs and livestock keepers who attend training are illiterate. The same training principles apply, but the training techniques may have to be modified. As a rule of thumb, when training illiterate people *avoid writing*. If written words are used, they should be used individually and considered as codes. They should be read out regularly so that the shape of the word can be associated with the spoken word. In this way individual disease names written on cards can be used successfully in disease ranking exercises with illiterate people. Writing phrases and sentences on a blackboard or flip-chart is meaningless for people who cannot read what is written, and may only serve to alienate them and make them feel uncomfortable about the training.

Experience from the field

A livestock project in Ethiopia was carrying out training where all but two of the trainees were illiterate. The trainer continuously wrote the key learning points down on the blackboard. His reason for doing this was so that the two literate people could take notes and explain any important points the rest of the group may have forgotten in the evening or at the end of the course. While this may have some use, the effect during the course was that the two literate people answered most questions and received more attention from the trainer than the illiterate participants. Despite his good intentions, the trainer had inadvertently discouraged the participation of most of the trainees. Also, because of his need to write everything down on the blackboard, the trainer tended to keep falling into a lecturing mode. After considering this issue, and attending a Training of Trainers course, the trainer decided not to use any writing at all, to use a wider range of training tools and visual aids, give everyone handouts prepared as pictures, and give additional printed notes to literate trainees. The quality of the training and satisfaction from trainees improved immensely.

Some of the training techniques described in this chapter can be modified for people who do not read and write. Instead of writing key points on the blackboard the trainer can make short notes on what people are saying in a notebook, and refer to these to help facilitate and summarize. Issues raised by participants in sessions can be discussed one after the other, rather than gathering them all together first on a flip-chart and then discussing them. The trainer should also make plenty of use of pictures and other visual aids to reinforce key points.

Box 4.2 Lack of literacy is not a barrier to training

A variety of educational aids have been specially designed by us at ANTHRA to make the training of CAHWs more appealing and enjoyable. These aids include posters, flip-charts, slide shows and cloth banners. Our trainees come from different educational levels. In fact, many of them have no literacy skills. The absence of literacy skills has never been a barrier to learning and we have always encouraged women to join our programme, despite many of them possessing no reading and writing skills. Theatre/role plays have also been important learning and teaching tools especially for those who do not read and write. Interestingly, we have observed that many women who do not write retain information much better because they can only rely on their memory. Concurrently, many who joined our training programmes have been inspired to develop these skills and become proficient in reading and writing by the time they have completed their training.

Since the approach is participatory, we encourage the trainees to share their experiences and knowledge. This lateral sharing of information has proved extremely beneficial for farmers. We have also organized farmer exchange programmes from one region to the other. This gives them an opportunity to observe how different farmers cope with the same or similar problems.

(contributed by ANTHRA, India)

A final consideration is that when training literate people the key points of each lesson are often summarized by the trainer at the end of the lesson by writing on a flip-chart. With illiterate trainees, this summary has to be done verbally, perhaps by reference to training aids that have been used and by asking trainees about the key lessons learnt. If attending a Training of Trainers course, make sure it covers working with illiterate people in detail.

4.4   The CAHW trainer

The role of the trainer

The role of the trainer in CAHW training is two-fold:

- ◆ to facilitate a learning process in which participants analyse livestock problems faced by the community, and develop appropriate strategies to deal with these problems;
- ◆ to instruct trainees in new knowledge and skills.

In both these roles, the trainer aims to build on the existing experience of the participants and emphasis is on a mutually respectful partnership between the trainer and participants. Here the flow of information is a two-way process – the trainer often has as much to learn from the participants as there is to teach. This approach increases participants' confidence and motivation to learn. The trainer should have good facilitation skills and be an experienced user of participative training approaches and methods, or be willing to learn these skills.

a. Creating a learning environment

During a participative training course, the trainer uses dynamic methods such as role play, group discussions, pictures, games, drama and song to create a *learning environment*. A learning environment is very different from a conventional teaching environment and is known as 'trainee-centred' rather than teacher-centred.

In a learning environment, participants are encouraged to share ideas, analyse problems, develop their own solutions, and to question and challenge each other and the trainer. Participative methods help trainees to discuss and review their understanding of particular topics, and identify the strengths and weaknesses of what they know and do. As they are involved in identifying weaknesses themselves, they are more likely to acquire new insights and knowledge. Skills are taught using practical methods where participants have plenty of opportunity to practise the new skills.

In a good learning environment, the trainer constantly checks the understanding of the participants by asking questions, setting tasks and observing how the participants behave. At times when CAHW training has not gone well, a trainer might say: 'Yes, but I went through the manual and taught them all that was in the notes. The trainees should now understand.' The problem here is that the trainer was

---

Box 4.3 Teaching and learning environments

Teaching environment

- lecture is the main method of teaching
- trainees have no role in design of course
- assumption that teacher has all knowledge
- teacher tells trainees what they need to know
- information passed from teacher to trainees only
- one-way flow of information
- teacher dictates
- training is rigid and fixed
- trainees are passive and quiet
- little participation
- emphasis on examinations
- trainer's role is to 'teach'
- the most important person is the teacher

This environment is trainer-centred.

Learning environment

- no lectures
- trainer responding to learning needs of trainees
- flexible

- two-way flow of information

- participative techniques encourage trainees to think

- discussions, plays, pictures, exercises
- demonstration and practice
- discover, experience, invent, create
- identify, analyse and solve problems
- trainees gain knowledge and skills
- trainer's role is to facilitate the learning process of the trainees

This environment is trainee-centred.

---

focused on getting through the manual, rather than making sure that the trainees acquired the necessary skills and knowledge. Sometimes it may be better to cover fewer topics in the course, but to cover these topics well so that the trainees can actually put into practice the skills they have learnt. They should be able to do this competently and with confidence.

b. Motivating the participants

Motivating participants to learn is an important role of the trainer. The CAHWs will come to the course with a variety of feelings and expectations: some may feel nervous, others will be unsure of their ability to acquire the necessary knowledge and skills to be a CAHW. Most will probably expect to be lectured to. The trainer can motivate trainees by aiming to build their confidence throughout the course.

Participants also need to know why they are attending the course, what the course will cover and what is expected of them. They need to feel that they are taking an active role in the learning process and that their experience, insights and opinions are respected and taken into consideration. The content of the course needs to be set at the level of the trainees' experience, so that they feel they are learning something useful (rather than something they already know or will never use). Much of the motivation of participants depends on the behaviour and training style of the trainer, and a well-designed course.

What makes a good trainer?

A key factor for effective training is the behaviour, attitudes and facilitation skills of the trainer. For example, when CAHWs are older than the trainer, correcting mistakes needs to be done sensitively and positively so that the trainees do not feel embarrassed or ashamed in front of their peers. Harsh criticism can quickly make trainees feel discouraged and lose confidence.

The trainer needs to create an environment where trainees feel free and confident enough to make mistakes, and to learn from their mistakes, as well as to ask questions when they do not understand. Encouraging trainees and focusing on what they can do (rather than what they cannot do) is an important way of increasing motivation to learn. Often, the best CAHW trainers are people of the same ethnic

---

Box 4.4 The qualities of a good CAHW trainer

A good CAHW trainer:

- is humble and approachable;
- has a warm, open, friendly and polite personality;
- considers him/herself on an equal level to trainees;
- is not arrogant about his/her professional qualifications or experience;
- respects the culture, traditional beliefs and practices of the trainees, even if he or she does not share these beliefs;
- respects the experience, knowledge and skills of the trainees;
- is able and willing to listen to trainees;
- is able and willing to learn from trainees;
- has a genuine desire for trainees to learn;
- is able to create a safe learning environment so that trainees feel confident to express their views and to ask for help if they do not understand something;
- is able to put participants at ease and to gauge the mood of the group;
- is flexible and able to respond to participants' needs;
- is able to see when trainees are having problems and to take appropriate action;
- is well-organized and a good planner;
- is constructively self-critical, so that his or her own training skills are constantly improving;
- has good technical knowledge of animal health and husbandry;
- is enthusiastic about animal health and husbandry, and able to share this enthusiasm with trainees.

---

group as the CAHW trainees. These trainers know the local language and understand the local culture and sensitivities.

Good facilitation skills come with practice and with awareness of how your behaviour affects others. Being able to receive constructive criticism from other trainers as well as trainees enables us to improve our training skills. The qualities of a good trainer are summarized in Box 4.4. In addition to facilitation skills, the trainer also needs to learn participative training techniques, how to design courses and how to write session plans. It is best to learn how to use these techniques on a Training of Trainers course.

Training the trainers

a. Why train the trainers?

CAHW trainers who have not received training in participative approaches tend to rely on conventional training methods such as lectures because this is the approach they are familiar with. They often learn through experience that farmers and CAHWs prefer more practical training, but lack the skills to carry out such training. This can be frustrating for both the trainer and the trainees, and hampers the progress of the project.

> ### Experience from the field
> *Poor training technique was evident in a CAHW project with the Boran people of northern Kenya. In this training course, the trainer used demonstrations, lectures and visual aids to train CAHWs. The groups of trainees were large (15 to 20 trainees) and the trainer had limited equipment such as one syringe and needle to teach the group how to inject goats. He was trying to incorporate practical sessions into his training, but was unaware of the principles of practical instruction and how to plan sessions in a structured way. He thought that, if he demonstrated what to do, trainees would then be able to inject goats correctly themselves. He found this was not the case and that when trainees returned to their communities they were often confused about even how to withdraw medicine from the bottle properly or how to read the markings on the syringe. After attending a course on participative training techniques this trainer was able to develop effective training for CAHWs and share his technical skills with the community in a very constructive way.*

Designing and running CAHW training courses requires a considerable range of skills and experience. Therefore, one of the first stages in developing effective training programmes for CAHWs is to ensure that the trainers themselves have the skills and support they need to carry out the job being asked of them. Responsibility for training CAHWs usually falls on the shoulders of the person qualified in animal health and husbandry, such as the project vet. However, it is unrealistic to expect a livestock professional to design and run CAHW courses without any prior training in how to do this. We cannot assume that, simply because a person has technical training, that person will automatically know how to develop courses to train others, especially livestock keepers with little formal education. If the trainers do not have the skills they require to design and run appropriate courses for CAHWs then the training may not be effective, resulting in CAHWs not being fully competent to carry out the work for which the community has selected them. CAHWs may then not be able to treat animals properly, leading to disappointment and dissatisfaction in the community.

b. Who should carry out CAHW training?

Training of CAHWs, including the design and planning of courses, should be carried out by people who are technically qualified in animal health and husbandry to a level sufficient to train the CAHWs. This group of people includes veterinarians, qualified livestock production specialists and animal health technicians. In all cases, a qualification is required which is recognized by government and professional veterinary bodies, and which permits people to treat animals using scheduled drugs (for example, Animal Health Assistants in Kenya attend a two-year diploma course at college).

It is usually better not to ask CAHWs from neighbouring projects or unemployed field staff from old projects (such as a previous vaccination campaign) to train new CAHWs. Dealing with animal health problems effectively is a complex process requiring considerable technical know-how, for example developing a strategy for controlling diseases like intestinal helminthosis or trypanosomiasis. These issues require the attention of professionals working alongside livestock keepers.

Even though the trainers need not necessarily be veterinarians themselves, the training programme should be supervised by a veterinarian. This ensures that the CAHWs are trained competently from a technical viewpoint, the content of the training meets with government regulations concerning the treatment of animals, and that the training is credible in the eyes of professional veterinary boards. Trainers may be government staff or staff from a collaborating organization such as a non-government organization (NGO).

c. Training of Trainers courses

Although there are many training manuals available, the most effective way for livestock professionals to become good trainers is to attend a Training of Trainers course. The course must be carefully chosen to ensure that trainers actually receive training in *participative* training techniques as opposed to formal teaching methods (such as lecturing). The best option may be to recruit a professional course facilitator to design a Training of Trainers course to meet the specific needs of the CAH project, and for that facilitator to run the course locally for all the project trainers.

A good Training of Trainers course will usually last at least three weeks and consist of two parts:

1. principles and methods of participative training;
2. how to design a CAHW course.

It is important to ensure that plenty of time is provided for the new trainers to practise the training techniques they are learning, as well as design a CAHW training programme with the support of the course facilitator. Emphasis should be placed on practising techniques, rather than simply observing them being carried out by the course facilitator. In other words, the Training of Trainers course should itself be run in a participatory manner. The best way to learn how to be a trainer is to practise designing, planning and running training sessions. The specific contents of a Training of Trainers course are summarized in Box 4.5.

Box 4.5 Example of a Training of Trainers course

Part 1. Participative training approaches and methods

Principles of participative training

◆ introductions and expectations for the course;
◆ course objectives;
◆ course timetable and outline;
◆ principles of adult learning;
◆ lectures and participation;
◆ training environments – teaching and learning environments;
◆ types of training needs – skills, behaviour and attitudes, knowledge;
◆ principles of designing training for illiterate people;
◆ using questions in training and listening skills;
◆ facilitation skills.

Participative methods: practical skills

◆ principles of training someone in a practical skill;
◆ how to plan and run practical skill lessons;
◆ participants each plan and run a practical skill lesson.

Participative methods: knowledge, behaviour and attitudes

◆ how to plan and use a range of techniques: pairs discussion, group discussion, role plays, picture codes, brainstorms, games, stories, case studies, drama, exercises, farm visits;
◆ participants practise planning and running sessions using each technique.

Training aids

◆ use of training aids: visual aids, models, pictures and use of appropriate images, live animals, plants, equipment such as medicines.

Learning needs

◆ assessing the learning needs of trainees. What do the CAHWs need to know in

---

order to do their work? What are the existing skills and knowledge of the CAHWs? Know your trainees' background.

Lesson planning

◆ lesson planning: principles, setting objectives, breaking down the lesson into easily digestible steps, following logical steps, timing, materials, writing lesson plans.

Course design

◆ principles of designing courses based on learning needs: setting objectives, writing a course outline, length of course, selecting appropriate training methods for the topic and for the needs of trainees, timing of sessions.

Logistics of course organization

◆ logistics of organizing courses: location of course, the building for training (or under a tree?), training materials and equipment, food and accommodation, per diems and so on.

How to evaluate training

◆ methods for checking whether the trainees have met the training objectives: have the right knowledge and skills been acquired?

Part 2. Design a CAHW course

Using the principles and methods learnt in PART 1, the participants design a CAHW course for their project including writing session plans.

4.5　Some participative training techniques

During a typical training course, three broad types of learning needs can be identified (see Box 4.6).

Box 4.6　Three types of learning needs

1. Skills

Skills are things that we are able to do *practically*. For example:
◆ inject a cow;
◆ plant a tree;
◆ cook chicken balti;
◆ drive a motor bike;

- organize a meeting;
- write a report.

2. Knowledge

Knowledge is something that is *in our heads* that we know or understand. Knowledge is what we have learnt from courses, reading and life experience. For example:

- dose of an antibiotic for a sheep of a given size;
- the best time to plant wheat;
- the ingredients needed to make chicken balti;
- the theory of relativity;
- which drug is used to treat which disease;
- theory of how people learn.

3. Attitudes and behaviour

This is *the way we relate to other people*. Attitudes and behaviour are determined by many factors, such as our belief system, life experience, culture, religion, personality and so on. Of the three types of learning needs, challenging people's attitudes and behaviour is the most difficult. Attitudes and behaviour desirable in trainers include respectful, approachable, humble, gentle, patient, trustworthy, punctual, friendly, empathic and culturally sensitive.

There are numerous training techniques available for the trainer to use on CAHW courses to assist the participants with their learning, and to make the training stimulating and effective. Although they are generally flexible and adaptable, in some cases specific techniques are required. For example, if participants need to learn a skill, then we must use *practical* instruction. It is not very helpful to teach someone how to deworm a goat using a discussion. If participants are learning about communication issues then plays, drama and group discussions are appropriate. Box 4.7 lists some of the more common participative training techniques and indicates how to use specific techniques for particular learning needs.

Box 4.7 Some participative training techniques and when to use them

The participative training techniques described in this chapter include:
- warm-ups and energizers;
- use of questions; question and answer;
- practical instruction;
- discussion techniques: pairs discussion (hum), group discussion (buzz), brainstorm;
- plays and drama: problem play as a discussion starter, role play for practice, puppets;

- problem pictures and picture codes;
- exercises;
- training visits;
- case studies;
- stories, songs, fables, poetry;
- games;
- presentations and talks.

Examples of how and when these techniques can be used include:

To teach skills	practical instruction
To teach knowledge	discussions, question and answer, plays and drama, picture codes, exercises, case studies, training visits
To teach communication skills	drama, role plays, picture codes
To examine behaviour and attitudes	drama (e.g. problem plays, role plays, puppets), case studies, discussions
To stimulate and relax participants; for fun	warm-up exercises and energizers

Trainers need to feel comfortable with the methods they are using and learn which techniques work well for them. Remember that attitude and skill at helping trainees to enjoy and benefit from the training is more important than the number of different techniques you know.

Warm-ups and energizers

Warm-ups and energizers are not training techniques but they form an essential part of training. They are used to change the tempo of a session and encourage participants to move about and relax after spending some time sitting in discussion. Energizers should be active and humorous. The trainer should always be aware of the mood of the participants. If people look tired then it is better to stop and have a break, rather than push on with the lesson and end up making people feel frustrated and demotivated. Warm-ups and energizers can also be used at the beginning of a course to help participants get to know each other in a relaxed fun way. Two examples of energizers from CAHW training courses in southern Sudan are described in Box 4.8.

Use of questions during training

The effective use of questions is one of the most important skills needed by trainers.

All the techniques described below involve asking questions. By asking questions, the trainer helps the participants to think for themselves and stimulates a process of discovery. If participants think about a problem and come up with an answer themselves, they are much more likely to remember the information than if they were just told that information by the trainer. Questions can be used to probe and analyse issues or problems in detail.

Using questions is an art and a skill, which ties in closely with facilitation skills and requires much practice. Some questions need to be carefully prepared when planning sessions in order to reinforce the key learning points for the session. As far as possible the trainer should use 'open questions'. Open questions are those questions that start with the words 'what', 'when', 'how', 'where', 'who' and 'why'. These types of questions encourage people to think and analyse. Examples include: 'What are the causes of poor growth in animals?' and 'How can the existing veterinary services be improved?' 'Closed questions' are those questions where the answer is either 'yes' or 'no', such as: 'Do you understand?' and 'Do you think animals get thin from poor-quality feed?' In general, such questions should be avoided because they do not stimulate much discussion or thinking, and can often invite a specific, misleading answer.

Question and answer

This is one of the most basic training techniques, and is usually used during sessions when the whole training group is together. Here the trainer asks a series of questions of the whole group. Key learning points for each question may be written up on flip-chart paper or a blackboard. A question and answer session is used for short topics and lasts ten minutes or less; it is often used as a link between one major topic and the next.

Practical instruction

Practical instruction is used to teach participants a *skill*, such as how to give injections or how to mix and apply acaracide. Practical instruction is based on the principle that people learn by doing. All too often trainers believe that, if they just demonstrate a skill – for example how to give an injection – and then allow one or two participants to have a go, then the class as a whole has received adequate instruction. This is not the case.

Despite having observed the trainer carrying out a skill, it is often not until the trainees try it themselves that they and the trainer suddenly realize all the intricacies and steps involved in the skill.

Practical instruction in CAHW training in Somaliland

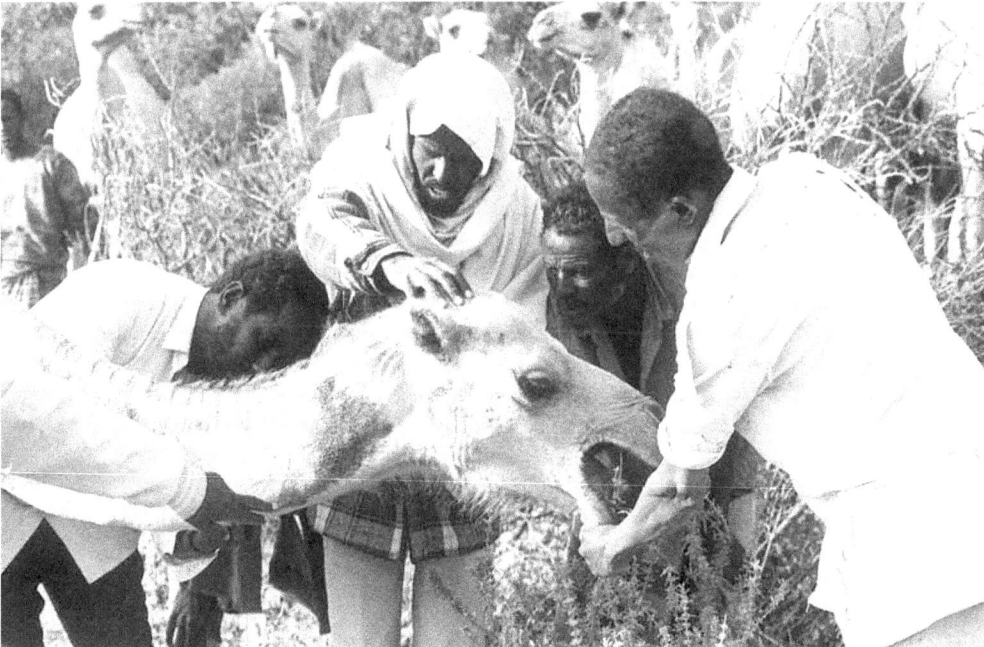

Plate 4.1 CAHW training really comes alive when trainees start to handle and examine animals, and practise new procedures. (*Andy Catley*)

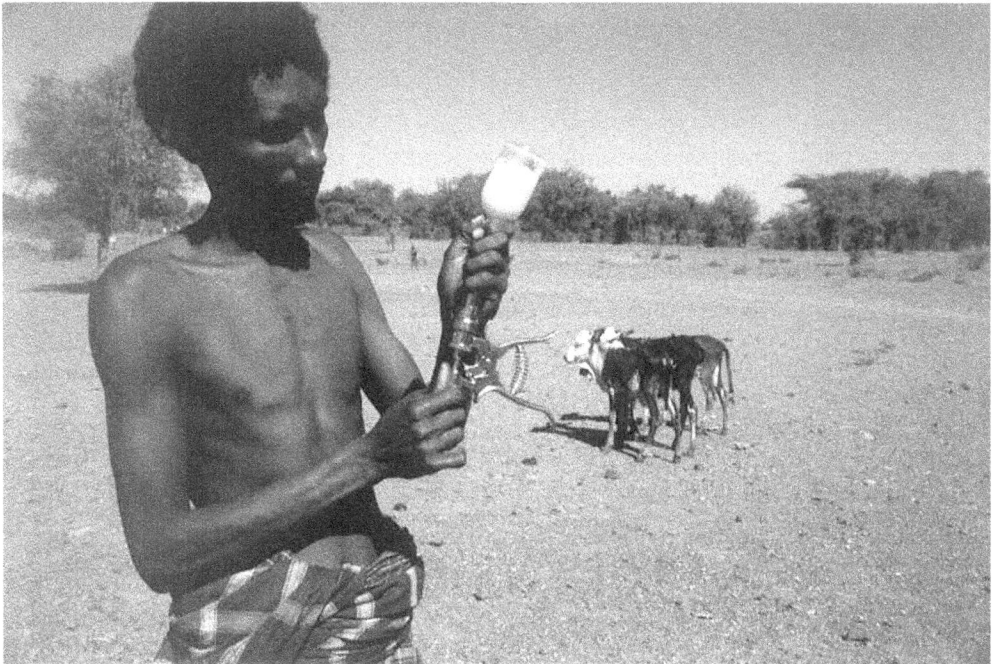

Plate 4.2 In this picture a CAHW in Afar region, Ethiopia, learns how to use an automatic vaccination syringe. (*PARC Communications Unit*)

Experience from the field

When teaching how to fill a syringe with medicine and inject a cow, questions and comments from trainees typically include: 'How do I get the bubble out of the syringe?'; 'What angle should I hold the bottle at when drawing out the medicine?'; 'I can't pull the medicine out of the bottle – it feels like something is preventing it.'; 'How do I know I have pushed the needle into the cow deep enough?'; 'Why is there blood in my syringe when I withdraw it a little? Is this OK?' And so on.

Practical instruction provides the trainer with a framework to design and conduct sessions in such a way that all the intricate steps of a skill are taught to trainees in a clear, logical sequence to avoid confusion. Practical training may also involve the use of training aids or other techniques such as role play.

Practice time for every trainee forms a major part of the session. The trainer is on hand to assist, correct and encourage each individual trainee in a safe, controlled environment. If trainees do not practise in the session, when they try to put their new skill into practice with farmers they will make mistakes, try and correct themselves, and may pick up bad habits and carry out the skill incorrectly.

Important features of practical instruction include:

Practice time

At least 70 per cent of the lesson time should be spent on participants doing things and practising,

Practical instruction in CAHW training in India

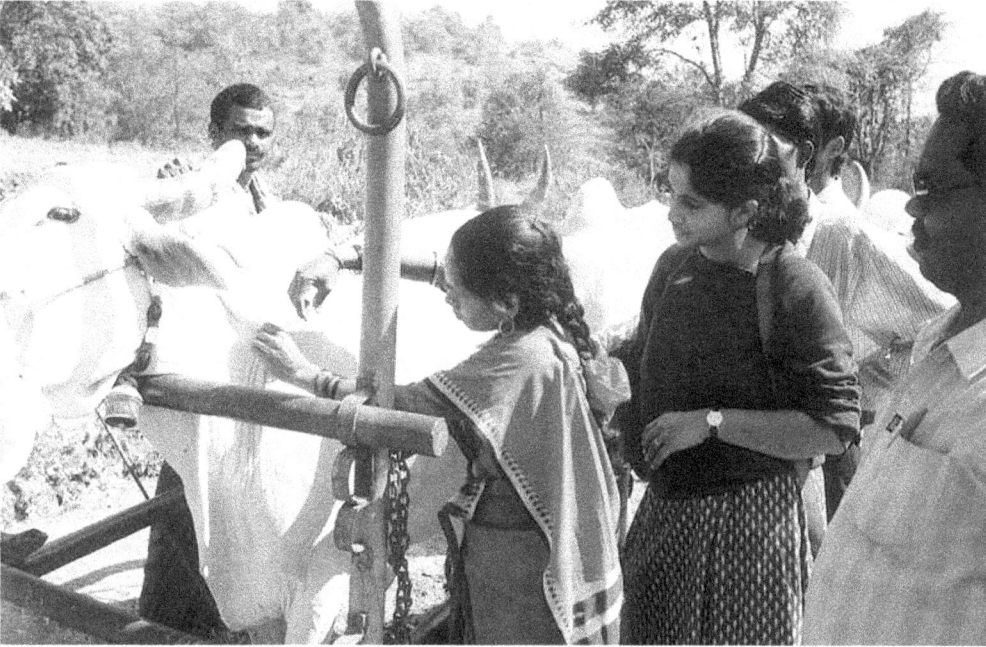

Plate 4.3 If trainees are made to handle equipment and practise techniques such as injection, problems can quickly be corrected by the trainer. (*ANTHRA*)

Supervision of CAHW training

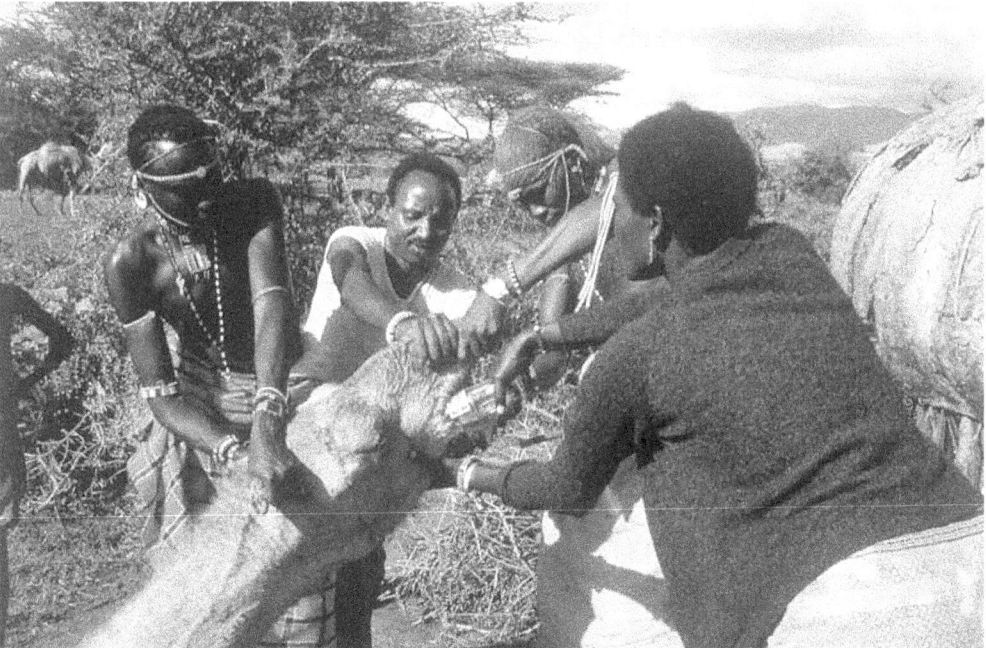

Plate 4.4 A trainer from ITDG closely supervises CAHWs in Samburu, Kenya. (*Stephen Blakeway*)

with 30 per cent of the time spent with the trainer providing explanation and demonstrating. The lesson should not consist of a long explanation and demonstration by the trainer followed by a quick five-minute practice for the participants at the end.

Planning

Practical instruction lessons need careful planning to ensure that all the important points are covered and that the lesson is clear and easy to understand. Long explanations and lecturing should be avoided. If long explanations are required then the trainer may want to consider holding a theory lesson first, using other techniques like group discussion, and then run a practical instruction class.

Ask questions

As much as possible the trainer should ask questions to help participants think and remember, rather than just tell them everything. Specific questions should be planned, written in the session plan and linked to key learning points.

Logical sequence

Some skills are quite complex and need to be broken down into a series of steps. Participants should be taught one step at a time so that each step follows on from the other in a clear logical sequence.

Sufficient equipment and animals

It is absolutely essential to have enough equipment and materials for everyone to practise adequately. If there are 12 people learning to drench calves with anthelmintic, we need 12 drenching guns, enough bottles of medicine for everyone to practise drenching and plenty of animals to practise on (plus the equipment used by the trainer). The trainer should also supply the same type of equipment and medicines in training that the CAHWs will themselves use when they begin their work.

Practical instruction involves four main stages as detailed in Box 4.9.

Box 4.9 Practical instruction

Practical instruction is used to train participants in a skill. The overall objective of a practical instruction lesson is that by the end of the lesson each trainee will be able to carry out that skill (e.g. inject a cow) correctly and safely without the aid of the trainer.

There are 4 stages in a practical instruction lesson:

1. Introduction
The introduction allows participants to know what is happening in the lesson and covers:

◆ what skill the participants are going to learn;
◆ how they are going to learn this skill;
◆ why they are going to learn it.

This is done by:

- ◆ stating the objectives of the lesson: what, how, quality, equipment;
- ◆ asking the participants about their previous experience of that skill;
- ◆ asking them and discussing what use the skill will be to them.

2. Demonstration

During the demonstration part of the lesson we show and demonstrate to the participants the skill they are about to learn. This includes several steps. For example, for a complex skill:

- ◆ show the equipment to the participants;
- ◆ ask them to watch while you demonstrate the whole skill;
- ◆ explain that the participants are now going to learn the skill step by step;
- ◆ discuss and encourage participants to handle the equipment;
- ◆ go through the skill again, this time step by step, demonstrating each step, asking participants questions, and letting them practise each step;
- ◆ if participants are making mistakes, ask questions to help them learn from their mistakes, and give encouragement.

3. Practice

- ◆ This is a very important part of the lesson. Approximately 70 per cent of the lesson should be spent with participants practising (including practice during the demonstration part of the lesson).
- ◆ Let the participants practise the skill until they have learnt to do it correctly without any help from the trainer.
- ◆ If trainees are making mistakes, ask questions to help them learn from their mistakes.

4. Summary

Summarize at the end of a lesson to find out:

- ◆ whether or not the trainees have learnt the skill;
- ◆ if the trainees have understood the lesson (*do not ask*: Do you understand?);
- ◆ if we have achieved our objectives for the lesson.

Summarize by asking three or four open questions that check the understanding of the trainees. These questions need to be carefully prepared. A summary is not for the trainer to explain the lesson again. Do not introduce new information in the summary.

Discussions, hum groups and buzz groups

There are various types of discussion techniques used in participative training courses. The most common are the pairs discussion (sometimes called a hum) and the group discussion (sometimes called a buzz). A pairs discussion involves dividing participants into pairs and asking them to discuss a problem or task such as: 'List the factors affecting the availability of feed for livestock.' The key points from each group are written on the flip-chart and the trainer facilitates a general discussion on the points raised. For the group discussion technique, participants are divided into groups of three to five, and asked to discuss a problem such as: 'What problems do people face with keeping animals?' Each group writes its key points on flip-chart paper and presents them to the rest of the group. The trainer facilitates a general discussion in the plenary on the points raised.

Box 4.10 Pairs discussion

A pairs discussion has 5 parts:

1. Write up the question or task on flip-chart paper.
2. Divide trainees into pairs and ask them to discuss the question for five minutes. Go round the pairs to check people are discussing the right thing.
3. Write the responses on the flip-chart.

   ◆ Move around the pairs and take one point per pair.
   ◆ Go round a second time taking another point from each pair (from a different person, so that everyone has a chance to speak).
   ◆ There should be no discussion at this time – simply write down the points.
   ◆ Do not ignore a point.
   ◆ Avoid paraphrasing. Write what people say in their own words.

4. Discuss

   ◆ Using a different coloured pen, circle one point, ask the person who made that point to explain what it means, to give reasons, to expand on the point, for example: 'What made you say this?', 'How do you mean?'
   ◆ Ask the rest of the group what they think about this point. Do people agree or disagree, or have a different opinion?
   ◆ When the discussion on the first point is finished, circle another point with a coloured pen, and repeat the process. Continue until five or six points have been covered (or how ever many the trainer wants to cover).
   ◆ It is not necessary to discuss every point on the list. The trainer can decide which points it is important to discuss.
   ◆ When the discussions have been finished on five or six points, summarize each point briefly.

5. Explain how this lesson will lead in to the next lesson.

A pairs discussion should be run in 20–30 minutes. It can be used:

◆ at the beginning of a training session as a 'warm-up';
◆ to set the scene of a new topic;
◆ to establish previous experience of a topic (e.g. training experience);

During the plenary discussion for both hum and buzz groups the trainer asks probing questions to stimulate debate, share experiences and encourage participants to come to a consensus on issues, or agree to differ.

Practical tip

A common mistake here is for the trainer to take over the discussion and start explaining the points to the trainees or tell them the 'correct' answer. Suddenly the group discussion turns into a lecture. Trainers should avoid this temptation, and encourage the trainees to explain their own reasoning. If the trainees fail to mention important points then the trainer can often draw these out of the group through careful use of probing questions. Finally, the trainer may add other key points from experience. At the end of the session, the trainer can ask the question: 'Who spoke the most during the discussion?' If the answer is 'Me', then clearly the session was not very participative.

Using participatory techniques such as group discussion does not automatically make the training participative. The trainer must also implement the *principles* of adult learning and participation. This means creating a learning environment through activities and tasks, encouraging trainees to express their opinions and a genuine willingness on the part of the trainer to listen to trainees and respond to what they say.

Discussion techniques are used to explore a range of opinions and to allow participants to share their experiences, knowledge and ideas. The group discussion takes longer than the pairs discussion and so is used for more in-depth analysis of an issue. Discussion techniques are most often used when participants are learning knowledge, or addressing behaviour and attitudes issues.

Brainstorming

One type of discussion method is brainstorming. This is a lively method used for gaining a rapid overview of participants' knowledge or ideas on a particular issue. The brainstorming method is described in Box 4.11.

Box 4.11 How to use brainstorms

Brainstorms should be short, fast and lively.

1. Write a short title or question on flip-chart paper. (e.g. 'How do you know when an animal is sick?')
2. Ask for one-word contributions from the group (e.g. diarrhoea, lameness).
3. List the contributions. Write down every contribution. Write very fast. Do not worry about spelling. Keep your back to the trainees. Encourage them to make many contributions.
4. Group the contributions. Explain that you want to categorize the contributions into groups. The trainer must decide what these groups will be before the session. After explaining what the first group is (e.g. 'signs of disease affecting the head') the trainees are asked to shout out which words fit in that category. The words are grouped, for example, by drawing a circle round them with a coloured pen or putting a symbol by them.

   Then the trainer should explain the second category (e.g. 'signs of disease affecting the skin') and ask the trainees to put the relevant words into that group. The trainer circles these words with a different coloured pen or by using a different symbol. Continue until all words have been put into the categories. With this example, other categories might be 'signs affecting the limbs', 'signs affecting the chest' and so on.

   No discussion is necessary. The trainer should not question why people put certain words into a group – just accept what the trainees say.

5. Link into the next session. For example, 'In the next session we will discuss why different diseases cause different signs of disease.'

A brainstorm should be run in 10–15 minutes. It is used to:

◆ switch to a new subject;
◆ examine a subject very broadly;
◆ obtain 30–40 ideas quickly;
◆ create a lively atmosphere and wake people up.

Examples of brainstorms are:

◆ 'signs of livestock disease' which can be grouped into signs affecting the head, chest, limbs and so on;
◆ 'spread of livestock diseases' which can be grouped into direct contact, vectors, wildlife and so on.

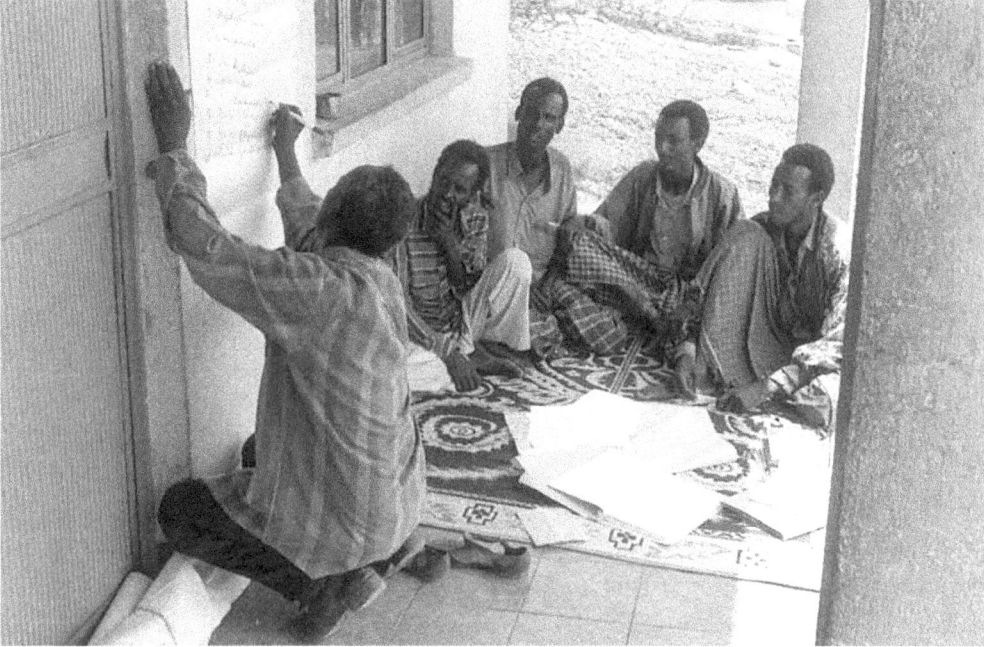

Plate 4.5 A brainstorm allows ideas and information from the trainees to form the basis for discussion. In this example, trainees in Ethiopia have provided a list of clinical signs for the disease of camels called *gendi*. (*Andy Catley*)

The debate

The debate is useful for encouraging participants to think for themselves and identify key points for and against a particular issue. The participants also have to work as a team, decide which points to present during the debate and select a speaker to forward their views. An example of a debate on traditional veterinary practice in southern Sudan is described in Box 4.12.

Box 4.12 Using debates

During a CAHW training session among Nuer communities in southern Sudan, the CAHWs were divided into a 'right' proposers' group and a 'left' opposers' group to debate the motion 'Traditional livestock care is better than modern, scientific veterinary care'. Each group was given ten minutes to discuss among themselves and then present their arguments in turn through key speakers.

Some of the main points were as follows:

Rightists (proposers)

◆ We have cheap medicine for killing ticks, by fermenting urine for ten days and applying it to cows.
◆ Traditional medicine has been used by our ancestors for many years and is part of us.
◆ Traditional medicines are inexpensive and, usually, there is no cost.
◆ Traditional doctors can treat many different types of disease compared with the modern doctors.
◆ Modern drugs come from far away. If there is insecurity, a flight ban or the airstrips are unlandable, CAHWs will cease to work.
◆ Traditional medicines are readily and locally available.
◆ There are many traditional medicines for a wide variety of diseases.
◆ Modern medicine does not cure at all times.

Leftists (opposers)

◆ Traditional treatments are risky, especially in regards to the correct dosage. One can easily overdose.
◆ Animals treated with modern drugs recover quickly.
◆ Traditional medicine is seen as backward by the members of the community, who are ready to use the CAHWs' drugs.
◆ We have medicines (vaccines) for rinderpest and CBPP, unlike the traditional doctors.
◆ Traditional doctors treat with beliefs in strange powers, like 'the evil eye', and sometimes their treatments do not work.
◆ Modern drugs are scientifically proven and therefore more effective.
◆ CAHWs have good knowledge on dosage, maintenance and mode of action of modern veterinary drugs.

After the debate, the facilitator emphasized that, because of some of the possible advantages of traditional veterinary medicines, VSF-B would not try to replace those traditional medicines that seemed to work well. Instead, the organization would try to assist with scientific validation of the medicines and promote their use as well.

(contributed by Dr Ashford Gichohi, VSF-DZG, Belgium)

Plays and drama

Plays and drama are extremely effective training techniques because they can be used to focus on real-life problems in an active way, especially where participants are encouraged to act out issues themselves. There are various ways of using plays in training, all of which have quite different learning objectives. Confusion arises when all types of plays and drama are simply referred to as 'role plays', and so each method will be discussed in turn.

Problem plays

These are used specifically to pose a problem or issue. A short play depicting a problem and lasting only two or three minutes is enacted at the beginning of the session. Participants are asked to draw out and analyse the causes of the problem, discuss how it relates to their life situation, and then to suggest solutions or strategies for tackling that problem. This play should only show the problem/issue in question and not possible solutions. It should be short and simple (see Box 4.13).

Box 4.13 Using problem plays

1. Prepare a short play of two to three minutes.
2. Brief a few participants on the play you want them to enact.
3. Ask these participants to act out the play. Ask the rest of the participants to watch and listen to what happens in the play.
4. When the play is over, ask questions as follows:

General feedback	What did you see and hear happening in the play?
Problem questions	What are the problems you saw in the play?
	Why is this a problem?
Real-life questions	Does this happen in real life? What are your experiences?
Causes questions	What are the causes of these problems?
Solutions question	How can these problems be solved?

   The trainer should ensure that everyone contributes to the discussion.
5. Summarize the problems identified and the suggested solutions.
6. Link into the next session.

There are important points about using problem plays:

◆ A problem play session can last from 30 minutes to an hour.
◆ This technique is used to *identify problems* and help people *find solutions*.
◆ The play should concentrate on one problem only. Remember, most of the problem play technique involves discussion, which is started by asking the questions. The short play is only to set the scene.
◆ The actual play should be short (only two to three minutes) and simple.
◆ The trainer must carefully plan the play before hand, and must be very clear what problem needs to be brought out.
◆ Solutions to the problem must not be shown in the play.
◆ The actors must be properly briefed, away from the rest of the group, and given time to practise.
◆ The main points from the session can be recorded on a flip-chart, for example causes of the problem and possible solutions.

Examples of issues that can be discussed using the problem play technique are:

◆ poor listening skills – where a play shows two people arguing and not listening to each other;
◆ poor facilitation skills – where a play shows a trainer lecturing to students.

Problem plays are ideal for addressing behaviour and attitudes with participants, for example interview technique with farmers, facilitation in training, body language in training, types of behaviour in groups, and listening skills when working with livestock owners. They can also be used to explore complex concepts such as vaccination. For example, trainers working with an ITDG CAHW project in Kenya used plays to help explain vaccination of chickens by discussing the reasons for vaccinating children, a topic which trainees already understood well.

Practice plays

Practice plays involve participants either being themselves or taking on the role of others such as farmers. Here the participants can be divided into groups to practise communication skills such as listening, asking questions, chairing a meeting and interview technique.

Box 4.14 Using practice plays

Practice plays are very different from problem plays. A practice play has the following characteristics:

◆ It is used for trainees to practise something they have learnt, for example interviewing a farmer about herd structure using the progeny history method.
◆ It is used by the trainer to explain how to do something, for example how to interview a farmer for life status ranking.
◆ It does not illustrate a problem.
◆ It is sometimes called a role play, because the trainees or trainer take on the role of other people, for example one pretends to be a farmer.
◆ It can last from five to 30 minutes or longer.

Examples of practice plays are:

◆ Trainees are divided into groups of three and practise listening skills.
◆ Trainees are divided into pairs and practise asking open questions.
◆ The trainer demonstrates good facilitation technique.
◆ The trainer demonstrates how to interview a farmer.
◆ Trainees practise how to use ranking methods by interviewing each other (where one is the farmer and the other is the CAHW).

Drama

Drama can be used to encourage participants to act out their experiences, and explore difficult issues. Examples include the problems people face getting animals treated, fears participants may have about their work as CAHWs, and difficulties participants have faced speaking at public meetings. Participants are asked to discuss a certain issue in groups of four or five and then to create a play to illustrate it. They may act out just the issue, or act possible solutions as well. Alternatively they can just act the issue and ask the rest of the group to suggest solutions. During the whole process of the drama the trainer facilitates discussion, making sure that the key learning points are brought out.

Puppets

Puppets are another way of presenting drama. Puppets are small models of people and animals that are used to tell a story. The puppet story can be told by the trainer or by participants. Puppets can be used to help participants discuss sensitive issues more easily, because the discussion can be focused on the puppet character rather than directly on a particular person. However, the discussion must link in with a real-life situation and focus on ways the situation can be changed. Such topics might include illegal traders selling livestock drugs in market places, or the role of traditional healers in a community-based animal health programme.

There are various types of puppets, ranging from simple finger puppets where faces are painted on fingers, to puppets made from cloth, sticks, socks and vegetables like potatoes. Puppets are easy and fun to make using locally available materials, and are an effective way of encouraging participants to explore difficult issues in depth. As with all the techniques, the trainer needs to facilitate the discussion in a structured way so as to bring out the learning points.

Problem pictures and picture codes

Problem pictures are used in a similar way to problem plays, except a picture is used to pose a problem rather than a play. Problem pictures can be used to analyse issues that are difficult to depict in a play, such as overgrazing around water holes. Similarly, a chaotic scene of a poorly organized vaccination campaign can make a good problem

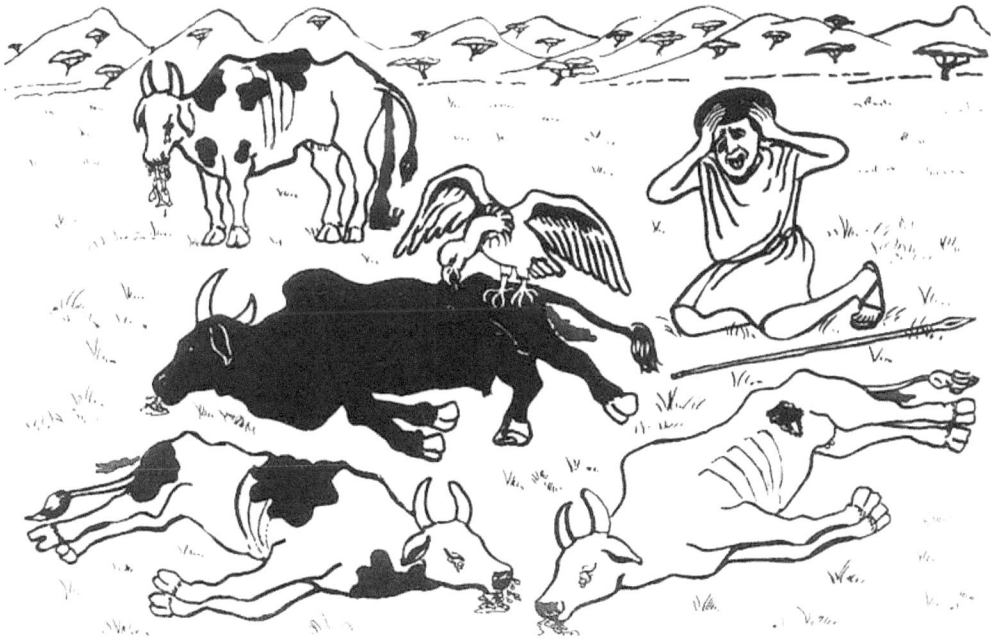

Figure 4.2 This picture was developed by PARC. It is a simple but dramatic line drawing.

133

picture. The picture used should show only one problem and should not show possible solutions. It should be a simple line drawing, avoiding too much shading and colour, and with no abstract symbols that might confuse the picture.

Pictures should always be 'tested' before the course to check the problem or issue is clearly seen. Testing can be done with colleagues or other trainers, where the trainer simply asks them what they see in the picture. Problem picture sessions are run in the same way as the problem plays described above, using the same set of standard questions (see section *Plays and Drama* above and Box 4.13).

Exercises

Exercises are used to give participants practice in certain skills and knowledge they have learnt. Examples include calculating correct dose rates for a given size of animal, number of vaccine vials and water required to vaccinate a given number of cattle, and keeping records of animal treatments or drugs sold from the CAHW kits. The trainer prepares hypothetical problems and tasks and then asks participants to work through

---

Box 4.15 Exercises

1. Brief the participants about what they have to do for the exercise, and give them an exercise sheet with the task written on it. Tell them what materials they should use and how much time they have. Divide them into groups or tell them to work alone.
2. Supervise the participants. Go around making sure everyone understands what to do. Give encouragement and assistance for those having difficulty, by asking questions to help them to think about their mistakes and learn for themselves.
3. Review the results of the exercise. Ask groups or individuals to present their results. Discuss the results and reasons why certain answers are correct and others not. Focus on areas where trainees were having difficulty and discuss reasons for this. The aim of exercises is for trainees to learn by doing something, including learning from mistakes. Discuss what went well and not so well. Encourage everyone to contribute.
4. Summarize the main points.
5. Link into the next session.

Exercises can last from 30 minutes to 2 hours. they are used:

◆ for trainees to practise something new they have learnt;
◆ to build confidence in a new skill and set of knowledge;
◆ to encourage trainees to accept a new technique or process.

An example is:

◆ filling in the record book.

---

them. Exercises can be used to test the skills and knowledge of individual participants and so each person is asked to work alone. When everyone has finished the exercise, the answers can be discussed in the plenary.

When exercises are used well, the trainer can identify which trainees are experiencing problems and provide necessary assistance and further explanation. Exercises are particularly useful for tasks that each participant will have to be able to carry out on their own after the course, for example record keeping. For this reason it is important to check that each and every person is able to do the task unaided. If exercises like this are done as group work, participants who do not understand can easily be missed by the trainer.

Training visit

During training visits, participants are taken to a specific site outside the training venue, such as a farm, livestock kraal, veterinary office or a public watering point for livestock. Training visits are very useful for putting theory into practice in a real situation. Here the trainer facilitates discussion around issues related to this site. It is important that the visit is well-structured with specific learning objectives, and is not simply aimless wandering around. The participants may be involved in planning the visit by preparing key questions or issues they can discuss with people at the visit site. Another way to make the session more structured is to give participants a training visit 'score chart', listing important aspects of the site which have to be examined for good and bad points, and then recommendations made for improvement. Each participant is given a score chart and asked to examine the site. Following this the trainer facilitates a discussion on the participants' findings. An example of a score chart is shown in Box 4.16.

Case studies

Case studies are used to analyse a situation that has occurred in real life and to learn lessons from this experience. The case study can depict a negative or positive situation. Examples include CAHW projects that were established in other areas, the problems they faced and the way these problems were overcome. Case studies are useful for looking at the wider issues, such as the approach taken by the project as a whole.

Case studies require careful research and preparation, and therefore they can take some time to put together. A case study should include: background to the project (size, location, history, aims and objectives), strategy and activities being carried out, progress so far, what the situation is now or at the end of the project. Participants are then given questions about the case study to discuss in groups, such as: 'Why did this project fail?', 'What made this project successful?' or 'How could the problems illustrated in this project be avoided?' The trainer then facilitates a discussion on the groups' findings in the plenary.

Stories, songs, fables and poetry

Many CAHW trainees belong to societies that have a strong oral tradition in which stories, songs, fables and poetry form an important part of cultural life. Stories can be told by either the trainer or the participants, and can be an effective way of raising important issues during training. Stories can be about people and situations that occur in everyday life, or can be fictitious. The stories should consist of characters and places with names, and a series of events with a beginning and an end.

Traditional fables and legends can be told, for example about how the hyena used all kinds of devious means to outwit the honest hare, and lessons can be drawn about various ethical or behavioural issues. Poetry and song can be used in a similar way, as well as to reinforce approaches and key learning points, for example a song written about the role of CAHWs, as often happens spontaneously on training courses.

Sometimes elders and holy men or women close a training session or course with a prayer, which often reinforces points agreed in the session and carries great weight with the participants. In Samburu, Kenya, women being trained to treat bloat added a blessing by using mud and dung to draw a circle with a cross in the middle on the side of the animal.

Games

Games can be used to raise issues about behaviour and attitudes, such as how people behave in groups, conflict resolution, co-operation and team work. Games can also raise participants' awareness about how their behaviour as individuals and as a group affects others in both a positive and negative way. Games are a useful way of introducing such issues by allowing participants to actually experience a real situation that is both fun and non-threatening. With games, all participants should take part. After the game, the trainer facilitates discussion on how people felt during the game, what frustrations arose, why people behaved the way they did, what implications this behaviour has for team work or the project, how they resolved problems as a group, and how such issues can be addressed in future. With games, as with all other training techniques, it is important that the session is well-structured with clear objectives. The trainer should ensure that the key learning points are drawn out.

cardboard box, cups, bottle, paper, pens, sticks, grass etc.), and tell them they have ten minutes to construct a tower 1 metre high. The first group to finish is the winner.

Presentations and talks

Presentations and talks do have a role to play in participative training but they should be used sparingly. It may be tempting for the trainer to try and *explain* everything to the trainees in an effort to give them as much information and as many facts as possible. The trainer may even use good visual aids – such as pictures, models, and animals – and deliver the talk in clear, appropriate language. The session may be well-planned and set at the level of the trainees. But no matter how well a trainer explains a topic, experience has shown that, unless trainees have been challenged to think about and work through problems *themselves*, they will not remember most of what has been said. Before deciding to give a presentation the trainer should ask: 'Is there another training technique I can use that will allow the trainees to be more involved and active?' When presentations are used the following principles apply:

◆ Presentations and talks are used to provide participants with knowledge, for example correct dose rates for medicines and which medicines to use for which disease. The trainer should avoid giving long lectures – talks should be kept to a maximum of ten minutes. With longer talks, the training quickly becomes boring and ineffective. When giving the presentation, avoid 'talking' to the flip-chart. Stand and face the participants, and talk to them – this will make what you have to say far more effective, and make participants feel they are part of the session.

◆ The talk should be well-planned with a clear structure and it should make use of visual aids such as pictures and examples of medicines and equipment (but note that this is not a substitute for *practical* instruction). Flip-charts should be carefully prepared with clear, bold writing. Don't write the whole talk out on the flip-chart and cover the paper with lines of detailed notes. This is difficult for people to follow. Only write the major headings and key points for each heading. Detailed notes for the talk can be written out on small cards or A4 paper for the trainer to refer to. Notes can also be written lightly in pencil on the flip-chart, so only the trainer can see them, as a way of helping the trainer remember important points. Use flip-charts in imaginative ways, such as covering up the words or pictures and slowing revealing them as the talk progresses. Adding pictures or words to the flip-chart as the talk develops can help maintain interest.

◆ A presentation does not mean that the trainer just has to tell participants what they need to know, like a mini-lecture. To make presentations more effective incorporate the question and answer technique so people are encouraged to participate, and think about the information being presented. This will help them to remember what has been said.

4.6   Training aids

Training aids are used to help illustrate and reinforce key learning points during training. They can be used with any of the participative training techniques described above. A wide variety of training aids are available such as flip-charts and coloured markers, chalkboard and chalk, photographs, pictures, models, animals and medicines. Computer presentation systems, video, slides and overhead projectors can also be used. The choice of training aids depends on many factors such as cost, electricity supply, literacy of the participants and the subject being covered in the training.

Within a participative training approach, there is considerable scope for trainers to develop their own training aids according to local animal health problems and local languages.

Experience from the field

The concept of immunity is a difficult issue to explain to CAHWs. Working in southern Sudan

Using pictures

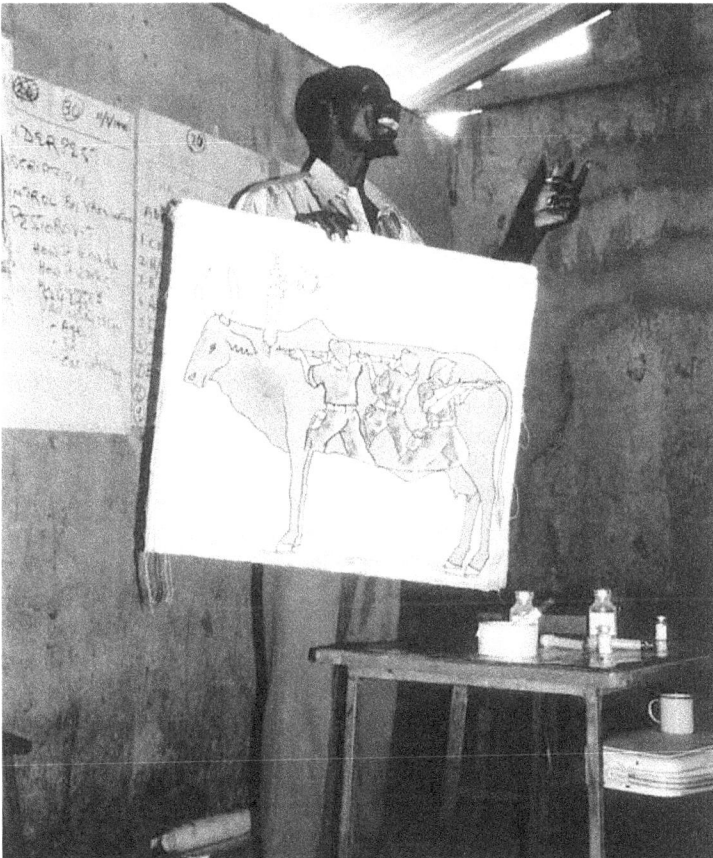

Plate 4.6 The design of pictures can be creative and based on local situations. In this example, Dr Darlington Akabwai uses three well-armed warriors inside a cow to explain how three doses of rinderpest vaccine can protect the cow. (*PARC Communications Unit*)

In the following section, information is provided on some of the most useful training aids for CAHW courses. Each of these can be adapted to meet local needs – be creative.

The real thing

As far as possible, real objects as opposed to pictures should be used as training aids. For example, rather than use a picture of medicines, show participants samples of real medicine. When discussing signs of disease or how to examine a sick animal, try to use a live animal with that disease, rather than a picture of a sick animal. In the case of diseases, it is often difficult to show all the detailed variations of signs in a picture, whether this is a drawing or a photograph, whereas a live animal presents a far more accurate and realistic view. This is particularly important in CAHW training, where a major part of the work is being able to recognize diseases and conduct clinical examinations. If you are discussing the components of a balanced diet for livestock, then show participants examples of real feed samples, rather than just talking about feeds or showing pictures. Using real objects may take more time to prepare, but is worth the effort.

a. Live animals

Live animals are an essential training aid for CAHW courses. They are used for learning about how to handle animals, the signs of health and disease, clinical examination, diagnosing specific diseases, correct administration of medicines and sample collection. The use of live animals during training requires careful organization and attention to animal welfare. The various issues to consider are explained in Chapter 5.

b. Post-mortem examination

Animals can be purchased for slaughter and post-mortem examination. This is a useful way of learning about internal organs and, in the case of sick animals, participants can see how organs are affected by disease. Animals that die within easy reach of the training venue can also be examined by the trainees. Whenever an animal is killed during training, the killing should be an example of the most humane method of slaughter locally available.

Experience from the field
The ITDG/Oxfam livestock project in Samburu, Kenya made use of post-mortem examinations when training CAHWs in the use of anthelmintics and helminth control. Animals were

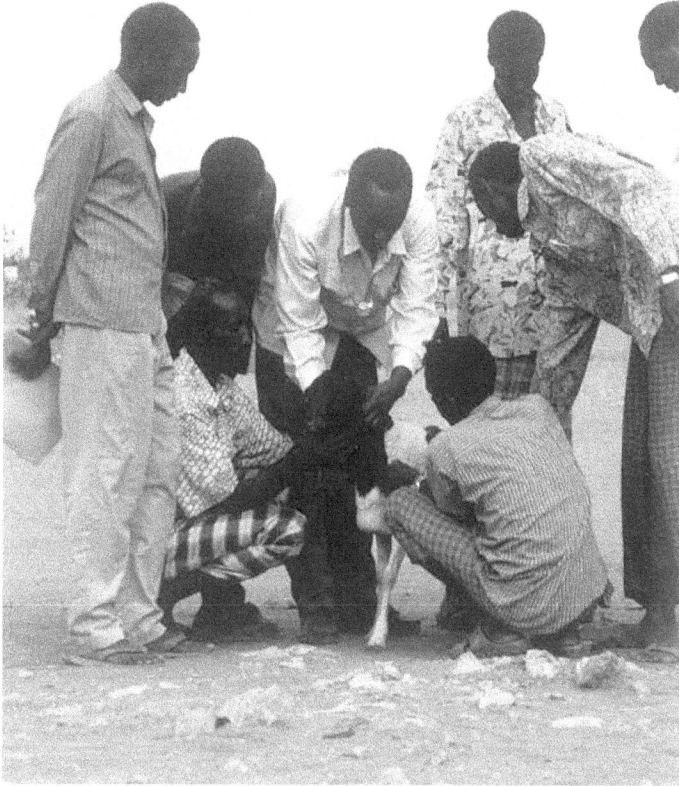

Plate 4.7 Live animals make the perfect training aid in CAHW courses. (*Andy Catley*)

examined for common helminths and, by reference to the post-mortem materials, the trainees described their understanding of where helminths came from, how they affected animals and local treatments or preventative measures taken. These ideas were quite different from current western knowledge. Trainers were then able to build on the local perceptions and provide trainees with more information on helminth life cycles, sources of infection, methods of treatment and appropriate management measures.

Abattoirs can also be visited. The local abattoir may be able to keep samples for you if this is arranged in advance. Trainers with the ITDG CAHW project in Kenya worked closely with the local abattoir to provide specimens of diseased organs for trainees to examine. This proved particularly effective in helping people understand the effects of diseases such as fasciolosis.

c. Preserved specimens

Pictures of small objects such as ticks, lice, flies, worms and flukes can be confusing to trainees because pictures often depict objects on a scale which is much larger than

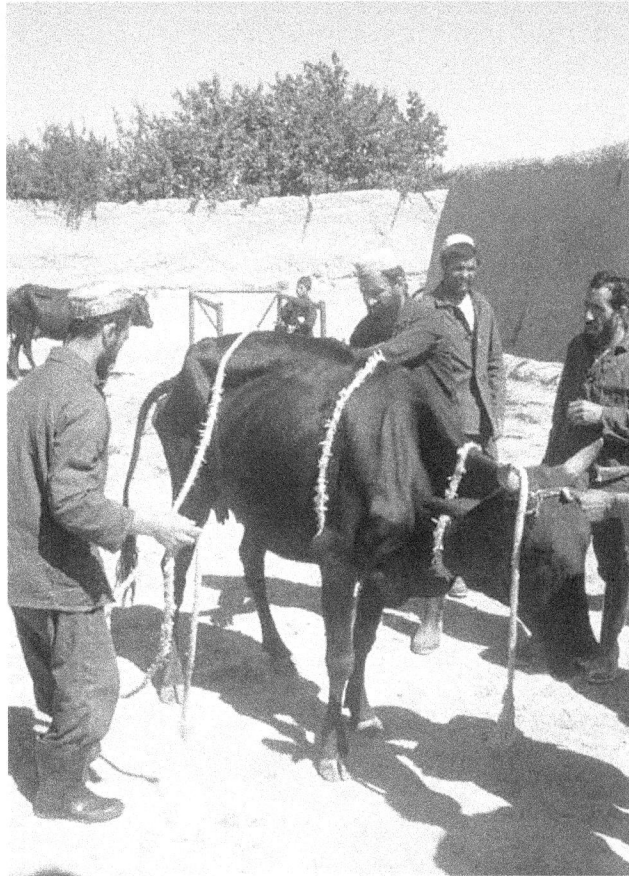

Plate 4.8 CAHWs in Afghanistan learn how to cast a cow. (*Lex Ross*)

real life. Hence, a tick which people are accustomed to seeing as a few millimetres in length can suddenly acquire giant proportions! This problem can be overcome by using preserved specimens. These specimens are very effective training aids and can be collected during the initial participatory surveys (Chapter 2) or from a local slaughter slab or abattoir. Collect specimens which can be seen with the naked eye and collect a sufficient number of each type to ensure that each trainee has the chance to look at the specimens properly. Parasites and flies should be preserved in 70 per cent alcohol and stored in clear bottles so that the specimens are easily viewed.

Chalkboards and flip-charts

Chalkboards are probably the most easily available training aid. They are usually cheap to obtain or make and can be used repeatedly. Flip-charts are more expensive and more difficult to obtain in remote areas. Both are useful for noting down key points in training to reinforce important ideas and information. A few useful guidelines for using chalkboards and flip-charts are:

Using preserved specimens in CAHW training

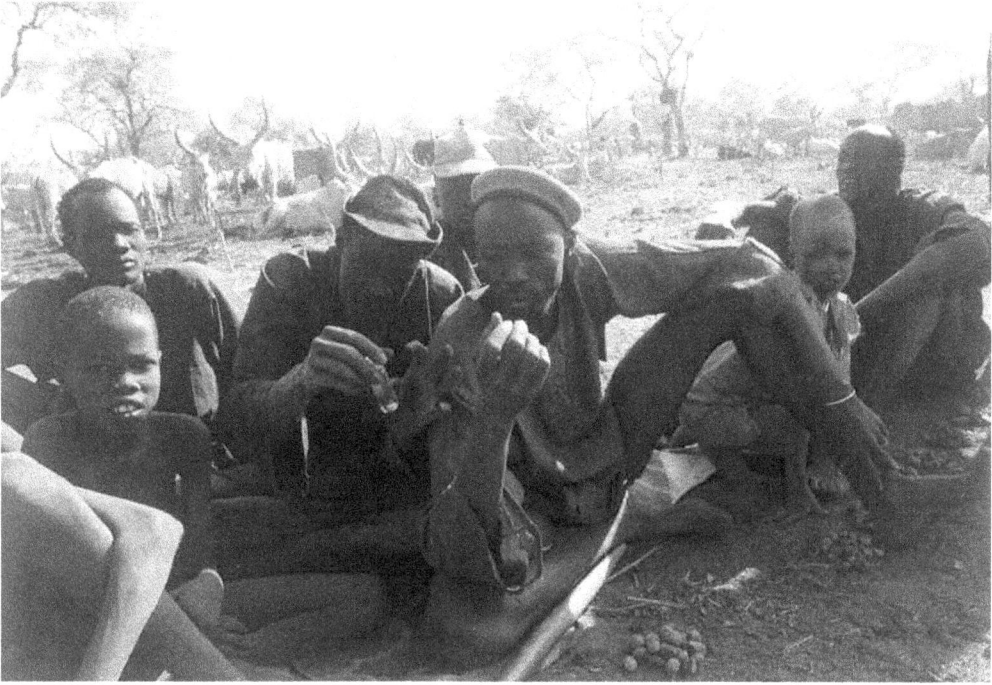

Plate 4.9 Preserved specimens of flies, ticks, worms or other parasites enables trainees to see the 'real thing' rather than a picture. (*Andy Catley*)

Three pictures from the PARC Communications Unit

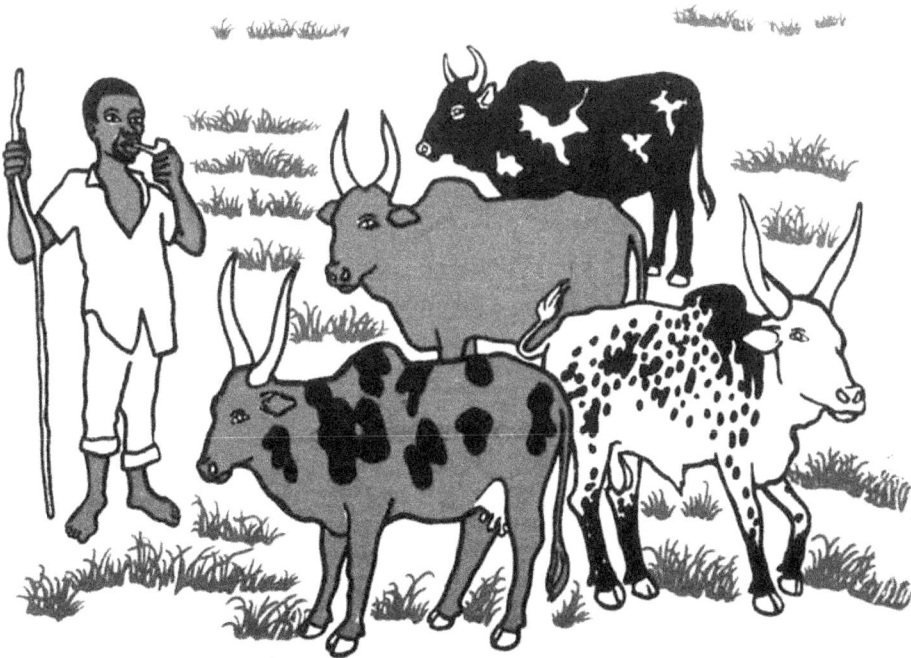

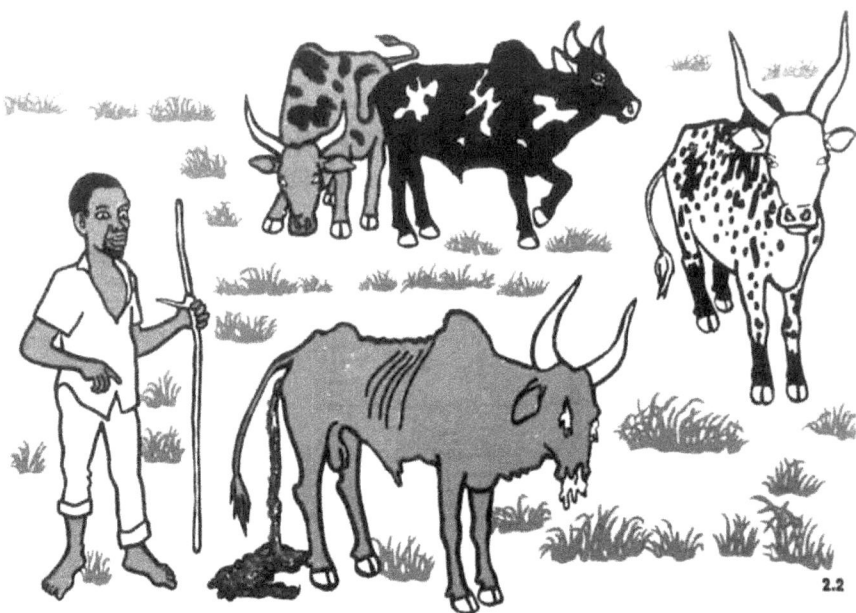

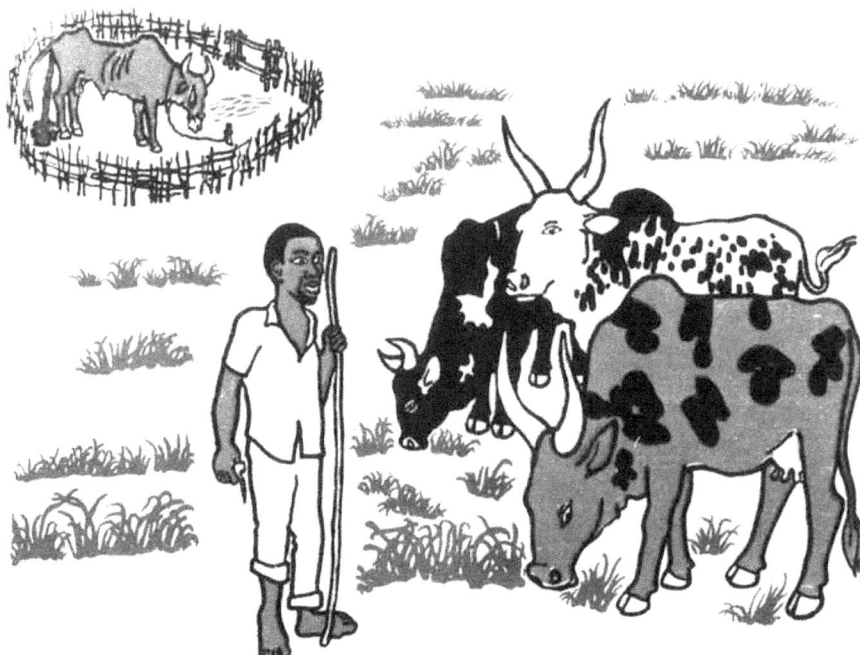

Figure 4.3 These pictures help to explain the value of separating sick cattle from healthy cattle. Note that the pictures contain no writing and the drawings are simple and clear.

- ◆ The trainer's writing must be clear and large enough for participants to read.
- ◆ If coloured pens are used, try to make the use of colour meaningful rather than random. For example, write all the points for one topic in green, then the points for the next topic in blue.

◆ Avoid writing down everything that is said and focus on the key words, headings and points.

Pictures

Pictures are a very useful training aid. They are usually inexpensive to make and easy to transport. Pictures can be used in situations where real objects are not available, or where the trainer wants to illustrate a complex idea such as the life cycle of a parasite. When discussing contagious or zoonotic diseases it is easier to use pictures instead of live animals due to the risk of disease transmission. If an opportunity arises for participants to see an outbreak of disease, this is better than using pictures provided that appropriate sanitary measures are taken.

Some guidelines for designing and using pictures are as follows:

◆ Use simple line drawings, with a minimum of shading and colour, because they can often obscure the meaning of the picture and confuse people. Avoid unnecessary detail and decoration, for example around the edges of the picture. Keep the picture simple.

◆ If the picture is for use with illiterate people, do not including any writing (see Figure 4.2 and Figure 4.3).

◆ Be cautious of perspective and size, for example drawing a tick the size of a dinner plate on the back of a cow may seem very unrealistic to participants. It may be better to use actual specimens of ticks first of all, and then explain any pictures that show ticks 'larger than life'.

◆ Avoid using strange symbols such as arrows, flow diagrams, tick marks and crosses. Such symbols are only meaningful to people who have learnt what they mean.

◆ Always test the picture before training, by showing it to colleagues and farmers, and asking them what they see in the picture. If people do not describe what you expect then the picture must be revised.

◆ If possible, produce pictures specifically for the project, rather than copying them all from other areas or books, so that you get the precise images you need for the particular training course.

◆ Use culturally appropriate images – people wearing local dress, local style of houses, local breeds of animals and agricultural scenes typical of the area. Avoid pictures of animal health workers wearing white laboratory coats and carrying clipboards looking like officials, or images of CAHWs sitting behind desks in offices;

◆ When using pictures that you want to show to the whole group, make sure that it is large enough for everyone to see clearly.

When producing pictures it is often best for the trainer to work with a local artist. This gives the trainer the opportunity to explain to the artist exactly what is required, and provides more flexibility to test the pictures and make the necessary alterations.

Pictures can be produced on a variety of materials including paper and cloth, and can be drawn, painted or printed. Cloth pictures are useful because they are durable and easy to transport, and pictures can be grouped together for specific training lessons. They can be hung on a tree, vehicle or other convenient place. Large cloth flip-charts also have the advantage of enabling pictures of some animals (e.g. sheep and goats) to be shown near to 'life-size'. This can help to overcome some of the difficulties of illustrating small objects (e.g. ticks) in an unrealistic way because the ticks can then also be drawn on the animals as life-size. Relative to cloth pictures, paper pictures are easily damaged. Although they can be laminated to make them more durable, this is expensive.

Electronic development picture libraries are now available. These include large collections of simple black and white pictures on subjects such as livestock and show, for example, different species and breeds of livestock from around the world, different disease signs, veterinary equipment (syringes etc.) and people from different cultures handling and treating animals. These pictures are copyright-free and can be downloaded from the internet (free of charge) or purchased on disk (small charge).

Computer equipment and scanners now make it possible to reproduce complicated pictures such as labels from medicines. These images are particularly useful for making 'drug information leaflets' for either literate or illiterate CAHWs.

Using flip-charts

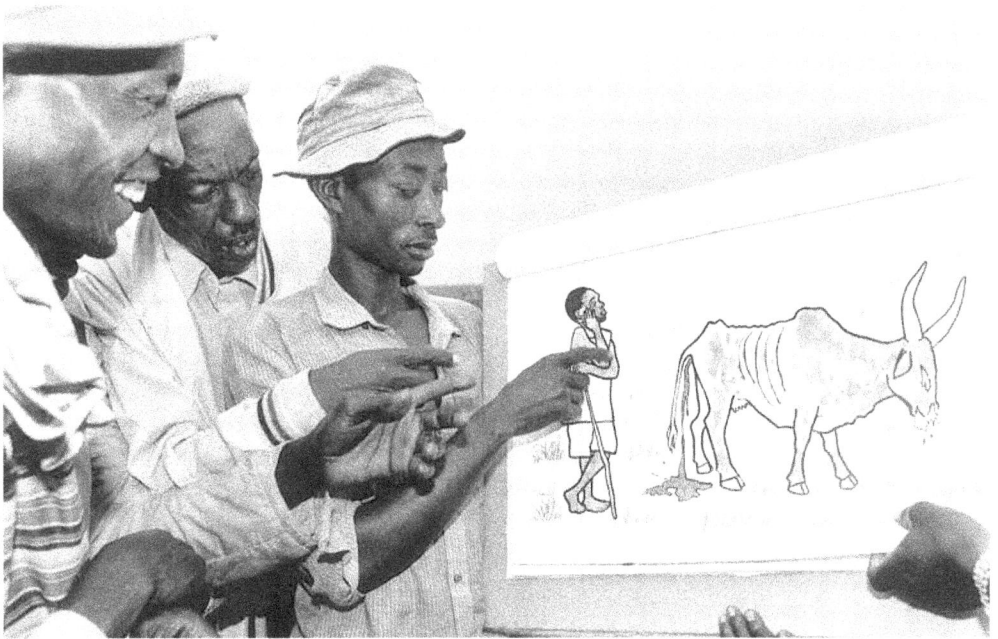

Plate 4.10 Flip-charts made of paper or cloth are excellent training aids. They are cheap and easy to produce, and cloth flip-charts are very robust and will survive frequent use in the field. (*PARC Communications Unit*)

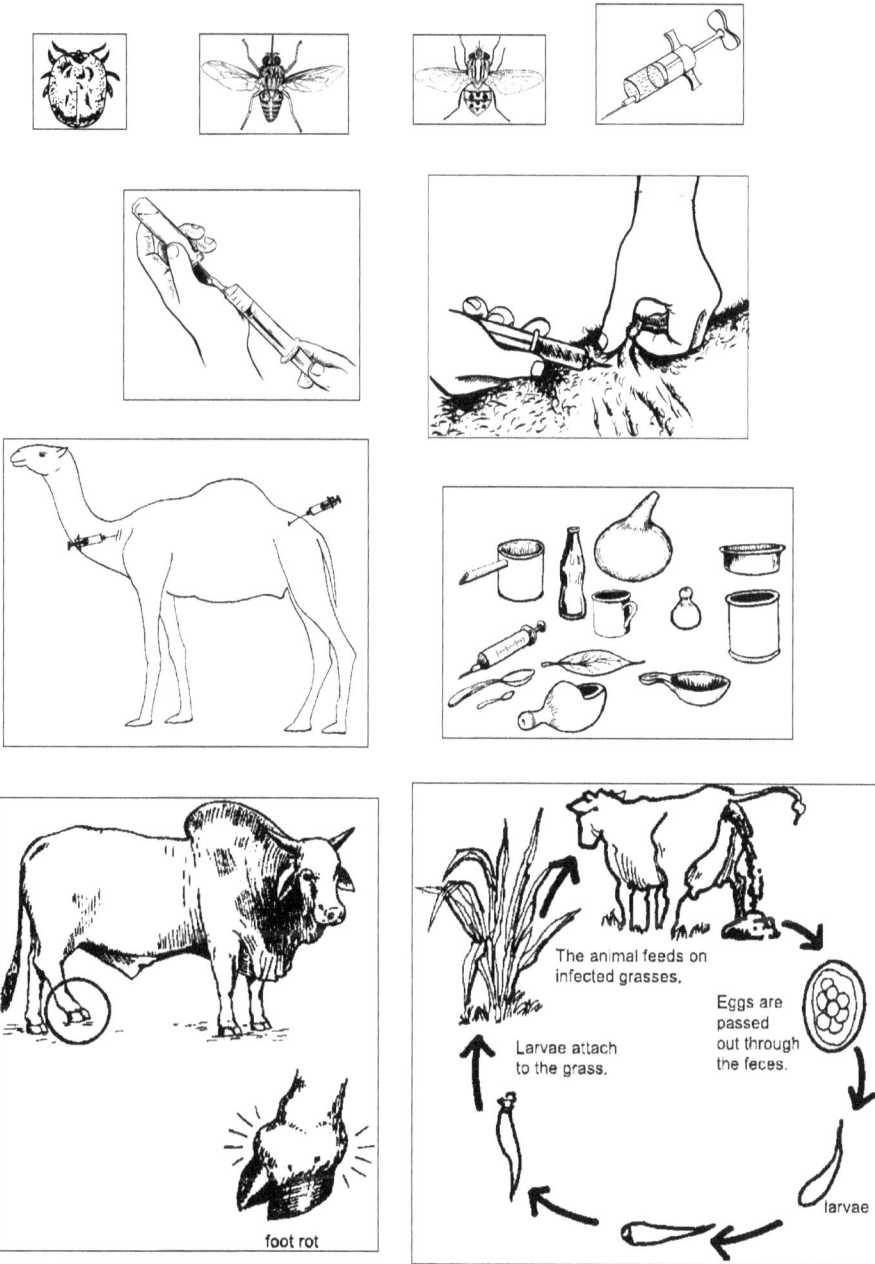

The animal feeds on
infected grasses.

Eggs are
passed
out through
the feces.

Larvae attach
to the grass.

larvae

foot rot

Figure 4.4 The pictures above and many more like them can be obtained from the internet. The pictures can be inserted directly into all kinds of training aids for CAHWs, such as handouts, drug information leaflets, posters and flip charts. See 'Some useful internet and other contact addresses'.

Photographs and slides

Photographs and slides can be effective training aids because they show images of real situations, particularly if these are not directly available during the training course, for example animals with specific diseases. Some points to consider when using photographs are as follows:

- ◆ Taking a good, clear photograph (or slide) requires skill. We need to consider what exactly it is we want to show in the photograph, and the composition of the picture.
- ◆ A common problem with photographs is that the object, for example a cow, is too far away and so appears too small in the picture for specific details to be easily seen.
- ◆ Another common problem is caused by photographs with too many images in them; the picture becomes confusing and people are unclear what it is they are supposed to be looking at.
- ◆ If a trainer wants to use photographs and slides as training aids, some basic instruction in how to take good photographs can be beneficial.
- ◆ Another factor, of course, is the cost of buying a camera and film, film processing and presentation. For slides, a slide projector is needed with a source of electricity. Solar-powered slide projectors are available; some projectors can be powered from 12-volt car batteries.

Using photographs in CAHW training

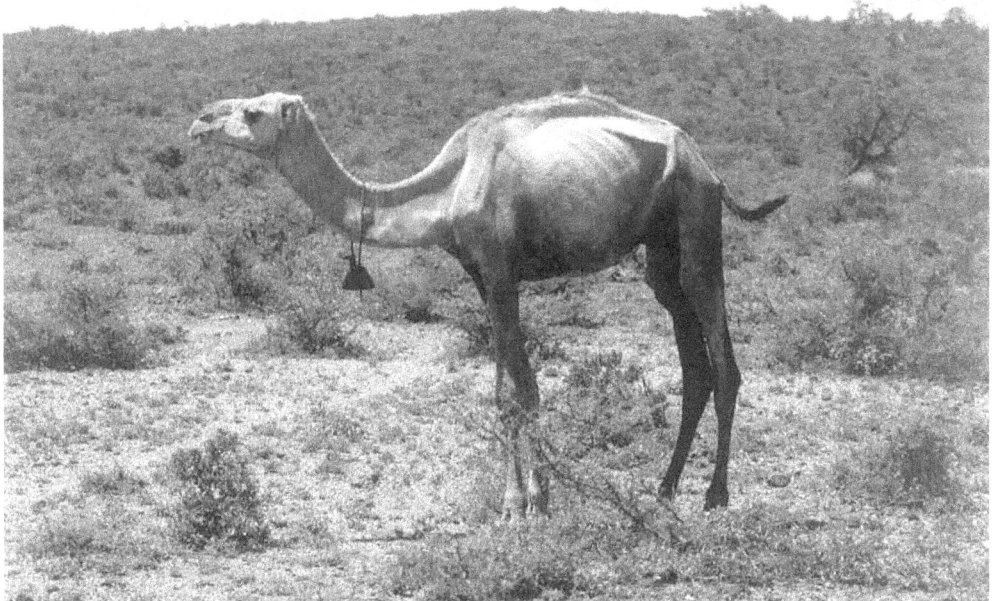

Plate 4.11 A good photograph of trypanosomiasis in camels. The picture clearly shows the emaciated body condition of the camel. (*Andy Catley*)

Models

Models may be used when it is not appropriate to use a live animal. For example, when first learning how to inject, trainees can practise on an orange or other thick-skinned fruit. Similarly, if materials and craftworkers are available, it can be simple to make a model to practise the skills needed to assist in birthing problems.

Computers, videos and overhead projectors

More high-tech training aids are available in some areas. Such technology is expensive, requires considerable training to use properly and requires electricity. Also, because CAHW training frequently takes place in rural areas and is highly practical, the use of computers, videos and overhead projectors may not be appropriate. If funds and conditions allow, videos can be useful for showing examples of projects from other areas, the progress of certain livestock diseases or other topics.

Handouts

Handouts are notes given to participants that contain the key learning points from the course. They can be in written form or as pictures if the participants are not literate. Handouts need careful preparation. They should not simply be a copy of the trainer's notes, but should consist of a summary of important information – such as dose rates for medicines – which are presented in a way that is easy for participants to refer to. Each topic should have clear bold headings, with just the key points listed.

4.7 Summary

This chapter has introduced some of the important principles of training and learning, and has explained the advantages of participative learning approaches and methods. A key factor in effective CAHW training is the proper use of the participative training approach and this requires investment in training veterinarians and other livestock professionals before training CAHWs. Also, the costs of participative training courses for project staff need to be considered when project budgets are being formulated.

A wide range of dynamic and innovative participative training methods are available. The training approach is very flexible and provides scope for trainers to improvise and develop their own methods according to local circumstances. Although participative approaches and methods are a central theme in successful CAHW projects, CAHW training also requires careful design and planning. These issues are discussed in the next chapter.

How to design and implement training courses

Karen Iles

CONTENTS

5.1 Introduction

This chapter begins at a point when project staff are ready to design and implement a community-based animal health worker (CAHW) training course. The chapter assumes that project staff have conducted participatory assessments with the community (Chapter 2), considered the long-term sustainability issues of the project (Chapter 3) and have been trained in participative training approaches and methods (Chapter 4). As the process of designing and organizing the training begins, the trainer needs to address a number of key questions, as listed in Box 5.1. This chapter will discuss each of these key questions in turn.

Box 5.1 Key questions when designing and organizing a CAHW training course

◆ What are the skills, knowledge, behaviour and attitudes the CAHWs need in order to carry out the job they are being asked to do?
◆ What are their existing skills, knowledge, behaviour and attitudes?
◆ Where are the gaps between what the CAHWs need to know in order to do the job and what they already know?
◆ How can the course fill these gaps?
◆ What training techniques should be used?
◆ How long should the course and sessions be?
◆ Where should the course be run and how should it be organized on a practical level?
◆ Who is going to pay for it all?

The gaps between what the CAHWs need to know in order to do the job and what they already know are called the 'learning needs'. When the learning needs have been defined, the 'training objectives' for the course can be set and a detailed course developed. The major steps for designing and implementing a CAHW course are illustrated in Box 5.2.

It is important that the training is designed and carried out systematically. Also, the CAHW curriculum should not simply be copied from a textbook, nor be based on a formal animal health and husbandry course. Each geographical area and community is unique and so a CAHW course curriculum should be designed specifically for that area. The content of the CAHW training will also be heavily influenced by the roles of the CAHWs agreed during the initial participatory survey, as described in Chapter 2.

In some countries, nationwide CAHW training courses are being developed that are endorsed by professional veterinary bodies. However, these standardized curricula are still being refined and specific lessons about their value have yet to

Box 5.2 Steps for designing and implementing CAHW courses

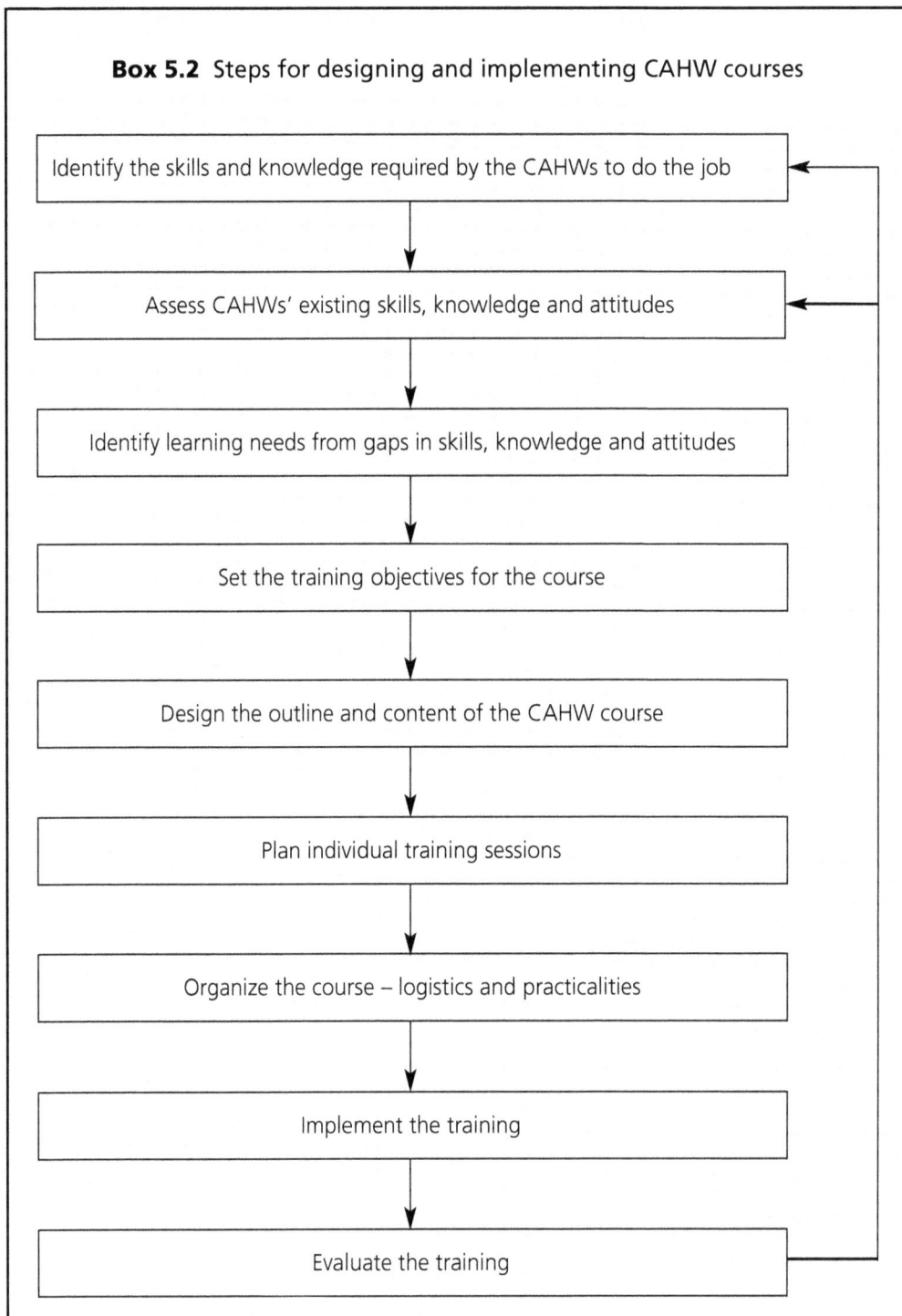

```
┌─────────────────────────────────────────────────────────────┐
│ Identify the skills and knowledge required by the CAHWs to    │ ◄───┐
│ do the job                                                     │     │
└─────────────────────────────────────────────────────────────┘     │
                          │                                           │
                          ▼                                           │
┌─────────────────────────────────────────────────────────────┐     │
│ Assess CAHWs' existing skills, knowledge and attitudes        │ ◄─┐ │
└─────────────────────────────────────────────────────────────┘   │ │
                          │                                         │ │
                          ▼                                         │ │
┌─────────────────────────────────────────────────────────────┐   │ │
│ Identify learning needs from gaps in skills, knowledge and    │   │ │
│ attitudes                                                      │   │ │
└─────────────────────────────────────────────────────────────┘   │ │
                          │                                         │ │
                          ▼                                         │ │
┌─────────────────────────────────────────────────────────────┐   │ │
│ Set the training objectives for the course                    │   │ │
└─────────────────────────────────────────────────────────────┘   │ │
                          │                                         │ │
                          ▼                                         │ │
┌─────────────────────────────────────────────────────────────┐   │ │
│ Design the outline and content of the CAHW course             │   │ │
└─────────────────────────────────────────────────────────────┘   │ │
                          │                                         │ │
                          ▼                                         │ │
┌─────────────────────────────────────────────────────────────┐   │ │
│ Plan individual training sessions                             │   │ │
└─────────────────────────────────────────────────────────────┘   │ │
                          │                                         │ │
                          ▼                                         │ │
┌─────────────────────────────────────────────────────────────┐   │ │
│ Organize the course – logistics and practicalities            │   │ │
└─────────────────────────────────────────────────────────────┘   │ │
                          │                                         │ │
                          ▼                                         │ │
┌─────────────────────────────────────────────────────────────┐   │ │
│ Implement the training                                        │   │ │
└─────────────────────────────────────────────────────────────┘   │ │
                          │                                         │ │
                          ▼                                         │ │
┌─────────────────────────────────────────────────────────────┐   │ │
│ Evaluate the training                                         │───┴─┘
└─────────────────────────────────────────────────────────────┘
```

emerge. Some courses comprise both a 'core curriculum' and an 'adaptive curriculum'. The core curriculum is common to all geographical areas in the country and includes topics such as the signs of healthy and sick animals, modes of disease transmission and how to handle medicines safely. The adaptive curriculum is formulated in response to area–specific needs and variations in livestock production systems, disease incidence and community needs.

5.2 Training needs assessment for CAHWs

What is a training needs assessment?

Learning needs can be identified by carrying out a training needs assessment (TNA). In practice, much of the information required to design a training course for CAHWs will have been gathered during the surveys and investigations carried out in the initial

---

Box 5.3 Training needs assessment for CAHW training

A training needs assessment (TNA) forms an integral part of designing appropriate and effective CAHW courses. A TNA is used to:
- identify learning needs;
- set course and session objectives;
- ensure that the training is learner-centred and not teacher-centred, i.e. focused on what the participants need to know to do their work;
- make the training bottom-up, not top-down;
- identify appropriate training methods to use on the course by choosing:
  - suitable techniques for educational background (e.g. literacy level);
  - appropriate visual aids;
  - the correct speed at which training can take place;
  - meaningful technical terms;
  - appropriate content and level at which subject can be taught;
- plan sessions and organize the logistics of the course;
- motivate trainees to learn, because they feel the trainers are really trying to tailor the course to their learning needs, for example training must be related to daily life and address real livestock problems;
- ensure the training is interesting and relevant;
- make the training effective;
- build on experience and knowledge of trainees – follow the principles of adult learning;
- monitor development of trainees' skills, knowledge, behaviour and attitudes;
- evaluate the effectiveness of training;
- make the most effective use of time available for training;
- make the best use of scarce resources.

---

stages of the project (Chapter 2). The issues described in this section provide trainers with an outline of the type of information they need to ensure that the planned training is effective.

During a TNA, the trainer attempts to gain an understanding of the general background of the trainees and their existing technical knowledge (see Box 5.3). When combined with the results of the general project survey, this information enables the trainer to determine which topics should be covered on the CAHW course. The information can be used to set realistic objectives that provide the participants with the skills and knowledge they need to carry out their work as CAHWs. The TNA also allows the trainer to select the most appropriate training methods to use on the course. For example, if the CAHWs have poor reading and writing skills then the training methods should cater for this situation.

The trainer can design the course (length, number of sessions per day, best time of year to run the course, and so on) to suit the work schedule and commitments of participants. TNAs also provide a baseline for evaluating the effectiveness of the training by assessing how much the trainees have learnt from the course.

A TNA has three parts:

General background of participants

Get to know your participants – including ethnic, cultural and religious background, level of education and literacy, age, gender, family, work and other commitments, major source of income such as livestock herding, farming or trading.

Technical knowledge and skills

Assess the experience of livestock keeping, treatment of sick animals, use of drugs and experience of indigenous medicines. Are any of the trainees traditional healers?

Attitudes

What are the prospective CAHWs' attitudes towards such issues as livestock keepers' experience and traditional beliefs, use of traditional approaches to dealing with livestock problems (e.g. plants)? How effective are their present communication skills?

Approach and methods for training needs assessment

A TNA can be carried out using a variety of methods including interview using a checklist, visiting the prospective CAHWs at their homes and places of work, observing them carrying out livestock husbandry tasks and treatment of animals, and observing the way the CAHWs manage their own animals. To assess precise knowledge of drugs and their uses, a short questionnaire can be used with carefully thought-out questions, for example: 'What is the dose of the project flukicide for a large adult goat?'

It is also important to assess the indigenous knowledge and skills of the prospective CAHWs. How much do they understand about local strategies for disease control and prevention, such as movement of animals to deal with a disease outbreak? How well do they understand the traditional grazing patterns? Do they have any experience of using traditional treatments such as plants, local methods of vaccination or bone setting? How much do the CAHWs understand about local perceptions of disease, including local beliefs about the causes of disease and how they influence approaches for dealing with disease problems?

All this information is useful baseline data or a 'profile' for each trainee and helps the project to assess the effectiveness of training on building the skills and knowledge of CAHWs. Also, as projects progress, an early documented profile of each CAHW enables the CAHW's performance to be assessed in relation to personal attributes of the CAHW such as gender, level of education and ownership of livestock. This kind of assessment is a useful component of monitoring and evaluation systems for CAHW projects, as described in Chapter 6.

During the TNA, it is important that the CAHW trainees do not feel that they are being examined or feel under pressure to 'get the answer right' for fear of being deselected. The TNA should be carried out in a sensitive and participative way, with the trainer carefully explaining why the TNA is being done. CAHWs should be reassured and put at ease.

Confidentiality

Information given by individuals during a TNA needs to be treated with respect. The project must develop a system for storing and using the information collected through TNAs (and all other participatory processes) that safeguards its confidentiality.

Gaps in skills, knowledge and attitudes: the learning needs

When the information on the general background, skills, knowledge and attitudes of the CAHWs has been gathered, it can be compared with the skills, knowledge and attitudes actually required for the CAHWs to fulfil their agreed roles and responsibilities. The gaps identified in this comparison are the learning needs of the CAHWs (Box 5.4). The learning needs are important because they are used to set the training objectives for the CAHW course, and design the course curriculum.

5.3   How to design the training course

Setting the training objectives

The training objectives represent what we want the participants to have achieved by the end of the course. As explained above, the training objectives are based on the learning needs of the CAHWs, and they also provide the basis of the course curriculum. In keeping with the principles of using a *learning* approach as opposed to

Box 5.4 Examples of learning needs of CAHWs: skills, knowledge, behaviour and attitudes to be covered in a typical CAHW course

The curriculum for a CAHW course is based on the learning needs of CAHWs. An example includes:

Skills

At the end of the course CAHWs should be able to:

◆ build a long-term rapport with livestock keepers;
◆ diagnose common livestock diseases by clinical examination;
◆ handle and restrain animals safely;
◆ administer drugs to animals safely using the correct dose rate and administration route;
◆ store drugs safely under optimum conditions;
◆ manage drug kit (storage, hygiene and maintenance of drugs and equipment);
◆ replenish drug kit when required (stock control, drug purchasing);
◆ keep records (animal treatments, vaccinations, drug sales) using writing or pictures;
◆ prepare vaccine correctly and under suitable conditions;
◆ store vaccine under correct conditions;
◆ administer vaccine using correct dose and correct administration route;
◆ maintain vaccine equipment;
◆ advise farmers of husbandry matters (e.g. housing, feeding);
◆ give clear explanations of, for example, follow-up treatment of animals the livestock owner must carry out, such as changing a wound dressing;
◆ mix a balanced feed ration for all classes of livestock.

Knowledge

At the end of the course CAHWs should know:

◆ which drug to use for which livestock disease;
◆ dose rates of each drug for each species and class of livestock;
◆ signs of common livestock diseases;
◆ causes, treatment and prevention of common livestock diseases;
◆ strategy for disease control, for example, time of year animals should be dewormed;
◆ strategy for reducing onset of drug resistance;
◆ law on drug use and treatment of animals;
◆ which vaccine to use for control of which diseases;
◆ reasons behind record keeping;
◆ calculation of profit/income/remuneration from treatments/sale of drugs;
◆ why good communication skills are essential for building a successful working relationship with livestock keepers;
◆ where to buy drugs and equipment to replenish kits;

◆ purchase and sale price of drugs, vaccine and equipment;
◆ principles of feeding livestock;
◆ principles of providing a suitable environment for animals (housing, kraals, etc.);
◆ role of ethnoveterinary medicine in animal health.

Behaviour and attitudes

CAHWs should be:

◆ able to communicate effectively to discuss livestock issues with farmers;
◆ friendly, open, approachable, empathetic, good listeners;
◆ respectful of livestock keepers' way of life and experiences.

a *teaching* approach (see Chapter 4), training objectives are written from the point of view of the participants and not the trainer. Training objectives include skills, knowledge and attitudes. An example of training objectives for a CAHW course is provided in Box 5.5.

Box 5.5 Example set of training objectives for a CAHW training course

By the end of the course the participants will be able to:

◆ diagnose common livestock diseases and conditions by clinical examination, including helminths, pneumonia, bloat, foot-rot, wounds, mange, eye problems, fleas and lice, ticks, mastitis;
◆ treat each of these common diseases using the appropriate medicine, with the recommended dose rate and administration route;
◆ prepare and administer rinderpest vaccine to cattle;
◆ carry out routine livestock tasks such as foot trimming;
◆ handle livestock safely using various methods including casting and rope halters;
◆ store and use a given number of medicines effectively, including preparation and spraying of livestock with acaracides;
◆ keep records on work done (animals treated and vaccinated, and drugs sold);
◆ know what action to take in the event of an unusual disease outbreak;
◆ maintain and replenish drug and equipment kit;
◆ explain ways of improving communication with livestock owners;
◆ explain ways in which advice can be provided to livestock owners on livestock feeding and housing.

Once the training objectives are known, the training course content and approach are developed.

Course content and approach

The training course content (curriculum) and approach should be developed methodically as follows:

◆ List the topics that will be covered in order to meet each of the course objectives.
◆ Decide how many sessions are required to cover each topic. A session usually lasts one to two hours. A single topic may need several sessions.
◆ Decide how many days are required to run the course, and how many sessions will be covered each day (see *Some practical considerations*, below).
◆ Decide on the most appropriate training approach to take. If most of the participants are illiterate, then training methods that do not rely on reading and writing are required. This will also affect the way training materials are prepared.

What is the ideal number of trainees?

Because of the practical nature of CAHW courses, the number of participants should not exceed 12. Any more than this and it becomes difficult for the trainer to manage the course to ensure that each participant gets enough individual attention. The quality of the training then suffers. If more participants need to be trained – say 16 or 18 – then a second trainer should be employed for the course or, preferably, an additional CAHW course should be organized. The number of participants also affects the time required to run each session, and the number of animals and amount of equipment required.

Some practical considerations

a. Course length

In part, the length of the course depends on how many days are needed to cover all the topics necessary to meet the course objectives. Course length also depends on the other commitments of the participants. The final decision on the length of the course should be made in consultation with the CAHW trainees to fit in with their work schedule. For example, some trainees might have important agricultural or herding tasks to perform at home. As these tasks are often seasonal, it is usually possible to identify the most convenient time of year to conduct the training (also see *Gender and cultural factors*).

b. Course structure and availability of training aids

The availability of training aids can influence how a CAHW training course is structured. For example, if animals are available for use in training every day, then the course may be structured so that theory sessions take place in the morning and

The number of trainees should be kept to a manageable size.

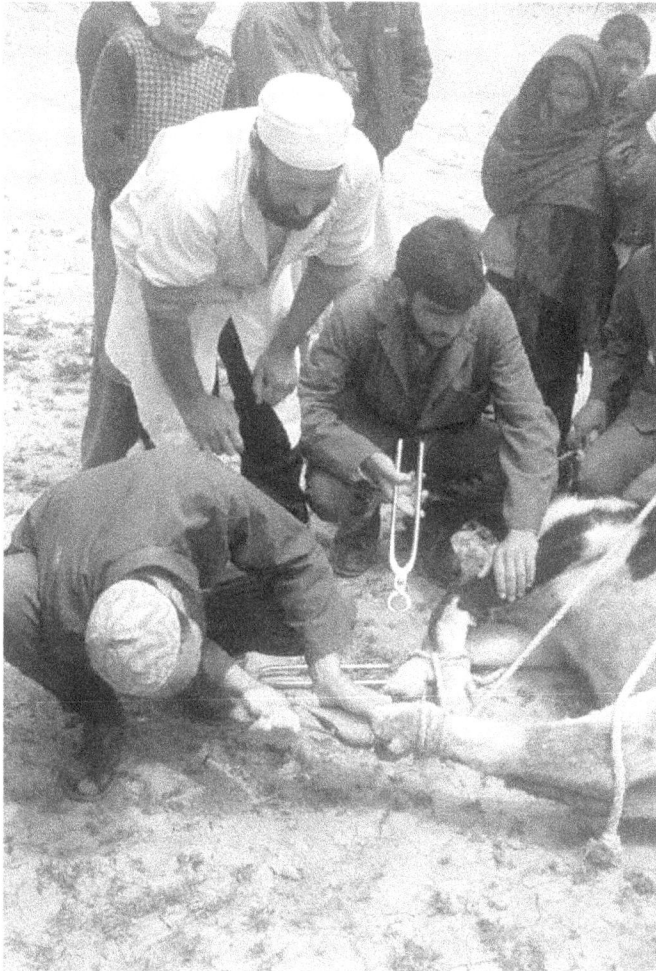

Plate 5.1 During practical sessions, can everyone see what is happening? Will everyone have a chance to practise new procedures under the supervision of the trainer? This trainer (dressed in white) in Afghanistan is able to keep a close eye on the trainees and offer guidance when needed. (*Lex Ross*)

practical sessions in the afternoon. If animals are only available on certain days or at specific times of day, then the course will need to be structured accordingly. Alternative ways of structuring a CAHW course include:

◆ theory in the morning, practicals in the afternoon;
◆ each disease is covered completely, theory and practical, one after the other, so that practicals take place at any time during the day, each day;
◆ theory lessons are carried out in the first half of the course, and the practicals in the second half.

159

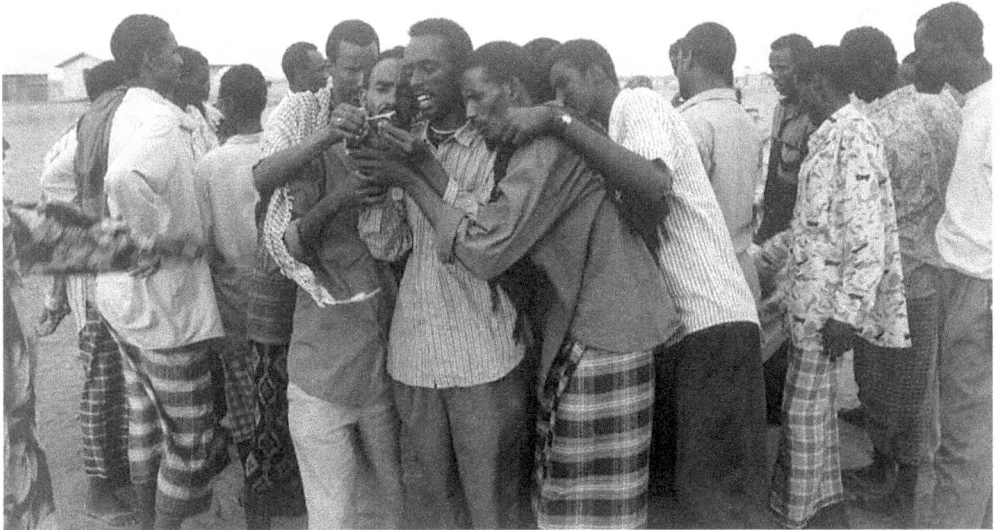

Plate 5.2 This training session is very overcrowded. There are too many trainees and not enough trainers or equipment. The trainees are struggling to see a thermometer. (*Andy Catley*)

In addition to the practical sessions linked to specific training sessions, a whole day should be set aside towards the end of the course for participants to practise treating animals with all kinds of disease problems. This gives them the opportunity to practise again all the skills and knowledge they have acquired on the course.

5.4 Planning the individual training sessions

The importance of proper planning for each training session

During the design stage of a CAHW course the trainer needs to prepare a detailed plan for each session. Inexperienced trainers sometimes make the mistake of assuming that, if they can carry out a skill themselves, or have a deep knowledge of a subject, then they can easily teach it to another person without planning.

Experience from the field

In a project in Afghanistan, a trainer prepared a few quick notes on how he was going to teach a group of farmers to take the temperature of a sheep. He said: 'This is so simple – it'll only take me a few minutes to teach!' He started the lesson, taught the participants how to shake down the thermometer, insert it into the sheep and hold it there for three minutes. He then

160

asked the farmers to read their thermometers and tell him if the animal's temperature was normal. The farmers could make little sense of the markings on the thermometer, did not know the significance of the mercury and were not aware of the normal temperature of a sheep. The whole lesson soon became meaningless to them with the trainer backtracking and trying to give a hurried theory lesson on animal body temperatures, the workings of a thermometer and the relevance of the markings on the thermometer.

Had the trainer in this example taken the time to think through all the steps of the skill in detail, he may have come up with the broad outline of a plan that looks something like this:

◆ theory session on normal and abnormal temperatures of sheep, and the role of temperature in an animal's health;
◆ practical session on how to use a thermometer and take the temperature of a sheep, which might include examining the parts of a thermometer and what they are used for, how to read and interpret the markings on the side, safe handling, how to shake down the mercury, how to insert it safely into the anus, how long to keep it there and why, how to read the temperature and so on.

The trainer would have developed these notes into a detailed session plan, with a clear sequence and proper introduction, main part and summary. He would use appropriate training techniques such as group discussion, a short talk with visual aids and practical instruction. Questions and key learning points would be written down.

It is these session plans that the trainer will follow while running the course, and which form the nuts and bolts of the training. Taking the time to plan the sessions carefully is essential and helps to ensure that important learning points are not missed.

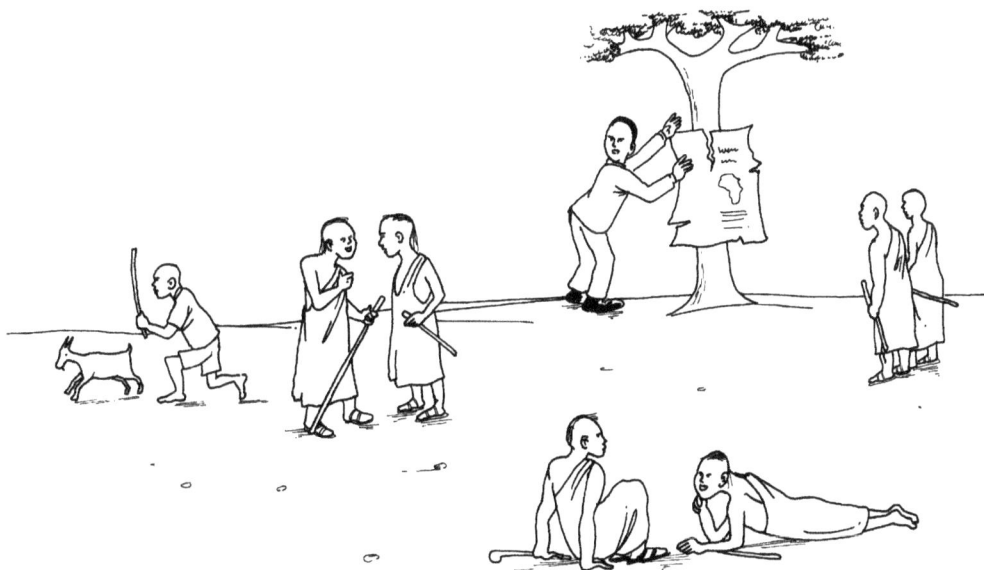

A hopelessly disorganised training session

Despite this, trainers often neglect to plan the sessions properly and, when standing in front of a group of participants, can forget important aspects of the session. The end result is poor-quality training. Training is not as easy as it looks.

How to plan the training sessions

Planning a session should be carried out methodically, and follows a four-stage process:

Stage 1 Set objectives for each session

As explained in section 5.3, the objectives of a session define exactly what it is we would like the participants to be able to do by the end of the session. It is important to set objectives for each session to ensure that the session remains focused, all the important learning points are covered, and the trainer can assess how much the participants have learnt. Setting objectives also greatly assists with planning the content of a session. Box 5.6 provides more examples of training objectives according to the need for participants to acquire a practical skill, learn new knowledge or recognize and practise appropriate behaviour and attitudes.

An important aspect of writing training objectives is to ensure that the

---

Box 5.6 Training objectives for different types of training sessions

Practical skill session

An example of an objective for a practical skill session is:

By the end of the session the participants will be able to administer the liquid anthelmintic, Nilzan, to goats, sheep and cattle, with the correct dose rate, by mouth, using a syringe and a 300 ml soda bottle, without injury to the animal or the participant.

Knowledge session

An example of an objective for a knowledge session is:

By the end of the session the participants will be able to describe the signs of foot-rot in goats and sheep, list the causes of foot-rot, explain ways in which foot-rot can be treated, and describe husbandry measures that can be taken to prevent foot-rot.

Behaviour and attitudes session

An example of an objective for a behaviour and attitudes session is:

By the end of the session the participants will be able to list the characteristics of a good listener, and be able to demonstrate effective listening skills while discussing a topic with another person.

---

objectives are *measurable*. This means that the objective should detail a specific action that the trainees will be able to perform at the end of the training session. With this in mind, objectives should include action words like 'list', 'explain', 'describe' or 'construct'. For example, if a participant can list the signs of foot-rot correctly, then the trainer is sure that the participant has understood that part of the session. Try to avoid using words like 'know' and 'understand' because these are rather ambiguous. For example, 'By the end of the session the participants will "know" the signs of foot-rot in goats and sheep': it is difficult for the trainer to assess whether the participants 'know' something unless they can explain or describe what they have learnt.

Stage 2 Decide the content of the session

When deciding the specific contents of the training sessions, a useful approach is for the trainers and their colleagues to brainstorm all the important subjects and learning points. This can be done on rough paper so that alterations can be made easily and new ideas added as they occur. The next step is to arrange the subjects into a logical order. The session should be broken down into a series of clear, simple steps that can be assimilated easily by the participants. The trainer should also think about how each subject will be linked to the next, so that the whole session flows smoothly in a 'step-by-step' process. For each subject, the key learning points should also be written down.

Stage 3 Decide which training techniques to use during the session

As we have seen in Chapter 4, different training techniques are suited to different learning needs and situations. Throughout the training course as a whole, a variety of techniques should be used to make the training as interesting and stimulating as possible. Therefore, provided you feel comfortable with the methods, try role plays, exercises, games, case studies, drama and puppets, rather than relying on one or two methods alone. If a skill is being taught, practical instruction should be used – the principle of skills training is 'people learn by doing'. In cases where participants are illiterate then appropriate training techniques should be used which do not rely on reading and writing.

After deciding which techniques to use in the sessions, the trainer can now add more details to the session plans. They plan the questions (open questions) for the participants, write out the key learning points, note the timing for each section of the session, and list what equipment and training aids will be used.

Stage 4 Write final version of the session plan in detail

Once all the rough planning has been completed the session plan can be written out in full. As these are the session plans that the trainer will use when running the course, it is important that they are written clearly and neatly so that they can be read easily. Using a highlighter pen to make key points stand out and writing in capitals all assist in making the session plan easier to use.

An example of a lesson plan is shown in Box 5.7. This lesson plan covers knowledge about worms and flukes, and how to control these parasites.

Box 5.7 Example of a session plan for improving knowledge on internal parasites

Training objectives

By the end of the lesson the trainees will be able to explain:

- the signs, cause and transmission of roundworms and liver flukes;
- the treatment and prevention of worms and liver flukes.

Methods

Problem picture or animals, question and answer, summary

Time *90 minutes*

Materials

Real animals suffering from worms, picture of sheep with worms, young animal suspected to have died from worms for post mortem, examples of anthelmintic medicines (liquid and tablets).

Introduction

We are going to learn about internal parasites in cattle, goats and sheep.

Problem picture

Real animal or picture of a sheep with worms (if no live animal available). Bloated belly, swollen jaw, thin, weak, poor coat.

Questions

Question 1 *What can you see in this picture?*

Key points

- a sheep;
- the sheep is very thin;
- the sheep has a swollen belly;
- the sheep has a swollen jaw;
- looks unhealthy;
- it is weak;
- the wool looks rough.

Question 2 *What disease do you think this is?*

Key point

- worms.

Question 3 *Have you seen worms before in your animals? What is your experience?*

Question 4 *What are the signs of worms?*

Key points

- animals are thin;

- animals do not grow well;
- there may be diarrhoea;
- gums, lining of mouth and eyes become pale in colour;
- the coat is dull, dry and looks rough;
- sometimes animals produce swelling under the jaw;
- young animals can die before showing the above signs, when they go out grazing for the first time in spring;
- some animals may die suddenly.

Question 5 Why are worms in animals a problem?

Key points
- Worms can reduce production and growth.
- Young animals are very susceptible and can die from heavy worm burdens.
- Worms suck blood from the animal and eat its food, so making the animal weak.
- Even if the animal is given plenty of food it can still remain thin and not grow well.
- Worms cause a lot of damage to the animal (reduced production and growth) even before other signs are seen.
- Worms can reduce the economy of the farmer.

Tell

There are two major types of internal parasites that are important:

- roundworms found in the digestive system;
- liver flukes found in the liver.

Question 6a What is the life cycle of roundworms?

Key points
- Adult worms live in the digestive system of the animal, and lay eggs, which pass out in the faeces onto the pasture.
- The eggs grow into young worms (larvae) on the pasture.
- Another animal eats the larvae, which grow into adult worms in the digestive system, and start laying eggs.

Training aid

Explain picture showing simplified version of the roundworm life cycle. If available, open up a dead lamb/kid and inspect the digestive system for worms. Show the trainees any worms found.

Question 6b What is the life cycle of liver flukes?

Key points
- Liver flukes are shaped like the leaf of an apricot tree and are 2–7 cm long.
- The adult liver fluke lives in the gall bladder where it lays eggs that are passed out in the faeces.

- When the faeces are passed into water, the eggs hatch into larvae and are eaten by snails.
- The larvae grow in the snails and are passed out of the snails.
- When an animal drinks contaminated water, it drinks the larvae.
- The larvae migrate through the liver to the gall bladder, where they mature and start laying eggs.
- The snails are found in slow-moving water such as irrigation ditches, canals and ponds.

Training aid

Explaining picture showing simplified version of the liver fluke life cycle. If available, open up a dead lamb or kid and inspect the liver for flukes.

Question 7a How are roundworms spread from animal to animal?

Key points
- Larvae on the pasture are eaten by animals when they graze.
- The young worms grow into adults in the animal and lay eggs, and the cycle continues.
- In a short time the pasture can become infected with eggs and larvae.
- The eggs and larvae survive best when the weather is warm and moist.
- Spring and early autumn is the time when animals are most likely to be infected with worms.
- Young animals going to graze for the first time are very susceptible, and some can even die if heavily infected with worms.

Question 7b How are liver flukes spread from animal to animal?

Key points
- When animals drink water that has been infected with liver fluke larvae they ingest the larvae.
- If manure from infected animals is allowed to pass into the water supply then other animals will become infected.

Question 8a What is the traditional treatment for worms?

Question 8b What are the traditional methods for preventing worms?

Question 8c What is the modern treatment for roundworms?

Key points
- Use dewormers (e.g. fenbendazole).
- When worms are diagnosed treat all animals and move them to new pasture where there are likely to be few worms.
- As young animals are most susceptible, make sure at least these animals are treated.

Question 8d *What is the modern treatment for liver flukes?*

Key point

◆ When liver flukes are diagnosed, all animals in the herd should be treated.

Training aids

Show examples of liquid and tablet anthelmintics to trainees.

Question 9a *How can we prevent roundworms?*

Key points

◆ Worms is a disease which it is far better to prevent than to wait until seeing signs before treating.

◆ Do not wait until animals show signs of thinness, rough dry coat etc. before treating – the damage is already done, and treatment may be too late.

◆ Give all animals anthelmintics at the beginning of spring when they go out for grazing, before they show signs of sickness.

◆ Give anthelmintics again in autumn and at the beginning of winter.

◆ Do not keep animals on the same pasture all the time - move animals to new grazing areas to prevent build-up of worms.

◆ Take care of young animals – put them on new grazing ahead of the adults.

◆ Keep the stable and place where animals are kept clean and dry.

Question 9b *How can we prevent liver flukes?*

Key points

◆ Give animals clean water from wells and fast-flowing rivers.

◆ Do not allow animals to drink water from slow-moving ditches, especially if snails are present.

◆ Do not allow animal manure to contaminate water supplies.

Summary

◆ Why are internal parasites a problem for the animal and the farmer?
◆ Why is it important to prevent worms?
◆ How can worms be prevented?
◆ When should animals be treated with anthelmintics?

Link

In the next lesson we will learn about correct dose rates for worm medicines and how to give worm medicines to animals correctly.

Hints for ensuring a trainee-centred learning process

a. Appropriate language and terminology

The terminology used in the training should be pitched at a level that is appropriate for the participants. Use of complicated veterinary terms, such as Latin names for livestock diseases, is rarely necessary in CAHW training. Why say 'parasitic gastroenteritis' or 'haemonchosis' if we can say 'worms'? 'Fluke' is easier than *Fasciola gigantica* and 'germ' will do instead of *Pasteurella haemolytica*.

A further consideration when discussing livestock diseases is the use of local disease names. During the initial participatory surveys (Chapter 2), the project veterinarians should have documented local disease names and, as far as possible, clarified the associations between local terminology and western disease names. Where possible, the trainer should use the local names for diseases because the CAHW trainees will be more familiar with these terms. In some cases, a direct translation between a western and local disease name will not be possible. For example, a local name for a disease may be based on a clinical syndrome (like 'poor-doer'). In these cases, the veterinarian will have to decide how best to describe the disease and the various differential diagnoses for cases of 'diarrhoea', 'coughing' and so on. A comprehensive participatory survey backed up by laboratory diagnosis at the beginning of the project helps to define the links between local and modern disease terminology.

b. Building on indigenous veterinary knowledge and skills

Participative training is based on the principle of building on existing experience and, therefore, it is important to start from what the participants already know. In addition to using local names for livestock diseases during the training, traditional knowledge and practices should also be discussed. Sessions on livestock diseases and husbandry can begin with discussions on local perceptions of disease including signs, causes, how the disease is transmitted, whether or not people believe it to be contagious, types of livestock affected and indigenous methods for prevention and treatment. It is important to remember that, in pastoralist societies in particular, people have gained a huge amount of experience of livestock diseases and health problems.

When using a participative training approach, the task of the trainer is to combine indigenous veterinary knowledge with western veterinary knowledge to address livestock problems. The aim is not to replace one system with the other, but to recognize that, in a dynamic and ever-changing world, both indigenous and western approaches are valuable. In some cases, we can be confident that a disease is best tackled using a modern veterinary solution, for example rinderpest vaccine. However, this might be combined with traditional know-how on avoidance of infected herds. Furthermore, local expertise in disease recognition can be useful after vaccination has stopped and active surveillance has begun (see Chapter 7).

Despite the value of indigenous knowledge in the training process, a difficult area for many CAHW projects is the promotion of traditional treatments that have

Indigenous knowledge and skills are the basis for designing a CAHW training course. If we understand what people already know and do, we can build on this knowledge.

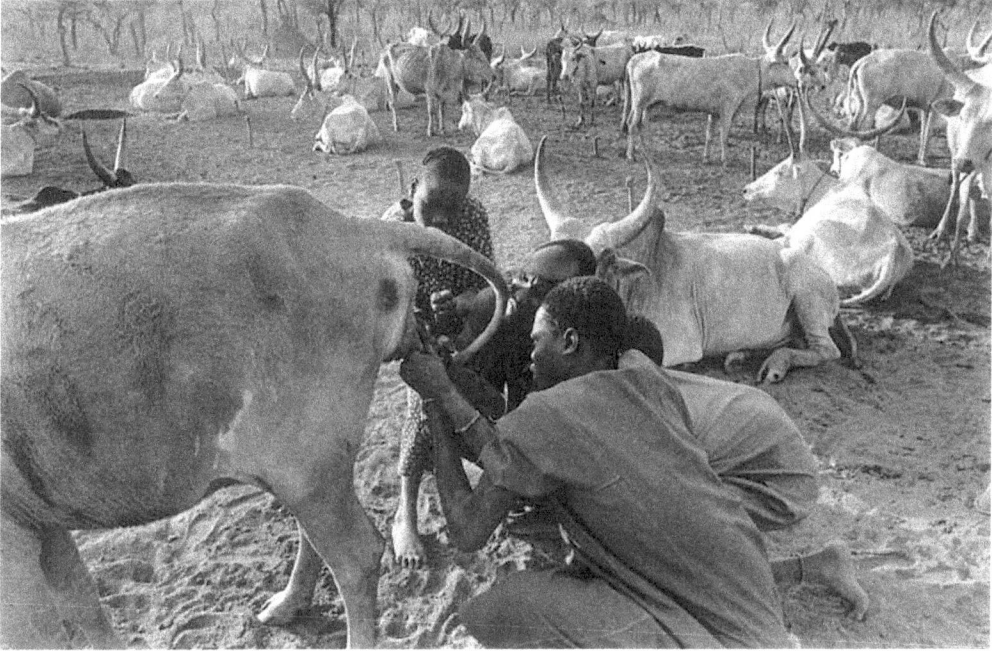

Plate 5.3 In southern Sudan, people are adept at assisting difficult calvings, but brucellosis or *cual* is a common problem. Introduction of hygienic measures during calving builds on people's existing knowledge and practice. (*Andy Catley*)

Indigenous knowledge of animal nutrition

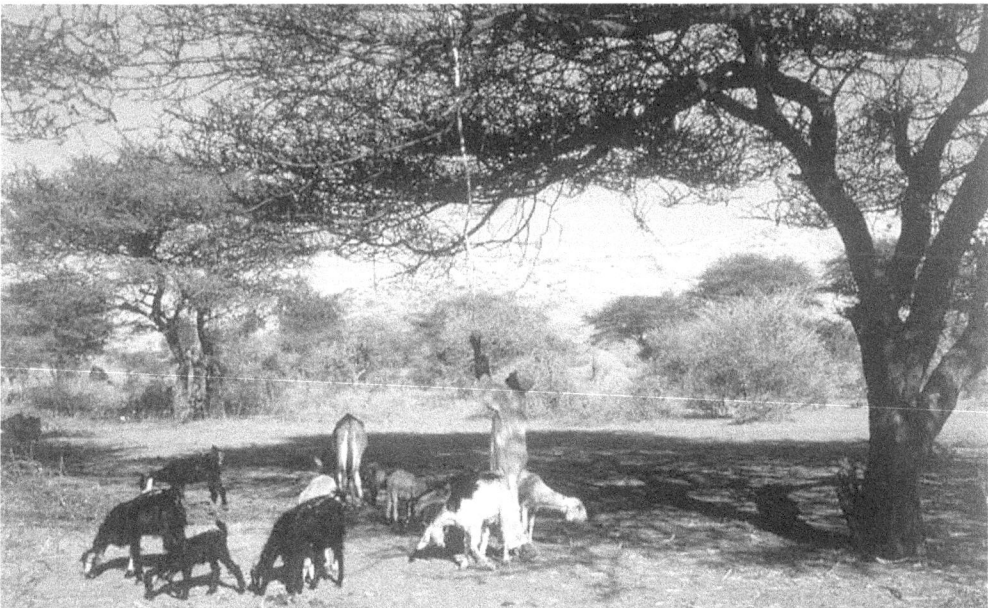

Plate 5.4 Using acacia pods as dry season supplementary feed. (*Stephen Blakeway*)

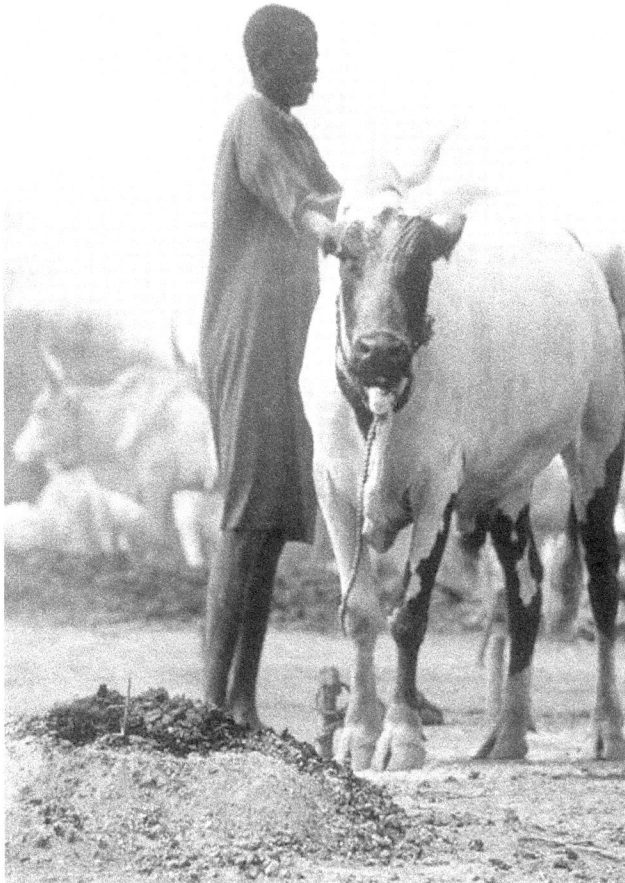

Plate 5.5 Using ash to protect cattle in southern Sudan. (*Stephen Blakeway*)

not been clinically or 'scientifically' proven. Scientific testing of plant remedies requires considerable resources and time, as any pharmaceutical company will testify. However, there are well-described methods for validating different treatments used within the community, based on local perceptions and identification of the most confidently used traditional treatments. The decision of whether or not to encourage a certain practice can be difficult and is often based on the technical knowledge of the veterinarian, the experience of livestock owners and, most importantly, the welfare of the animal.

Indigenous housing

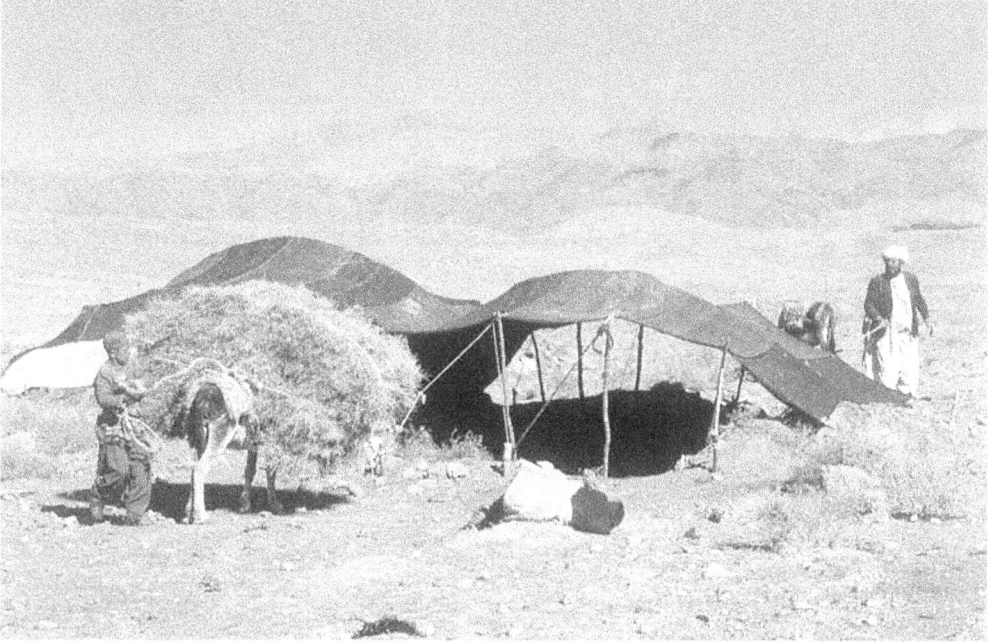

Plate 5.6 Preparing winter housing for livestock in Afghanistan. (*Stephen Blakeway*)

Use of branding to treat cattle diseases

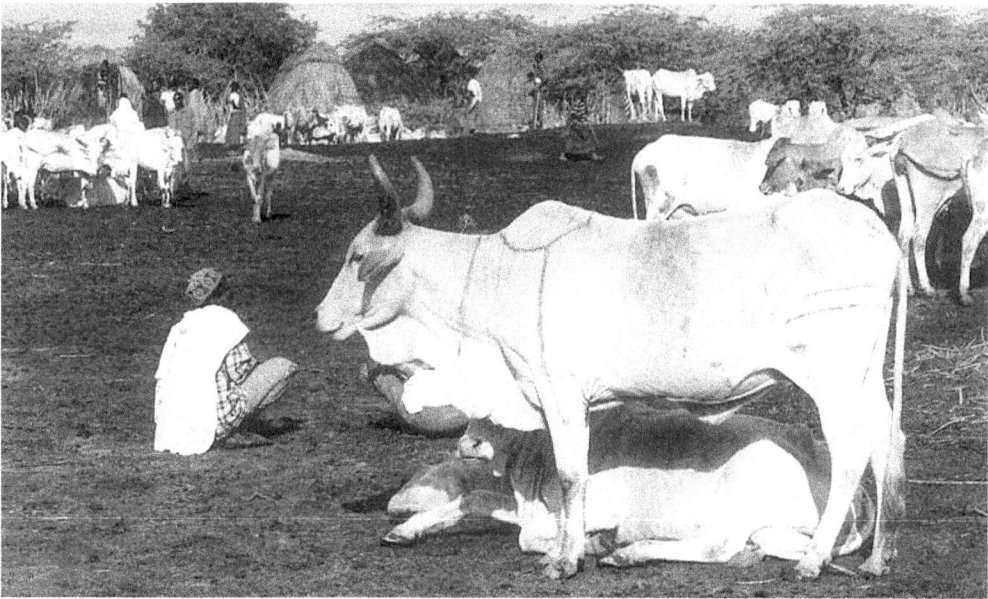

Plate 5.7 Some indigenous veterinary practices are difficult to validate from a western, scientific perspective. CAHW projects need to address these practices sensitively, support community-level evaluation of treatments and, if necessary, offer alternative solutions. (*Andy Catley*)

Box 5.8 Different types of indigenous animal health knowledge and their role in participative training

Local knowledge about disease signs, causes and epidemiology

This knowledge includes disease names, knowledge of vectors, seasonal variation in disease occurrence. It is very useful in participative training because we can build on this knowledge and/or correct as necessary.

Local disease prevention and control practices

These skills and knowledge include separation of sick animals from healthy animals; grazing animals on 'anthelmintic' plants; avoidance of ticky areas. This knowledge is also very useful in participative training. In some cases it is easy to relate these practices to western veterinary medicine and encourage them. Other practices can be discouraged, for example withholding colostrum from newborn animals.

Use of indigenous treatments

These skills and knowledge include a vast array of plant medicines, cautery and other treatments. This knowledge can vary from modern veterinary knowledge and it can be difficult to recommend in CAHW training without some process of validation (which can sometimes be done in the community). Some traditional treatments can be supported, for example use of salt to clean wounds.

5.5 Practical organization of the CAHW training course

As far as possible, the community should be involved in all aspects of organizing the CAHW course. This helps to ensure that local people take responsibility for the smooth running of the course and also instills a sense of ownership into the whole process. Decisions have to be made about issues such as who will cover training costs, where the course will take place, and how animals and equipment will be supplied.

Who will cover the cost of training?

Running costs for training courses include the cost of meals for participants, transporting the trainees to and from their homes, materials and equipment such as drugs, syringes and rope, as well as flip-chart paper, pens, visual aids, notebooks and handouts, and costs of the trainers. Ideally the costs should be split between the implementing organization and the community. The community will probably be able to make a contribution towards the running costs of the course in a variety of ways. For example, by providing goats for food for participants and trainers, or providing a training venue. The implementing organization may agree to pay for the training materials and trainers' expenses.

Gender and cultural factors

Gender factors and cultural sensitivities should be carefully considered when planning CAHW training. There are many experiences of women trainees taking a limited role in mixed-gender training sessions due to men dominating the training. In these situations, alternative arrangements should be made to ensure a separate course for women. Alternatively, separate sessions on the same course for men and women can be arranged. Residential courses involving men and women need careful consideration to ensure that participants and community are comfortable with the living arrangements. Men and women may also have different daily or seasonal timetables that might affect timing and organization of training.

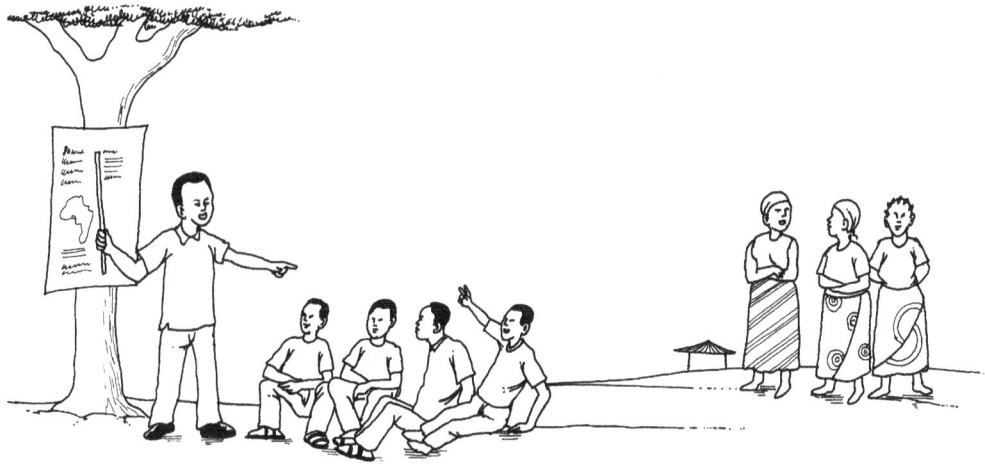

This is just typical! Another training course and we don't get a proper chance to join in.

Timing of the course

The training course should take place at a time of year when the trainees are not heavily involved in other work such as harvesting. In agropastoral or pastoral areas it is sometimes easier to conduct the training during the wet season when animals tend to congregate around permanent settlements and are easier to reach. Major religious or cultural events should be avoided. The daily timetable should be sensitive to participants' current commitments such as childcare and work at home. If the CAHWs are themselves farmers and livestock keepers, they may not be able to attend a full-time course. It may be more appropriate to plan the course to run only in the mornings, or to run the course in two parts with a break in between.

Location of the course

The best place to hold the CAHW training course is within the community. This allows the community to feel part of the training process, to see that the people it selected are really being trained and to monitor the progress of the training. The actual training venue should be discussed with the community. If a farmers' or pastoralists' training centre is located in the area this may be a good place to run the CAHW course because many of the facilities may already be there, such as crushes and animals.

Alternatively, the course can be run in the open air under a tree – Dinka communities in southern Sudan did just this. CAHWs were trained in cattle camps and were very comfortable with this arrangement. The community felt involved in the training and took an active role in ensuring that a suitable site was found away from the centre of community life; plenty of animals were provided for practice; and the training was not interrupted by casual onlookers.

If the training course is residential, provision needs to be made for accommodation of participants and trainers. Again, this should be discussed with the community and arrangements made accordingly. The advantage of residential courses is that everyone can focus on the training and not be distracted by events taking place at home. Residential courses may also be necessary if CAHWs from different areas are being trained. However, this is usually more expensive than if participants stay at home each evening. Another option is to ask members of the community to accommodate participants during the course.

Animals for practical training

Chapter 4 notes the essential role of live animals for practical training in CAHW courses. In order for participants to get enough practice it is absolutely essential that many animals of all species and ages be provided for the training. Organizing animals for training can be problematic and calls for careful planning with the community *well in advance of the course*. Try not to leave the planning of the live animals until the last minute because this usually results in insufficient numbers of animals for good practical instruction.

When using live animals for training, the welfare of the animals should be a prime consideration. Handling by a group of strangers will be stressful and will predispose to disease transmission. Also, practical training could result in injury to the animals so it needs to be very carefully supervised. As with all 'training aids' there have to be enough animals to minimize the stress on individuals and to provide adequate learning opportunities for all trainees. If live animals are going to be killed either for post-mortem examination or to feed the participants, the killing should be done with care and respect for the animal using the most humane local practice possible.

If animals from the community are used for the training, then clear agreements need to be made about who will pay for any veterinary drugs used. If livestock owners are given free treatments in exchange for allowing their animals to be used in training, then the project must make sure this is clearly understood by the community. Otherwise, confusion may arise, and the community might then expect the CAHWs to provide their services free of charge once the training is over.

There are several ways in which animals can be organized for training of CAHWs:

Livestock owners bring animals to training venue

Arrangements are made with the community to bring animals with specific diseases to the training venue on the days when those diseases are being covered in the course. This gives participants direct hands-on experience in examining, diagnosing and treating sick animals with the support of the trainer. The participants are also more likely to get experience of a wider range of diseases than if they just visit one or two livestock owners at home. The training venue should include provision for running practical sessions and treating live animals. Therefore a crush and proper livestock handling facilities will be needed, such as trees to tether animals to, possibly a corral and provision for watering stock. This approach was used by ITDG in Kenya and was found to be popular with local farmers. It was agreed with the community that the project would pay for medicines administered to animals, and that all treatments given by CAHWs would be strictly supervised by the trainer. However, caution needs to be taken with this approach, to ensure that contagious diseases are not spread between animals. Also, animals with some diseases will be physically unable to reach the training venue.

Take participants to livestock owners' kraals/farms

This arrangement can be made if animals cannot be brought to the training venue. However, care should be taken to ensure that a variety of kraals are visited, so that there is more chance of encountering different diseases. Also, the trainer should avoid just visiting the community leaders' kraals and providing free treatments because this may be viewed as favouritism by other members of the community. If animals are widely dispersed, the visiting method can be time-consuming.

Take participants to livestock gathering points such as water holes and public crushes

The advantage with this approach is that there will be many animals gathered in one place. However, problems and confusion may arise if the community is not forewarned and involved in the planning. For example, owners may refuse to have their animals handled if they do not fully understand what is happening. Also, as the water hole is a public place, it may be difficult to run practical sessions free of outside interference and disturbance.

Take participants to the local veterinary clinic

The advantages of this approach are that all the handling facilities are likely to be in place, the environment is conducive to treating animals, and sick animals brought to the clinic provide the CAHWs with good experience. However, only a few (or no animals at all) may be brought to the clinic on the practical days of the course, and there may not be enough animals for all participants to practise.

Training equipment and materials

In common with the use of live animals, it is essential that sufficient equipment is provided for practical training. This equipment includes medicines, ropes for restraining animals, syringes, foot trimming knives, cloths, buckets and other materials. There should be enough equipment for every participant to practise treating all the animal health problems taught on the course.

Certificates for CAHWs

CAHWs often ask for a certificate after completing the course. The advantage of issuing certificates is that they provide a formal record of the skills and knowledge the CAHWs have acquired on the course. This can be reassuring for the community, government and the CAHWs themselves that they are qualified to do the work for which they have been selected. Certificates can provide CAHWs with credibility and standing in the community. For certificates to have value, the trainer must make sure that each CAHW reaches the required standard and that those who do not are not given a certificate. One danger with certificates is that some people may agree to become CAHWs for the sole purpose of gaining a qualification, so that they can then move on to another job. However, these situations can be avoided if CAHWs are carefully selected in the first place.

5.6 Implementation of the training

Language of training and use of translators

The course should be run in the vernacular language of the participants using trainers from the area. Training tends to be much less effective when trainers do not speak the local language and therefore have to use a translator. Invariably, both subtleties and important points are lost in the translation process, and the whole training takes longer to complete. The project should carefully consider whether time and resources are better spent trying to recruit and train a local livestock professional to be the trainer, rather than use a person from outside the area simply to get the courses run sooner.

If it is absolutely necessary to run the course through a translator, then the translator should be chosen with care and, if possible, there should be more than one translator available. As any translator will testify, translating requires a great deal of effort and concentration. All too often, projects fail to give translation due care and attention and simply ask whoever happens to be around at the time. Translation is a skill. Remember, the quality of the training and the information that passes between trainer and participants rests on the translator, and so working with someone who is ill-prepared will result in poor-quality training. The translator, therefore, must be seen as a member of the training team, and be given some basic training skills and a brief overview of what will be covered on the course. The translator needs to be coached in how to translate for the trainer and participants, and should be someone who obviously has a good grasp of both languages, and is able to express complex ideas and technical terms.

Managing the training

During the training course, the trainer will be responsible not only for running the sessions, but also managing the logistics of the course such as equipment, animals and accommodation. For this reason, plenty of time needs to be allocated for planning a course. All training materials and preparations must be completed *before* the training begins. The trainer will not have enough time to start rushing around organizing such things as animals for practice in the middle of the course.

In many projects the participants themselves are also asked to take some responsibility for managing the training. For example, give some of the participants the responsibility for ensuring everyone arrives on time for training sessions, meals are served punctually, or organizing out-of-course activities and recreation.

If the course is run at a venue within the community, then the training is likely to attract a lot of attention. The trainer needs to ensure diplomatically that casual onlookers do not disrupt the training process.

5.7   Evaluation of training

Why evaluate the training?

The training must be evaluated to determine whether the course objectives have been met and how much the participants have learnt. If the training is not evaluated then the trainers cannot be sure that the participants have learnt the skills, knowledge, behaviour and attitudes to a sufficient standard necessary to do the work being asked of them. There are many reasons why participants may not have learnt what they were expected to from a course, and it is important to examine what may have gone wrong. Even though it is often tempting to blame the participants, the fault usually lies with improper planning and in how the course was designed and delivered (see Box 5.9).

Box 5.9 Reasons why participants may *not* have learnt what is stated in the course and session objectives

There are numerous reasons why participants may not have learnt what has been stated in the course and session objectives. These include:

◆ The trainer did not set clear session objectives so was not sure what he or she was trying to achieve in each session.
◆ The trainer did not write proper session plans so sessions were confused and illogical, and important learning points were missed when the trainer forgot what to say.
◆ The trainer did not use participative training methods and approaches – the participants were not actively involved in the session so they could not remember many of the learning points.

- The trainer did not use appropriate training methods, for example wrote key points on the flip-chart with illiterate participants.
- The content of the session was not pitched at the correct level because the trainer had not carried out a TNA and so did not know what the participants' learning needs were. The course may have been too complicated or too simple.
- The trainer did not attend a Training of Trainers course and so did not know how to plan lessons, or use participative training methods or how to facilitate effectively.
- There were not enough animals and equipment so the participants were not able to practise new skills adequately.
- The course was run through a translator, but the translation was not properly organized and many important points were lost in the translation process.

Courses are rarely perfect and there is always room for improvement. Evaluating the course provides invaluable information on how the training can be made more effective and should form an integral part of the training cycle.

How to evaluate the training

When embarking on an evaluation of CAHW training, two key questions can be asked:

- What do I want to know about the training from the evaluation?
- How will the information from the evaluation feed into the course, and help me to improve the training?

It is important that the evaluation of the training is carried out in a sensitive and participative manner so that the participants do not feel they are being examined. Explain to them and the community that you are evaluating the training to make sure the CAHWs have learnt what is required for them to carry out their work, to improve the course for next time and to arrange for follow-up and refresher training.

The training should be evaluated with reference to the CAHW course and session objectives. For example, if one of the objectives is 'The participants will be able to explain the dose rates of project wormer for sheep, goats and cattle', then the trainer needs to ask key questions like: 'What is the dose of liquid project wormer for an adult female goat, weighing 45 kg?' Training can be evaluated in a variety of ways at different times during and after the course:

During the course with the CAHWs

The trainer should continuously monitor the progress of participants during the course by asking questions, and assessing how well each individual answers questions, carries out exercises and tasks, and performs skills. For this reason it is important to ensure that each participant takes part in the training sessions. Avoid allowing a few extrovert people to answer all the questions, while the other participants remain quiet. At the end of the course, the trainer can organize a brief assessment where

Box 5.10 Example of how to evaluate CAHW training

Assessment of knowledge: questions list

1. What are the signs of rinderpest?
2. What is the control strategy for rinderpest in this area?
3. What are the signs and causes of foot-rot?
4. What medicine is used to treat roundworm in calves?
5. What is the dose of liquid project wormer for a weaned six-month-old goat?
6. What medicine is used to treat pneumonia in goats?
7. What is the dose of 5 per cent oxytetracycline for a local breed, mature three-year-old heifer?
8. What are the characteristics of well-constructed goat and sheep kraal?

Assessment of skills: observation

1. Watch the CAHW deworming goats. What medicine is used? What is the correct dose for the drug? How is the anthelmintic given? How is the animal handled? Note if any of these aspects are done incorrectly, and correct the CAHW if necessary.
2. Watch the CAHW giving an antibiotic injection to a cow. What medicine is used? What is the correct dose? How is the antibiotic given? How is the animal handled? Note if any of these aspects are done incorrectly, and correct the CAHW.
3. Check the CAHW's record book to note how records are being kept, including any aspect not done correctly.

Assessment of behaviour and attitudes: observation

Observe the CAHW working with a livestock keeper. Make a note of the CAHW's communication skills, how well the CAHW asks questions and is able to gather a history of the case from the livestock keeper, and the CAHW's general behaviour towards the livestock keeper (open, friendly, respectful).

participants are asked questions about key learning points such as signs of important diseases, dose rates for medicines and which medicine to use for which disease. If a practical day is organized towards the end of the course (where participants practise treating animals using all the skills and knowledge they have learnt on the course), then the trainer can assess skill levels by observation and asking questions of each individual CAHW.

After the course with the CAHWs

When the CAHWs have been working for some time – say three months – the trainer can again assess their skills and knowledge. The assessment should be carried out in a structured and methodical way, with each CAHW being asked the same questions. The assessment needs to be carefully prepared so that the information gathered can feed directly into modifying future courses and designing refresher training. Key questions related to medicines and dose rates, diseases and control strategies can be asked, as well as certain skills assessed, such as how well the CAHW handles animals. Box 5.10 explains how training can be evaluated with participants. The evaluation process can also be seen as an opportunity to answer any queries CAHWs may have and provides some informal refresher training.

After the course with the community

The evaluation can be carried out by holding a general meeting with the community to discuss how well the CAHWs are working, as well as by talking to individual livestock keepers who have worked with the CAHWs. The evaluation should take place three to six months after the course. It is important that the evaluation is not seen as a personal criticism of the CAHWs. The evaluation is an assessment of whether or not the CAHWs were given all the skills and knowledge they need to carry out their work and provide an animal health service to meet the needs of the community. Of course, any comments made by the community on the behaviour, actions or competence of individual CAHWs should be noted and addressed in discussion with the community. Example of issues that could be discussed with individual livestock keepers include:

- what prices the CAHW is charging for services;
- what medicines are being used to treat which diseases;
- whether or not the livestock keeper feels that the CAHW is able to provide a satisfactory animal health service that helps to address important livestock problems. Again, the evaluation of the training with the community should be carried out in a structured way, with the same questions being asked of a representative group of people (e.g. women, men, wealthy, poor, young, elders).

Box 5.11 The need for post-training monitoring of CAHWs: some lessons from Bangladesh

Context

I was working as a Technical Adviser in Prodipan, Bangladesh for a medium sized, local NGO called Prodipan. This NGO employed one veterinarian, one agricultural graduate, around 10 CAHWs.

Problem

Around 100 village poultry had been vaccinated by one of the CAHWs working for the organization. He had used government-produced vaccines against *ranikhet* (Newcastle Disease) and Fowl Cholera (Pasteurellosis). Within two days nearly 50 birds had died.

Cause

Post mortem examination revealed that main cause of death in these birds was gangrenous myositis associated with the injection site. This was probably caused by a dirty needle or injection of non-sterile material.

I spent some time observing the vaccination technique of the CAHWs. This revealed 21 deviations from good practice that could lead to failure of vaccination effectiveness or introduction of infection. The secondary cause was lack of practical expertise of the CAHWs. Like the other CAHWs, he had received training from the government *but had little experience and no post-training support from the NGO or government.*

Action taken

Training was given to the CAHWs and an attempt was made to set up a monitoring system. The villagers asked for compensation. The organization was reluctant to provide this in case it set a precedent and encouraged fraudulent claims.

Outcome

Most of the technicians who received training left the organization to better paid jobs elsewhere. Due to problems within management it was impossible to set up effective monitoring and supervision of technicians work. The villagers were compensated.

Learning experience

CAHWs should ensure competence in job requirements and include adequate practical training in topics such as vaccination procedures. Monitoring and follow-up training is a crucial component of vaccination programmes using CAHWs. When trained and supported properly, CAHWs can provide very valuable vaccination services.

(contributed by Delia Grace)

The post-training evaluations outlined above are very important components of a CAHW project. In particular, post-training evaluations with the community can help to identify any weaknesses in the system and allow problems to be solved promptly. Common problems include misunderstandings over prices of veterinary medicines and the financial incentives for the CAHWs.

5.8 Summary

Trainers should use a checklist of key points for effective training:

◆ Does the course curriculum cover the topics the CAHWs need to know in order to do their work? Are these in line with government regulations and policy on drug use and livestock disease control? Do they meet the needs of the community for animal health services, as agreed in the planning meetings with the community?

◆ Have you framed your course within local understanding and experience, and have you incorporated indigenous veterinary knowledge and the use of local names for diseases?

◆ Have you incorporated participative training techniques, especially those that can be used with illiterate people? Avoid lecturing and too much emphasis on writing on blackboards. Make the course as *practical* as possible. Use a variety of techniques that encourage discussion and analysis.

◆ Is the course pitched at the right level for the existing knowledge and skills of the CAHWs?

◆ Do the sessions follow a logical sequence, one session building on another?

◆ Have you planned each session in detail, including session objectives, timing of sessions, methodology and key learning points?

◆ Have you scheduled plenty of time in the session plans for trainees to practise their new skills?

◆ Have you organized enough training materials for everyone to practise, including animals, medicines and equipment?

◆ Have you prepared appropriate training and visual aids to help reinforce key learning points?

◆ Have you organized the logistics of the course – training venue, meals, transport, accommodation, trainer costs and certificates?

◆ Have you planned how the training will be monitored and evaluated?

Monitoring and assessment of community-based animal health projects

Andy Catley

CONTENTS

6.1 Introduction

When community-based animal health (CAH) projects are being implemented it is important to follow the progress of project activities, find out if the project has provided benefits and, if so, to whom and why. Monitoring and assessment help us to understand the impact of projects and answer specific questions such as: 'How are women using the services of community-based animal health workers (CAHWs)?' or 'How does the work of illiterate CAHWs compare with that of literate CAHWs?' By learning about the strengths and weaknesses of projects, inputs and activities can be modified in order to improve future work. Therefore, information derived from monitoring and evaluation activities can be used to learn about impact, correct problems, improve planning and ensure that animal health inputs are benefiting people as intended.

This chapter introduces some of the important principles of effective monitoring and project assessment, and explains how to design and implement monitoring and assessment activities for CAHW projects. The chapter discusses ways to ensure that communities are actively involved in measuring and assessing change on their own terms, and describes how participatory approaches can be used to enhance local measurement and analysis of changes that occur during a project. There are already a number of excellent books on monitoring, impact assessment and evaluation (see Further reading), and therefore the chapter focuses on experiences from CAHW projects in the field and the types of approaches and methods that seem to work well. The chapter also provides details of participatory tools that can be used to understand the impact of improved animal health on people's livelihoods.

Although monitoring and assessment are very important in community-based animal health services, they are often one of the weakest components. Field experience indicates that there are at least two important challenges facing these projects:

Looking more closely at 'real impact'
Many agencies consider CAHW training alone to be the key activity in a community-based animal health system. In these cases, success is measured according to the number of CAHWs trained rather than the long-term impact of these workers on animal health and human welfare. Consequently, project resources are directed at training CAHWs with limited attention to how they will be followed up and supervised. Training inputs are relatively easy to define, cost and implement relative to monitoring activities. Sometimes people forget to design and plan monitoring work, or underestimate the time and resources required. In large project areas, these inputs can be substantial.

Other CAHW initiatives are funded as 'emergency' or 'rehabilitation' projects that tend to be short-term in nature. In these projects, CAHWs can be a quick way to deliver vaccines or medicines to communities who are in need. Success is usually measured according to quantities of medicines or vaccines procured and delivered, and the number of CAHWs trained. When project life spans are only six months (e.g. emergency) to 18 months (e.g. rehabilitation), investment in proper monitoring of

CAHWs tends to be limited. In these cases, CAHW systems can quickly collapse because initial 'teething' problems are not resolved and there is no long-term support for the system.

Choosing appropriate methods

Veterinarians have experienced a university education and sometimes try to use scientific monitoring methods that cannot be applied easily in the field. For example, quantitative measures of disease prevalence by conventional means can be problematic in remote areas with limited resources. Therefore, monitoring is sometimes abandoned because technical staff cannot use scientific methods but, also, they are unaware of alternative approaches. And, finally, in community-based projects we can easily forget that local people have their own ways of assessing change and impact in the community. These perceptions matter a great deal. When using a community-based approach, it is desirable to encourage community-based organizations to develop their own monitoring and evaluation systems as part of the process of local institution building and local management of CAHW services.

As with most other aspects of community-based services, there is no rigid framework for monitoring and evaluating CAHW systems. Community-based monitoring and evaluation can be innovative and can evolve according to local needs with respect to both information requirements and data collection methods. In donor-funded projects, there are usually specific types of information that donors require in project reports.

6.2 Some basic concepts and meanings

Monitoring, review, impact assessment and evaluation

Various terms are used in relation to the monitoring and assessment of community-based animal health work.

- 'Monitoring' is the systematic measurement of a piece of work over time. Monitoring usually involves the continuous collection of information (e.g. on a monthly basis during a project). It allows changes to be made during the life of a project while also providing information for periodic reviews, impact assessments or evaluations.
- A 'review' is an assessment of a piece of work at a single point in time. The review can focus on particular aspects of a project and involves a more detailed analysis of issues than is possible by monitoring alone. Reviews are often conducted at the halfway stage of projects ('mid–term review').
- An 'impact assessment' looks at the effects of a piece of work on people, the environment or institutions. Impact assessment looks at changes that have occurred during a project and determines if and how these changes are related to project activities. Impact assessment is not necessarily related to project objectives.

◆ 'Evaluation' is a comprehensive, usually formal review of a piece of work. Typically, an evaluation relates project successes, failures and impact to project objectives. Evaluation can also assess the efficiency of work in relation to resources, particularly financial inputs, and can look at the sustainability and long-term implications of projects. Evaluations are performed fairly infrequently and usually take place at the end of projects.

This chapter uses the term 'assessment' to encompass common features of reviews, impact assessments and evaluations.

Although assessment is a very important activity in community-based animal health systems, people can sometimes feel threatened if they suspect that weaknesses and problems will be revealed. However, animal health projects are rarely problem-free and so assessment should be regarded as a *learning process* that enables everyone concerned to design and implement more effective work.

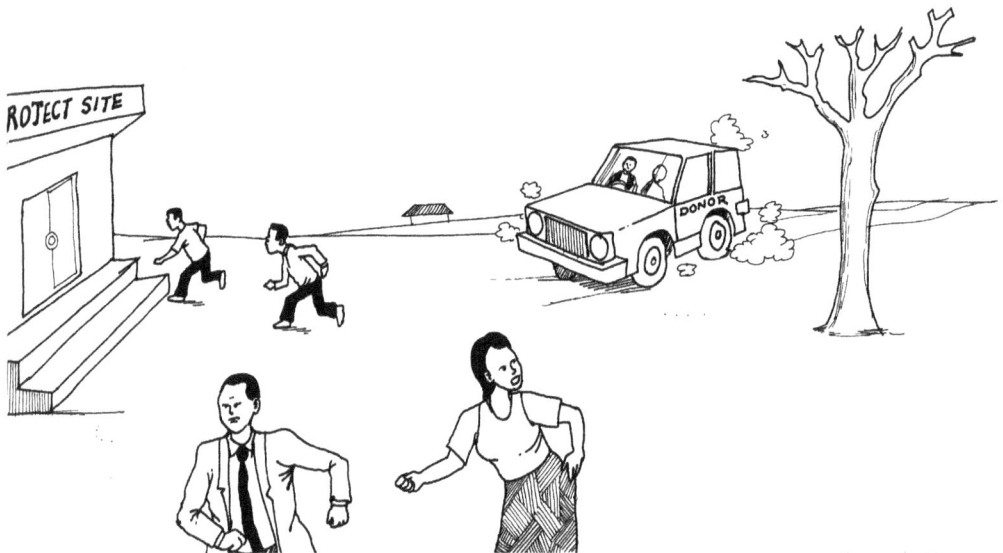

Oh no, the donors are coming!

Types of monitoring

In most CAHW projects there are two key monitoring periods:

Monitoring in the immediate post-training phase

This takes place between one and three months after the CAHWs have started to work. This monitoring is particularly important for identifying weaknesses or misunderstandings that have arisen between the CAHWs, project or community and is an opportunity to solve these problems before they escalate. Post-training monitoring requires an assessment of how the CAHWs are working in the community from both the CAHWs' and the community's point of view. It also needs project staff to be ready to engage in patient discussion at community level and be willing to help the community solve any teething problems that might have arisen. Essentially, post-training monitoring can require action to be taken 'on the spot'. Post-training monitoring is discussed in detail in Chapter 5.

Routine monitoring

This is the more regular collection of data that is required by the various stakeholders who are involved in the project. This type of monitoring is usually organized on a monthly or quarterly basis depending on the stakeholders concerned. In common with the post-training monitoring, routine monitoring should have the capacity to not only obtain information but also initiate action to solve problems and respond to opportunities.

In animal health projects, at least three types of routine monitoring are important:

Management and administration monitoring

This looks at factors concerning the day-to-day running of organizations, government departments or projects. This type of monitoring includes staff and personnel issues, supplies, logistics and vehicles. Management and administration monitoring is largely dependent on organizational procedures and rules. It is a topic that is covered in numerous other books (see Further reading) so will not be discussed in this chapter.

Financial monitoring

This looks at project budgets, income and expenditure, payments to staff, cash flow and other financial issues. Again, financial monitoring systems are usually determined by organizational procedures in government, NGOs or donors and this topic is also well-described in other books (see Further reading). In CAHW work, some projects become involved in monitoring CAHW income and revenues from drug sales. In these situations, there can be some overlap between financial monitoring and project monitoring.

Project monitoring

This relates to work activities, inputs and outputs. Project monitoring enables us to measure what has been done and achieved, and therefore forms the basis for this chapter. This type of monitoring includes both monitoring the work of specific projects and the context in which these projects are running, for example political, environmental or economic factors affecting the local population.

Project monitoring can be further subdivided into two main types:

◆ *'Process monitoring' looks at the implementation of project activities according to project proposals and work plans. Process monitoring notes whether or not things are being done, for example have veterinary medicines been purchased and delivered to the project area according to the work plan?*

◆ *'Impact monitoring' looks specifically at the impact of project activities on the community. For example, veterinary medicines have been provided to the CAHWs but what was the effect of this activity on the well-being of animals or the livelihoods of livestock keepers?*

Understanding the difference between process and impact monitoring is a crucial aspect of designing a useful monitoring system. In most animal health projects it is relatively easy to use process monitoring to see whether or not project activities are being implemented according to plan. However, it is often much more difficult to show whether project activities are actually affecting the lives of people in the community. It is sometimes assumed that, if CAHWs are actively treating sick animals, then people must be benefiting. However, who is benefiting and why? How do healthy animals improve human livelihoods in terms of economic or social benefits? Are there people who are not benefiting (or even suffering) as a result of the project? These questions can be answered by impact monitoring and evaluation.

Measurement and indicators

A key feature of all monitoring and evaluation work is that inputs, activities, outputs, change or impact are measured. The things that we measure are usually called 'indicators'. As project monitoring can be broken down into process monitoring and impact monitoring, so can indicators be either 'process indicators' or 'impact indicators' accordingly. Process indicators usually measure a physical aspect of project implementation such as the procurement or delivery of medicines, the number of training courses run by a project or the number of people trained. Therefore, process indicators are useful for showing that project activities are actually taking place according to the project work plan. However, this type of indicator may not tell us very much about the impact of project activities on beneficiaries.

- ◆ 'Process indicators' measure the implementation of project activities. These indicators are usually quantitative, for example 'quantity of veterinary medicines procured' is a process indicator which might be reported as '1000 bottles of oxytetracycline procured'.
- ◆ 'Impact indicators' measure changes that occur as a result of project activities. Impact indicators can be qualitative or quantitative, for example 'ability to use Albendazole correctly' is a qualitative impact indicator that might be used to measure the outcome of one part of a CAHW training course. In addition, 'milk production' is a quantitative impact indicator that might be used to measure the effect of anthelmintic treatments by a CAHW (though this is difficult to measure – see later).

Quantitative and qualitative data

As indicated above, monitoring and evaluation usually require attention to both quantitative and qualitative data. Quantitative data is derived from numerical indicators and counting things such as number of people trained or number of animals treated. This type of data is relatively easy to collect and present in project reports. While this is very important, other types of data are equally or more important. For example, how has the project affected people's knowledge, skills, attitudes, behaviour or well-being? This type of qualitative information can sometimes pose problems for veterinary workers who are not familiar with qualitative data gathering techniques.

When trying to decide which indicators are appropriate for a particular project, remember that virtually any subjective or qualitative information can be described numerically through the use of ranking or scoring methods. This approach usually requires people to describe the indicator in question according to an arbitrary scale, for example 0 to 5. As the project progresses we can then look at how the initial score changes and the reasons for change. This system is similar to a clinical trial in which a veterinarian scores the appearance of sick animals and then re-scores the same animals after treatment. In other words, a subjective assessment is captured using a numerical system. Some specific tools for applying this approach are described in *'Before and after' methods*.

CAHW work is often implemented in remote areas with limited resources and logistical constraints. In some cases, these problems can limit the use of conventional, quantitative measurements. For example, impact indicators such as 'milk production' need very careful thought before being included in a monitoring system, as discussed in Box 6.1. Although few CAHW projects have the capacity to conduct research using conventional, quantitative approaches, help is at hand in the form of participatory monitoring and assessment methods.

Box 6.1 Measurement and use of quantitative impact indicators: the case of milk production in a pastoral community

Imagine that the overall aim of a CAHW project is to 'improve the food security of the community'. At first hand, an indicator such as 'cattle milk production' appears to be highly relevant to this project and can be physically measured. However, the following questions need to be considered:

◆ Are we going measure total milk production from individual animals (calf consumption plus offtake) or only the milk collected during milkings (offtake only)?
◆ If we want to measure total milk production, how are we going to measure calf consumption if conventional methods require calves to be weighed before and after sucking?
◆ How are we going to calculate an appropriate sample size and identify the animals to be monitored?
◆ Do we have baseline or control data on milk production?
◆ Assuming that milk production changes during the project, how can we determine the role of animal disease control in the project in influencing this change relative to other factors (e.g. grazing practices)?

- ◆ Now imagine that the community in question are pastoralists in a remote area. Traditionally they milk their animals early in the morning and in the evening. Children herd the cattle during the day and usually take some milk from the cattle to feed themselves at this time. How do we measure this offtake?

Due to the aim of our project, we need to look not only at milk production, but also relate milk production to people's well-being. Therefore, we should look more closely at what happens to the milk after milking and consequently, various other questions arise:

- ◆ Is the milk consumed by the family, used to make milk products, sold or given as a gift to kinfolk? What is the relative importance of these or other uses of milk and how can they be measured?
- ◆ Within the family, how does milk consumption vary among the women, children, youths and men? For each group, how does milk contribute towards recommended daily nutritional requirements and are there important seasonal variations in consumption to consider?
- ◆ If milk or milk products are sold, what happens to the money or items received as a result of these sales? For example, do women control this money and use it to buy more food for the family, or do men control the money and use it to buy tobacco?
- ◆ What is the social significance of giving milk as a gift to less wealthy kinfolk?
- ◆ Is any milk wasted? For example, is there a convenient market to sell excess milk or milk products?
- ◆ Are there any negative effects from drinking milk (e.g. zoonotic disease)?

Suddenly, what seemed to be a simple matter of measuring milk production has become rather more complicated and we have a whole research project on our hands. This is an extreme example, but shows the complexity of measuring impact if conventional methods are used.

6.3 How to monitor community-based animal health work

This section describes indicators and methods for monitoring, and how to design and plan monitoring activities. Much of this information also relates to reviews, impact assessment and evaluation because these processes can involve a collation of monitoring data and use of methods similar to those used in monitoring.

Looking at the information needs of different interest groups: towards participatory approaches to monitoring and evaluation

If monitoring and evaluation are learning processes, we need to think about 'Who learns?' In particular:

- Who should be involved in monitoring and evaluation?
- Who uses the results?
- What are the information needs of different players?
- What methods should be used?

As different stakeholders can have different information needs in a CAHW system, identifying these needs is an important stage in setting up a monitoring system. Table 6.1 provides examples of needs according to different interest groups. Note that not all of the stakeholders mentioned in Table 6.1 are represented in all projects.

a. Community-based forums and institutions

Chapters 2 to 5 explain how local people can design and plan basic animal health services. Local participation in analysing problems and working to solve these problems are key features of community-based approaches. Most community-based animal health work involves a local group, forum or committee who act as a point of

Table 6.1 Examples of monitoring and evaluation information needs for different stakeholders in community-based animal health projects

Stakeholder group	Information needs for monitoring
Community-based organization (CBO)	Coverage and effectiveness of CAHWs, including relationship with community members and financial matters such as prices of veterinary medicines and incentives for CAHWs. Also information related to benefits derived from improved animal health.
NGO or government implementing agency	Coverage and effectiveness of CAHWs, including relationship with community members and financial matters such as prices of veterinary medicines and incentives for CAHWs. Might also need to monitor the establishment of a CBO(s), community participation and benefits derived from improved animal health.
Private veterinarian(s)	Information needs are likely to focus on financial matters related to volume of veterinary drug sales, types of drugs sold, seasonal variations in drug demand and profit.
Government veterinary epidemiology unit	Disease-specific information which is collected during the routine work of the CAHWs and reports of disease outbreaks.
Government regulatory body	Names, level of training and location of CAHWs and their supervisors.
Donor	Varied information needs depending on the donor concerned. Likely to prefer summaries and analysis of information.

contact between the community and an implementing or funding agency such as an NGO, government department or donor. In projects that aim to hand over the management of CAHWs to local groups, a useful way of building the capacity of these groups is to assist them to develop their own monitoring and assessment systems. This process is one way of encouraging local ownership of projects and information, and, ultimately, locally managed CAHW services.

Participatory monitoring and evaluation share many of the principles of participatory appraisal (PA – see Chapter 2). They assume that local people are well-placed to describe and analyse changes that take place in their community. Local people use their own methods for measuring and describing impact, and it is important for outsiders to understand and learn from these perceptions as projects evolve. Therefore, at least three important questions to consider are:

◆ *Is there a well-established community-based group that has the capacity to manage its own monitoring system?*
   The existence and capacity of such groups varies greatly between different CAHW projects, the approaches of development agencies and operational factors. In some NGOs, a key focus of projects is to develop community-based organizations (CBOs) that can take over local development activities. Other NGOs and government agencies prefer to retain control of all activities. In other situations, an NGO or government project might have an overall strategy of developing the capacity of CBOs but be unable to do so because of external factors, such as conflict.

◆ *Who controls the current monitoring and evaluation system with respect to the indicators, the methods used, and the ownership and use of information?*
   In many of the more successful community-based animal health projects, local people are actively involved in identifying needs, selecting CAHWs for training and contributing towards the costs of inputs such as starter kits for the CAHWs. However, it is common to find that, although community involvement in these initial stages of the project is high, as the project progresses this involvement begins to wane. When looking at this issue, it is useful to think about community participation in a project by reference to a typical project cycle, and describe types of participation at different stages in the project cycle. An example of this type of analysis is summarized in Box 6.2.

The non-government organizations Vétérinaires Sans Frontières Belgium and Vétérinaires Sans Frontières Switzerland have been implementing community-based animal health projects in southern Sudan since 1994 and 1995 respectively. These projects used typical monitoring and evaluation approaches that were based on information such as:

◆ numbers of meetings with communities;
◆ numbers of CAHWs trained;
◆ quantities of medicines and vaccine supplied to locations and CAHWs;
◆ numbers of animals treated or vaccinated;
◆ cost recovery from drug sales;
◆ disease outbreak reports.

In 1999, these NGOs decided to look at options for more participatory approaches to monitoring. During this process, project staff reviewed the current monitoring system and tried to describe levels of community participation during different stages of the project cycle. The results of this exercise are summarized below.

This analysis indicated that, as a typical project progressed through the project cycle, community participation decreased. Monitoring and evaluation needs and methods were focused on the requirements of NGO staff and donors. There was little scope for local players to access or use the monitoring information that was being collected.

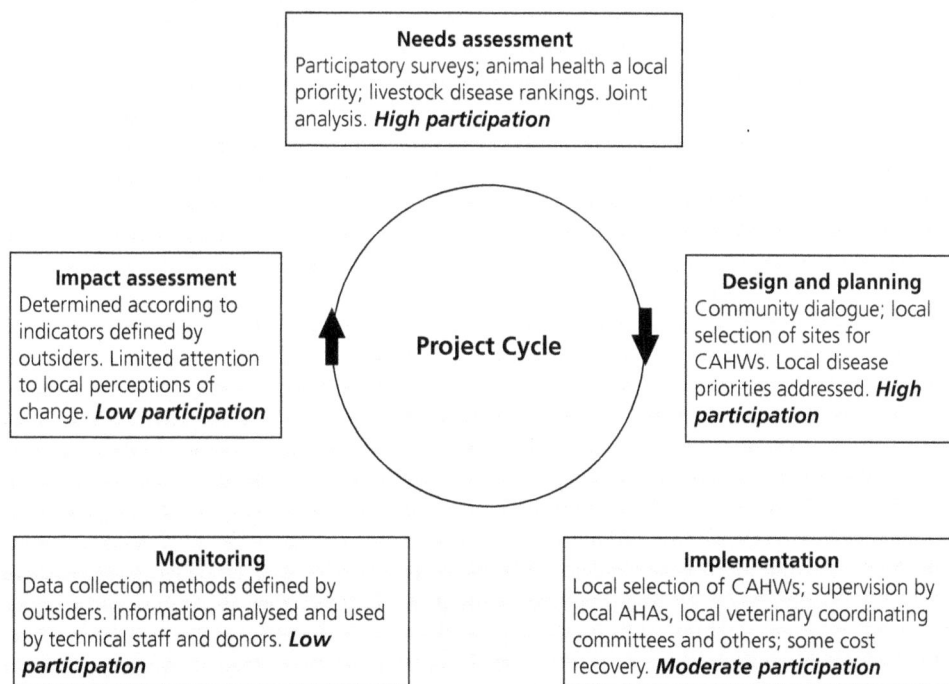

Needs assessment
Participatory surveys; animal health a local priority; livestock disease rankings. Joint analysis. **High participation**

Impact assessment
Determined according to indicators defined by outsiders. Limited attention to local perceptions of change. **Low participation**

Project Cycle

Design and planning
Community dialogue; local selection of sites for CAHWs. Local disease priorities addressed. **High participation**

Monitoring
Data collection methods defined by outsiders. Information analysed and used by technical staff and donors. **Low participation**

Implementation
Local selection of CAHWs; supervision by local AHAs, local veterinary coordinating committees and others; some cost recovery. **Moderate participation**

- *Assuming a community-based organization is in place, what kind of support or training might be needed in order to develop locally appropriate monitoring and assessment approaches?*

In some projects a CBO is involved in the project but its role may be restricted to project implementation only. In this situation, there may be opportunities to provide support to the CBO to develop a monitoring and assessment system which produces information that the CBO owns and can use to improve the project.

b. NGOs and government as implementing agencies

Both NGOs and government, or NGO–government partnerships, can be responsible for initiating or implementing community-based animal health work. As indicated above, levels of involvement can vary according to operational factors and the approach of the agency concerned. Therefore, information needs can also vary. In situations where the implementing body is controlling most aspects of a CAHW project, information needs are likely to be relatively comprehensive and will cover measures of both process and impact. This information is required in order to check the progress of the work, assess the results and produce reports for donors and government. Ideally, the information will also be used for organizational and institutional learning.

In situations where the implementing body is trying to hand over control of a project to local players (such as a CBO), monitoring and assessment systems can be developed with this organization. This approach reduces the information needs of the NGO because a local group takes over much of the responsibility for managing the project or service, and reporting. In these cases, the NGO might act as a channel for communicating experiences to donors and government, but in the long term the aim is for the CBO to interface directly with external agencies. Reviews and evaluations can produce information that is relevant to policy and legislative reform at central level.

c. Central or regional government

Regardless of whether or not government is directly involved in CAHW work, government bodies such as veterinary departments or NGO coordinating agencies will need information about the project. To date, typical government information needs for CAHW work are based on both process indicators and impact indicators. Veterinary departments may be interested in CAHW reports in terms of disease prevalence information and for news of disease outbreaks (see Chapter 7). In addition, government bodies may also be interested in experiences related to policy on rural development, animal health service delivery or disaster mitigation that emerge from the project. When designing a monitoring system it is useful to review existing government policies and consider which indicators in the project might be useful for policy makers in regional or central government.

d. Donors

Donors who support CAHW work usually have their own reporting procedures and guidelines that relate to both financial management of projects and project outputs and activities. There is considerable variation in donor reporting requirements in terms of the amount of detail required and the reporting periods. Although in the past donors have been particularly concerned with monitoring project expenditure and process indicators, some donors are beginning to look more closely at impact and demonstrating links between animal health inputs and human welfare. When designing monitoring and assessment activities, check that these activities will adequately cover the donor's requirements. Some donors like to place their own staff in project evaluation teams.

e. Private veterinarians

Although to date there has been limited involvement of private veterinarians in CAHW work, there is increasing interest in linking private veterinary facilities to networks of CAHWs (see Chapter 3). It is likely that monitoring and assessment approaches in these services will focus on financial indicators of success, as defined by typical business management procedures. However, for veterinarians who are developing business plans in areas where CAHWs are operating, information such as locally prioritized diseases, seasonal variations in demand for drugs, volume of drug sales and drug prices is relevant to the market research needs of a business plan.

Selecting the indicators

The careful selection of indicators is one of the most important steps in setting up a monitoring system. In CAHW services, project staff can work with communities or CBOs to select indicators according to both local and project information needs. Ideally, these indicators should relate directly to the objectives of the project, as defined in the project document. For example:

Project objective

'Develop a CAHW service in three districts linked to private veterinary pharmacies'.

Possible indicators

'Number of CAHWs working in each district by the end of year 3';
'Number of veterinary pharmacies supplying medicines and supervision to CAHWs per district'.

In some projects, monitoring and assessment indicators are defined when the project proposal is written. This is particularly true when the proposal uses a logical framework (logframe) to summarize project goal, objectives, activities, indicators and risks. Some indicators for CAHW systems are listed in Table 6.2 and these show how projects can measure both 'things happening' (process) and the 'result of things happening' (impact).

Table 6.2 Examples of indicators for CAHW systems

	Process indicators (measure 'things happening')	Impact indicators (measure the 'result of things happening')
Designing the system	◆ Completion of participatory survey and analysis ◆ Number of meetings with community	◆ Identification of the ten most important animal health problems in the community according to different wealth and gender groups ◆ Analysis of options for improving animal health ◆ Agreement on action to be taken
Formation of CBO	◆ Number of meetings with community ◆ Number of CBOs formed ◆ Number of CBO members ◆ Composition of CBO	◆ Terms of reference for CBO for implementation of the CAH system ◆ Selection criteria for CAHWs ◆ Selection of CAHWs ◆ Community contribution towards CAHW training course ◆ Community contribution towards CAHW starter kits ◆ Management of CAHWs
Links to drug outlets	◆ Number of meetings between private veterinarian and CBO	◆ Agreement between parties ◆ Number of CAHWs linked to private veterinarian
CAHW training	◆ Number of CAHWs trained ◆ Number and type of animal health problems covered in training course ◆ Geographical location of CAHWs ◆ Cost of training	◆ Improved knowledge and skills among CAHW trainees
CAHW activities	◆ Number of starter kits supplied to CAHWs ◆ Cost of starter kits supplied ◆ Quantities and types of medicines supplied to CAHWs ◆ Cost of medicines supplied to CAHWs ◆ Number of treatments per livestock type per CAHW ◆ Number of vaccinations per livestock type per CAHW ◆ CAHW income ◆ Number of monitoring forms submitted by CAHWs ◆ Number of disease outbreaks reported by CAHWs	◆ Incidence of ten most important animal health problems ◆ Prevalence of ten most important animal health problems ◆ Livestock mortality ◆ Geographical coverage of CAHWs ◆ Proportion of livestock-rearing households serviced by CAHWs ◆ Relative use of CAHWs by male and female-headed households ◆ CAHW drop-out rate ◆ Drugs and vaccines resupplied to CAHWs based on revenue collection ◆ Action taken according to disease outbreak reports ◆ Food consumption in community related to improved animal health and according to wealth and gender groups ◆ Income in community related to improved animal health and according to wealth and gender groups ◆ Influence on government policy

The indicators listed in Table 6.2 show how groups of indicators can be related to specific project activities or stages in a project. In some cases the indicators are linked to each other, with indicators used early in a project influencing things that are measured later in the project. For example, the identification of the ten most important animal health problems in a community will determine which diseases are measured in terms of incidence or prevalence. These kinds of links between indicators also show how, in many cases, information collected during the design phase of a project can be very useful for identifying the indicators in the monitoring system.

When considering indicators for a community-based animal health project, other issues are:

Availability and accessibility

Two important measures of service provision are availability and accessibility. Availability of a service is a measure of whether the service exists or not. For example, 'number of CAHWs per district' is an indicator of service availability. Accessibility of a service measures whether people can reach the service or not. For example, 'distance to the nearest CAHW' is an indicator of accessibility. Indicators that measure accessibility are useful for identifying problems that can prevent people reaching a service even though the service is available. These problems can include physical or geographical barriers or lack of transport.

Indicators do not tell us the whole story about a project

Indicators are specific, measurable aspects of a piece of work that can help us to communicate complex processes and trends to a wider audience. We cannot measure everything in a project and therefore a number of indicators are chosen to represent important activities and changes.

Avoid using too many indicators

It is a common mistake to select too many indicators that become difficult to measure or produce lots of data that is never used. It is always better to start with a small number of indicators and measure these properly, rather than identify many indicators but struggle to measure them.

Some indicators are difficult to measure in the field using conventional methods

As indicated in Box 6.1, some indicators seem simple on paper but can be very difficult to measure in practice. Unfortunately, this is particularly true for some important impact indicators such as those related to food consumption, income or social benefits for people in the communities concerned. This is one reason for developing participatory monitoring systems that use locally defined impact indicators to measure changes in the community, and often assess trends rather than precise quantities.

Baseline data

a. Using the results of the participatory survey

When selecting indicators for the monitoring system, review the information that the project has already collected. Reference to the initial participatory survey should reveal basic information on the geography of the project area, important livestock diseases, numbers of trained veterinary workers and the accessibility and availability of basic veterinary services. In many cases, there will be very limited modern services available in the project area and therefore baseline measures such as 'number of livestock owners reached by each CAHW' or 'availability of veterinary medicines' may be zero or very low at the start of the project. Hopefully though, these measures will increase as the project evolves.

b. Ranks and comparative data

Another type of baseline data is ranked data. For example, a simple livestock disease ranking could be included in the baseline information. If the project works well, monitoring should show that the top-ranked problems become less important as animals are treated and vaccinated. Ranking can also be used to compare preferences for different types of veterinary service as a project develops. An example of baseline data on treatment options is shown in Table 6.3. In this example, more urban-based livestock traders were using private outlets for veterinary drugs and government clinics to treat their animals. However, rural people – including women, herders and traditional healers – tended to use traditional practices.

A measure of the relative importance of treatment options at the beginning of a project can be used to follow changes in service preferences over time and, in particular, the uptake of services offered by CAHWs. This approach can also be useful for assessing the effect of increased use of modern veterinary medicines on traditional practices and beliefs.

Table 6.3 Relative importance of options for treating livestock among stakeholder groups in Jijiga, Degehabur, Shinile and Fik zones, Ethiopia

| | Ranking of options by stakeholder groups | | | | | |
| | Women | | Livestock herders and traditional healers | | Livestock traders | |
Options for treating livestock	Jijiga and Degehabur	Fik and Shinile	Jijiga and Degehabur	Fik and Shinile	Jijiga and Degehabur	Fik and Shinile
Use of Koran	1st	1st	1st	1st	nm	nm
Traditional treatments	3rd	2nd	2nd	2nd	2nd	nm
Private drug sellers	2nd	3rd	4th	4th	1st	1st
Government vets	nm	nm	3rd	3rd	3rd	2nd

Notes:
nm = not mentioned or ranked by informants
Traditional methods include plant-based medicines, cautery and soups/broths.

c. Baseline data forms

When baseline data has been reviewed, a simple form can be produced to record the key points. There is no gold standard form that suits all situations and projects can develop their own forms according to local needs and capacity. An example of a baseline data form is provided in Box 6.3. This form includes spaces for recording information on the predicted coverage of the CAHW in terms of number of households, the main livestock diseases and a space for a sketch map to show where the CAHW will be working.

Box 6.3 Example of a baseline data form for CAHW projects

Name of CAHW: ....

Village: ....

Parish: ....   County:.....................................

Nearest veterinary clinic or pharmacy: ....

Distance: .... km .... hrs

Estimated total number of households to be covered by CAHW: ....

Proportion of households owning livestock in CAHW target area: ....

Ranking of main livestock diseases in area:

Cattle	Camel	Sheep	Goat	Equines	Poultry
1.	1.	1.	1.	1.	1.
2.	2.	2.	2.	2.	2.
3.	3.	3.	3.	3.	3.
4.	4.	4.	4.	4.	4.
5.	5.	5.	5.	5.	5.

Geographical coverage of CAHW (sketch map):

---

d. CAHW profiles

Another component of baseline data is data on the CAHWs themselves. This information can be useful for learning about the personal qualities that make a good CAHW. For example, as a project progresses is might be possible to link CAHW performance to factors such as age, sex or level of literacy. A CAHW profile form can also record the initial expectations of the CAHW and, at a later stage, these expectations can be compared with actual experiences.

Box 6.4 Example of a CAHW 'profile' form

Name:..

Location:..

Age:...................................... Marital status:...

Family size:.................................. Number of years lived in village/area:...............

Education: ....

Languages spoken: ....

Languages written: ....

Current means of livelihood: ....

....

Livestock ownership (approximate):

Camels: .... Cattle: .... Sheep: .... Goats: ....

Equines: .... Poultry: ....

Expectations of working as a CAHW:

....

....

....

....

....

Date:

Monitoring the performance of CAHWs

Most CAHW projects develop some kind of system for monitoring the performance of CAHWs. Commonly, these systems are based on reporting forms that are completed by the CAHWs and submitted to the project at regular intervals. This approach enables individual CAHW activities to be checked and also allows information to be collated for the project area as a whole.

a. Designing a monitoring form for CAHWs

Many different monitoring forms have been used in CAHW projects and an example is shown in Box 6.5. This monitoring form uses simple, black and white diagrams of sheep. The top picture shows that the disease problem in this case is worms and the other two diagrams show different age groups of sheep (i.e. adults and lambs). Each time an animal is treated, the CAHW simply marks a circle. Spaces at the bottom of the form are for the name of the CAHW, area and reporting period, and are for completion by the CAHW supervisor. The supervisor might be a government or private veterinarian, or animal health assistant.

Box 6.5 Example of a CAHW reporting form for treatment of worms in sheep

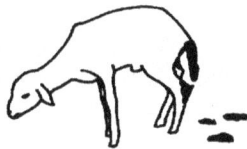

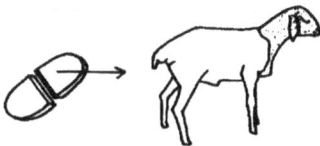

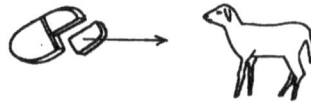

OOOOOOOOOO   OOOOOOOOOO
OOOOOOOOOO   OOOOOOOOOO
OOOOOOOOOO   OOOOOOOOOO
OOOOOOOOOO   OOOOOOOOOO
OOOOOOOOOO   OOOOOOOOOO
OOOOOOOOOO   OOOOOOOOOO
OOOOOOOOOO   OOOOOOOOOO
OOOOOOOOOO   OOOOOOOOOO
OOOOOOOOOO   OOOOOOOOOO
OOOOOOOOOO   OOOOOOOOOO

Name of CAHW: ....

Area: ....

Reporting period: ....

As with many aspects of designing a CAHW system, forms can be developed and adapted according to the local situation. Every format has strengths and weaknesses. The example in Box 6.5 is good for illiterate CAHWs because it contains no text and requires only a tick or mark in the appropriate circle. This format also reminds the CAHWs of the correct dose of anthelmintic for different sizes of sheep. The disadvantage with this form is that the CAHWs have to have a separate form for each type of livestock species and each disease. Therefore, the CAHWs may have to carry numerous bits of paper around with them and this can be cumbersome. Also, if new or different types of medicines become available in the project area, new forms will have to be designed.

An alternative reporting format is shown in Box 6.6. This is a more compact form for use with literate CAHWs and includes information on the livestock owners such as their names and locations. The form is produced in the local language. This form also allows the CAHW supervisor or project to check that the correct medicine has been used for different diseases and that the correct dose of medicine has been used. As the form includes the names and locations of people who have used the services of the CAHW, this type of form can also be used to identify people for interviewing during other monitoring or assessment work.

Box 6.6 Main headings for a monitoring form for use with literate CAHWs

Name of CAHW:

Area:

Reporting period:

date	name of owner	location	livestock type	disease	number of animals treated	medicine	quantity of medicine used	price of medicine

---

Whichever type of reporting form is used, it is usually beneficial if a draft version of the form is introduced to the CAHWs during the training course (see Chapters 4 and 5). This enables the trainer to check that the reporting form is clearly understood by the trainees and means that the form can be modified if necessary. In

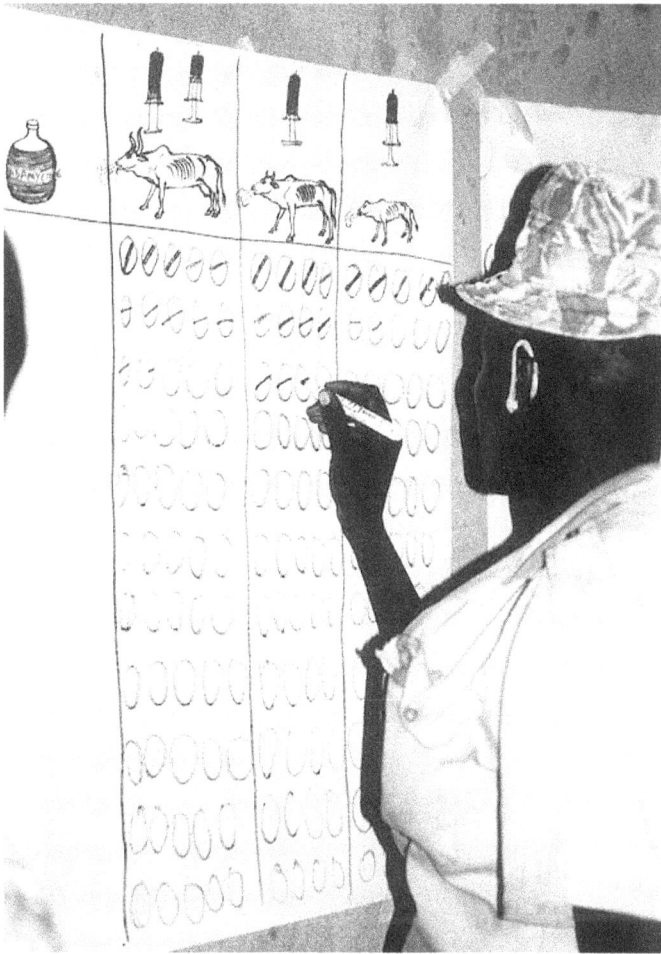

Plate 6.1 Poor literacy is not a serious constraint to developing monitoring forms for use by CAHWs. In this picture, a CAHW from Turkana in Kenya learns how to use a pictorial monitoring form. (*PARC Communications Unit*)

the case of pictorial reporting forms, it is especially important to check that the various pictures are understood by the CAHWs.

With computer equipment, it is now possible to create very realistic monitoring forms using scanned images of medicine labels. These forms are particularly useful for illiterate CAHWs. As a general rule, it is usually better to begin with a simple monitoring form and make sure that this form is completed properly rather than use a complicated form that is difficult to fill in.

b. Collecting the monitoring forms and deciding how often to monitor

Once the monitoring forms have been designed, the project will have to decide when and how to collect the forms. For CAHWs who are working in sedentary communities it may be possible for a project staff member to visit the CAHWs on a regular basis and collect the forms. Alternatively, the CAHW can visit a project office or private pharmacy, and this contact is an opportunity to collect monitoring information. In some cases, regular visits to CAHWs will be difficult because of factors such as heavy rainfall at certain times of year, or difficult terrain. These factors should be considered

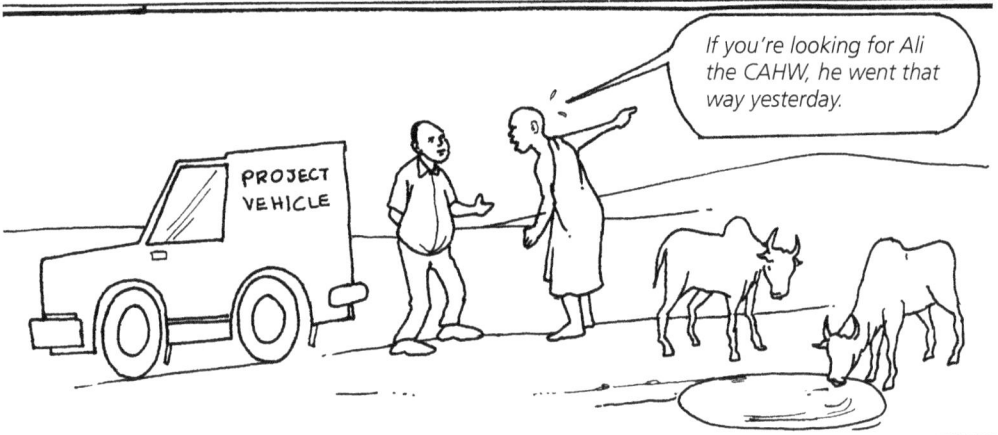

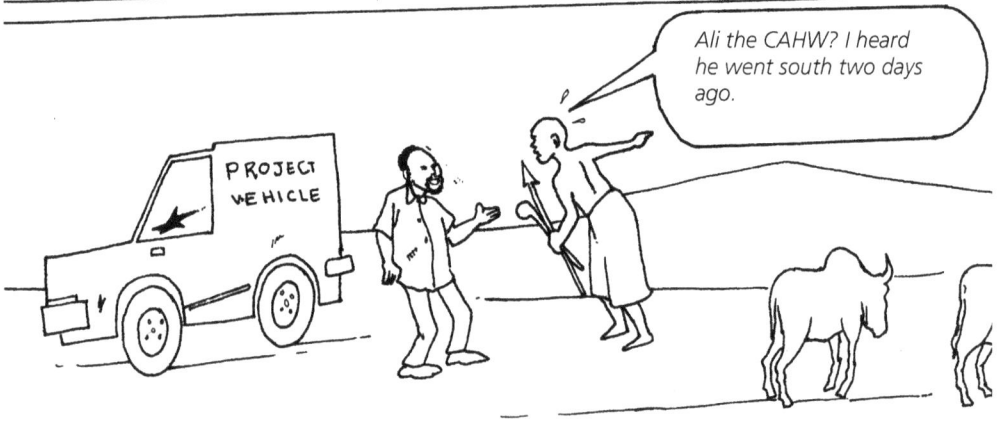

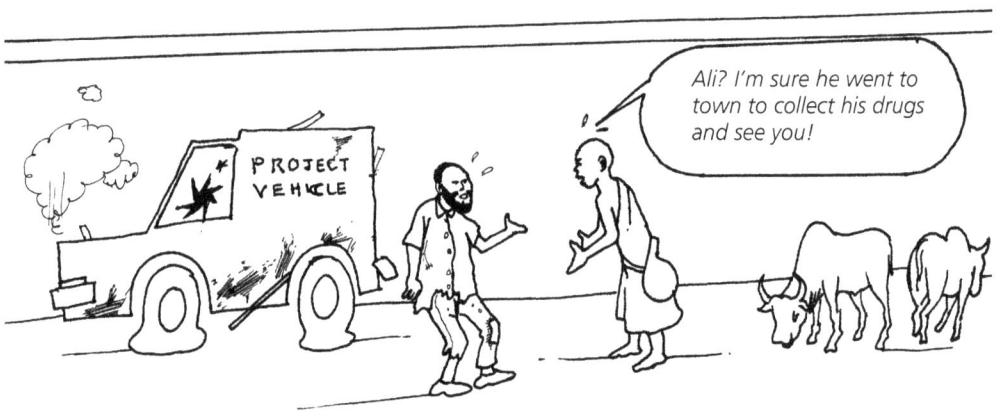

when planning monitoring events. Although reporting periods can vary, one month is usually an appropriate time period.

When working with mobile communities, monitoring can be especially problematic and, in many cases, a more flexible approach will be required. Rather than a project staff member trying to locate each CAHW, it is usually more practical if a fixed-point source of medicines is identified as a location where monitoring forms should be deposited. This source of medicines can be a private pharmacy, government clinic or project office.

c. Cross-checking CAHW performance with visits and interviews

In both sedentary and mobile communities, the CAHW reporting forms should be complemented with visits to the CAHWs to check that they are working correctly. This is particularly important during the immediate post-training period (as discussed in Chapter 5). In pastoral areas where communities and herds are mobile, CAHWs have their own animals and move with the herds. Even with good roads and vehicles, locating these CAHWs can be a long and difficult process. In these situations, implementing agencies need to be wary of trying to cover too large an area before learning about the number of CAHWs that can be properly supervised.

When visiting CAHWs to monitor their work, it is useful to develop a checklist of questions and activities (also see Chapter 5). For example:

Checking the technical knowledge of the CAHWs
Knowledge can be checked by asking CAHWs about livestock diseases they have seen and the medicines used to treat sick animals. Questions on drug dosages and drug safety are also useful.

Checking the equipment and medicines
The equipment and medicines that are used by the CAHW can be checked. For example, is the equipment clean? Are needles properly stored? Does the CAHW know how to sterilize the equipment? Are medicines being stored correctly?

Financial checks
Depending on the system that is being used by the project, the CAHWs may be required to keep basic financial records such as the amount of money collected from livestock keepers for drug sales, castration of livestock or other services. Information on drug prices can be checked during monitoring and levels of payment to the CAHWs can be discussed.

In addition to interviewing the CAHWs, it is often useful to talk to community members in both a formal and informal manner. A formal meeting with community representatives can be used to gauge their feelings about the CAHWs and this information can be cross-checked with more spontaneous, informal conversations. In both cases, it will be necessary to decide whether the CAHWs should be present during the discussions. People may feel inclined to talk positively about the CAHWs just because they are around. When meeting individual community members, open rather than closed questions tend to be more revealing. For example, the open question 'What do you do when your animals are sick?' is more useful than the closed question 'Do you use the CAHW when your animals are sick?'

The information provided by the CAHWs on their activities usually needs to be summarized before it is presented in project reports. These summaries can be prepared by project staff, CBO members or others depending on the roles and responsibilities of different people in the project. In some projects, CAHWs have specific disease surveillance activities and reporting forms are developed according to this role, as discussed in Chapter 7.

6.4 How to use participatory approaches and methods to monitor projects and assess change

In common with the use of participatory approaches and methods during the initial stages of project identification and design, participatory monitoring and assessment provide scope for local people and organizations to assess change on their own terms. The approach assumes that local perceptions of change and the reasons why change takes place are very important for informing the development of sustainable services. This section describes how to develop and use participatory methods for monitoring and assessing CAH services, and assumes that the use and ownership of information

Participatory review in Afghanistan

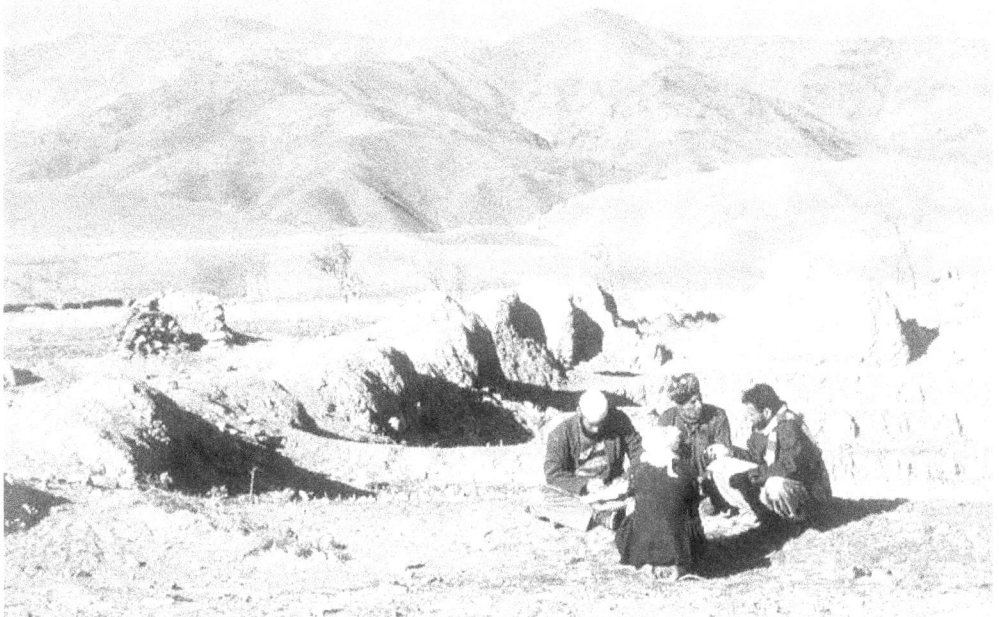

Plate 6.2 Participatory monitoring and assessment approaches are flexible and resource-friendly. (*Stephen Blakeway*)

by different stakeholders has already been defined within the project (see above, *Looking at the information needs of different interest groups*). Also, there are a number of excellent books that describe participatory monitoring and impact assessment methods (see Further reading) and therefore this section focuses on methods that are specific to animal health projects.

Although participatory approaches are still evolving and adapting to new situations, a couple of lessons learnt include:

Focus on key indicators of change as identified by different local groups

Focus attention on indicators of change that are locally identified and locally prioritized by different sections of a community. The comparison of views and opinions of people from different wealth or gender groups then allows exploration of key issues, the reasons why change is happening and the benefits perceived by different people in the community. Try to measure and analyse a few key indicators in some depth, rather than produce a superficial assessment of a wide range of indicators.

Participatory and conventional approaches are complementary

There is considerable scope to mix and combine methods. For example, 'formal' veterinary investigation data can be used to cross-check and complement participatory enquiry, and vice versa. Similarly, project activity reports that detail quantities of medicines used can provide indications of whether or not specific animal health problems should have declined during the project. Participatory methods can be used to determine whether local perceptions of changing disease patterns agree with the type of service provided by the project.

The process of methodology development

When using participatory methods during initial contact with communities and surveys, it is important that the facilitators have developed methods that suit a particular social and cultural environment (Chapter 2). For example, in some areas participatory diagrams work well whereas, in other places, there may be more emphasis on interviewing methods. Songs and drama might be useful in some communities but not others. A similar process of methodology development is required when using participatory methods for monitoring and assessing change. Project staff can work with communities to test different methods and identify those that work well.

Participatory methods that are used in monitoring and assessment work can be slightly more complicated than those that are used during surveys. In particular, some methods require people to compare two or more points in time and, for these methods, careful testing is required. The process of 'explaining the method' requires facilitators to develop and practise a logical and clear description of the method, and identify key open or probing questions that can be used to cross-check information or open up new lines of discussion. The time and resources needed to develop and practise new methods have to be considered when planning and costing monitoring activities.

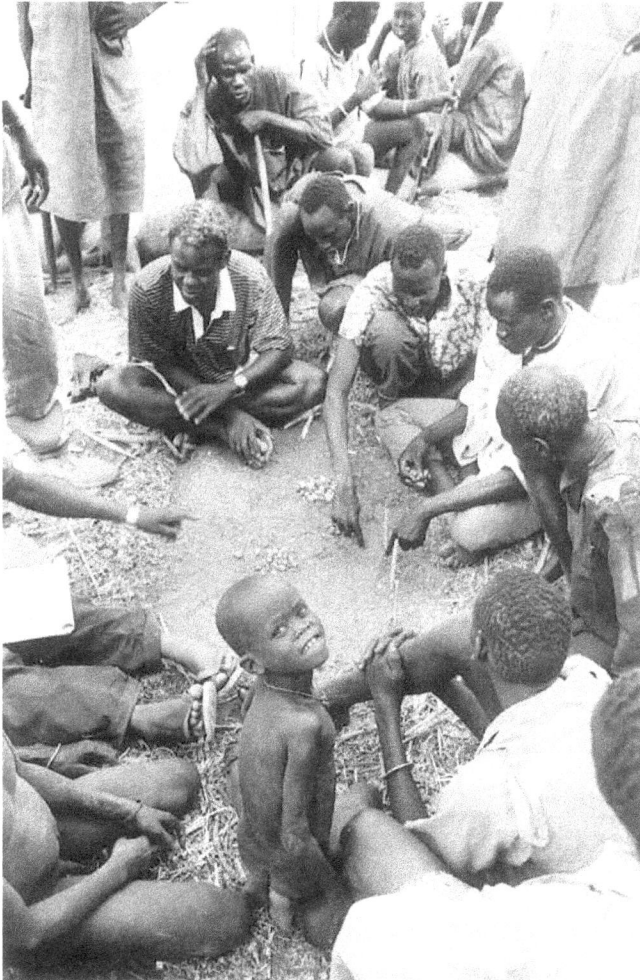

Plate 6.3 Participatory methods can be developed according to local practices. Traditionally, these livestock keepers place sticks in the ground to represent the key issues under discussion. This habit can be adapted into a scoring method to show the relative importance of livestock diseases, types of animal health services or other information. (*Andy Catley*)

As with initial surveys, during monitoring and assessments it is useful to identify different social and wealth groups within communities and repeat similar discussions and methods. This helps to understand different perspectives. For example, is it only the wealthier livestock keepers who are using the CAHWs and benefiting from the project, or are less wealthy people also using the service? Are women using the services of the CAHWs and if not, why not? How does the project affect people without livestock, if at all? During the initial participatory survey, methods such as wealth ranking can provide useful baseline information that can be used to identify people with different livestock holdings. Wealth ranking can also be used as a tool within a monitoring or evaluation process.

A summary of participatory methods for use in monitoring and assessment is provided in Table 6.4. This list is not exhaustive and other methods are described in publications produced by the International Institute for Environment and Development (IIED) and other organizations (see Further reading). As mentioned above, communities and project staff can also develop their own methods.

Table 6.4 Participatory methods for use in monitoring and assessment of community-based animal health projects

Method	Notes on usage
Mapping	Use to define the geographical boundaries of the project and physical features that can affect service accessibility. Work areas for different CAHWs can also be mapped out. Can be cross-checked using formal maps if available.
Timelines	Use to define the time boundaries of the project and, in particular, the period before the project relative to the period during or after the project. Therefore, timelines can be a useful method to precede 'before and after' type methods. Can be cross-checked using historical records and dated project documents.
Ladder diagrams	A simple visualization method for showing trends over time. Informants need to be familiar with ladders!
Pair-wise comparisons	Comparison of two or more things can be a useful way to identify indicators. Scoring of indicators then shows their relative importance and defines priority indicators for use in a monitoring system. In CAH projects, pair-wise comparisons can be used with livestock diseases, livestock species or different types of veterinary service.
Scoring methods	These methods can use various scoring procedures but, in general, a pile of counters is used to measure an indicator 'before and after' the project. If a scoring method indicates that animal health has worsened or improved during a project, the reasons for the change can then be discussed and also scored. Useful indicators to score include: – presence of important livestock diseases; – changes in use of livestock-derived products (e.g. milk); – changes in use of different service providers (e.g. CAHWs, drug vendors, government clinic, traditional healers). Scoring methods are fairly easy to standardize. This enables results from different social or wealth groups to be compared.
Flow diagrams	Flow diagrams are useful for understanding the various factors that can cause change (impact). For example, although animal health might improve as a project progresses, this improvement can arise for numerous reasons. Flow diagrams enable the factors that cause change to be visualized and discussed.
Venn diagrams	Venn diagrams are particularly useful for showing institutional and organizational relationships. If there are various players involved in a project, Venn diagrams show how these players interact and can be used to assist discussion on management, decision making and control of resources in projects.

Using participatory methods to identify indicators of change

Indicators that local people use to describe change in their communities can be identified and agreed with the community or CBO. A useful first step in selecting local indicators is to refer back to the initial participatory survey (see Chapter 2) and look for some of the fundamental reasons why people in the community keep livestock. In addition, the survey may also show how people prioritize different animal health problems and the reasons for the choices they make. This type of information can arise from the use of participatory tools, for example:

Proportional piling of benefits and problems

A very useful way to understand livestock-related indicators with communities is to prompt a discussion using questions such as: 'What are the benefits you receive from livestock?' and 'What are the problems of keeping livestock?' This type of discussion usually reveals lists of benefits and problems

---

Box 6.7 Benefits provided by livestock in Akop Payam, Tonj County, southern Sudan: potential indicators for community-based animal health work

The NGO Vétérinaires Sans Frontières Belgium decided to invest in participatory monitoring of a community-based animal health project in southern Sudan in 1999. This project was implemented with an agropastoral Dinka community. In order to understand local perceptions of the benefits provided by livestock, a simple proportional piling tool was used with five different groups of informants. The results are presented below in tabular form and the ten main benefits are shown visually in the pie chart. When discussing the results with informants, men in Toic Lou noted how 'Everyone depends on milk like a drug. It makes people fat and healthy', and women in Panhial explained that 'Milk brings health and if healthy, one can marry'. Milk and marriage seemed to be two key indicators of project impact for this community.

Stated benefits from livestock	Scores provided by different informant groups by dividing 100 seeds					Total
	Women in cattle camp, Panhial	Men in cattle camp, Panhial	Men from cattle camp, Toic Lou	Village-based women, Marial	Village-based officials, Marial	
Milk	37	27	41	49	19	173
Meat	9	1	7	5	9	31
Butter	–	–	7	–	6	13
Marriage	32	51	10	23	14	130
Ceremonies	–	1	4	–	–	5
Compensation	–	14	18	–	10	42
Kinship support	–	3	–	–	–	3
Manure	22	–	5	14	7	48
Ploughing	–	2	–	–	11	13
Hides & skins	–	–	–	–	8	8
Sales	–	1	6	9	16	32
Ash	–	–	2	–	–	2
Total	100	100	100	100	100	500

Method: proportional piling using 100 seeds per informant group. A dash means that the
benefit was not mentioned by the informants.

Notes: In this community, marriage required payment of cattle to the bride's father;
compensation payments (e.g. for injury caused to another person) involved fines of
cattle; kinship support included loans or gifts of livestock or milk to needy relatives.

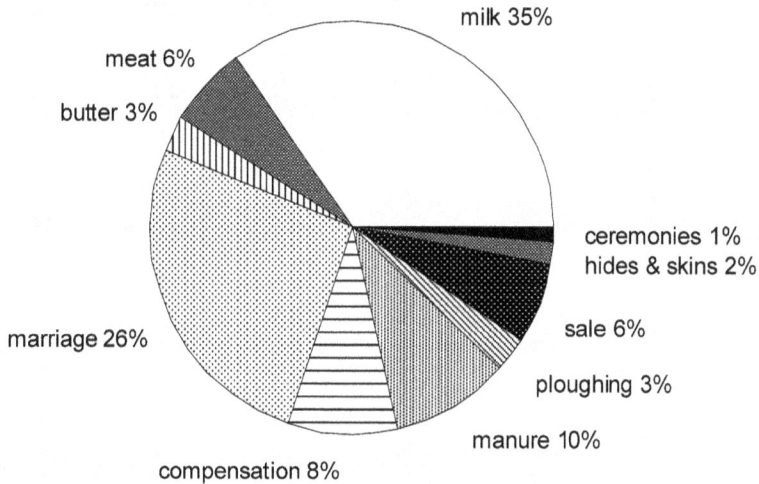

that can be weighted using proportional piling. An example of this approach is presented in Box 6.7
and shows how different people in southern Sudan identified and scored livestock-derived benefits. In
common with the livestock-species scoring tool (Chapter 2), this approach revealed both the social and
production benefits of keeping animals and highlighted the importance of milk and dowry payments
(with cattle) in the community concerned. Herein lies an important advantage of the participatory
approach – it recognizes both production and social impact indicators.

Livestock disease scoring

This tool uses a method similar to the livestock-species scoring tool. However, diseases are compared
and scored instead of livestock types, and indicators are produced which show how and why some
diseases are more important than others. An example is provided in Chapter 2 and this shows how
livestock keepers associate disease with indicators such as reduced milk yield, mortality, reduced sale
value of stock and even 'poverty'. All these indicators are potentially useful impact indicators for
animal disease control.

Regardless of whether we are thinking about conventional indicators (defined by
outsiders) or participatory indicators (defined by local people), when selecting
indicators it is often useful to bear in mind the overlaps and differences between
conventional and participatory indicators. When using participatory tools, livestock-
owning communities will often identify indicators that veterinarians also consider as
important, for example poor fertility or reduced sale value of livestock. However,
although livestock keepers and vets might select similar indicators, participatory

selection of indicators is important because it is part of the process of handing over the analysis and monitoring of projects to local people. Also, as shown above, participatory identification of indicators often reveals useful social indicators that might otherwise be overlooked by project technical staff. These social indicators are crucial if the project is seeking to gain a broad understanding of how healthy animals benefit people. For example, with reference to Box 6.7, how many vets would think of including 'cattle available for marriage' as an indicator of an animal health project?

'Before and after' methods

After the indicators have been identified, they need to be measured over time. Measurements do not need to be precise quantities, but can be qualitative comparisons and use simple scoring systems. Various 'before and after' participatory methods are shown in Boxes 6.8 to 6.11.

Ladder diagrams are a visual method for showing trends over time (Box 6.8). The other methods use a comparison of scores at the beginning (or before) a project with scores after the project has been operating for a few years (Boxes 6.9 to 6.11). Although these scoring methods produce numbers, the numbers themselves are not as important as the trends and relative size and direction of the trends.

In Box 6.10, a paired proportional piling method was used to assess local perceptions of changing patterns of important cattle diseases in Uganda. Informants were then asked to identify factors that had influenced the changes that they described, and score these factors in order of importance. This process revealed that from the informants' point of view, reduced cattle mortality was due to both 'project factors' such as the provision of drugs and vaccines, CAHW activities and cattle crushes, and 'non-project factors' such as peace and reduced raiding of cattle. The identification and scoring of these factors enabled project staff to learn about how the project had influenced change relative to other events.

Box 6.11 summarizes experiences from southern Sudan and, in particular, shows how the repetition of a paired proportional piling tool was used with different informant groups. This enabled perceptions of changing patterns of livestock mortality to be compared between groups.

One weakness of 'before and after' scoring methods is that they require informants to think back to the time before the project started. Consequently, these methods are subject to lapses in memory or 'recall bias'. There are at least two ways to reduce this problem. One approach is to use data that was collected during the initial participatory survey and ask people to compare these results with the current situation. Another approach is to use a timeline to highlight key historical events in the community and identify the precise time that the CAHW project began relative to other important events. This method helps people to recall the start of the project because they connect the project to other things that have happened in the community. An example of a timeline is shown in Box 6.12.

Box 6.8 Use of ladder diagrams to assess changes in accessibility to animal healthcare, FARM Africa, Kenya

FARM Africa works with farmers in Meru and Tharaka Nithi in Kenya where they implement a dairy goat and animal healthcare project. The project uses PRA methods during needs assessments and results are compared with questionnaires sent to government veterinary officers. The project also uses participatory methods during impact assessments.

Ladder diagrams were used to look at farmers' accessibility to animal health services over a five-year period. Three ladders were used to represent three different points in time. The base of each ladder was assigned a qualitative measure of 'low accessibility' whereas the top of the ladders represented 'high accessibility'. Stones or other markers are used to show changes over time as shown below.

The ladder diagrams can then be used to aid discussion on the reasons why accessibility changed during the life of the project.

The ladder diagrams were not used alone during impact assessment work, but were combined with an economic analysis of the performance of the CAHWs and other activities.

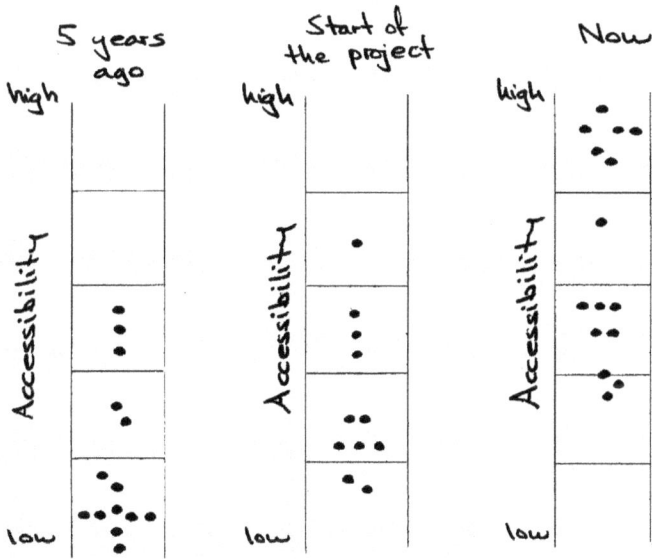

213

Box 6.9 Use of preference scoring to assess options for solving animal health problems in 1992 and 1998, ActionAid-Somaliland

In this method, informants gave each animal health problem a score out of 10 using stones. The scores show preferences for using five different ways to treat or prevent diseases, in two different time periods, 1992 and 1998. As with most other scoring methods of this kind, it is not the precise numbers that are important, but the trends that emerge during the method.

| Animal health problem | Different options for preventing or treating livestock | | | | | | | | | |
| | CAHW | | Traditional | | Religious | | Modern | | Cautery | |
	1992	1998	1992	1998	1992	1998	1992	1998	1992	1998
Nairobi sheep disease	2	7	8	2	5	5	1	3	0	0
Worms	2	7	4	1	5	5	1	5	0	0
Dhaleeco	2	7	1	1	5	5	0	5	6	6
Pox diseases	2	7	2	2	5	5	0	4	3	3
Foot-rot	2	7	3	3	5	5	0	3	0	0
Goat respiratory problem	2	7	2	2	5	5	0	2	4	4
Anthrax (young stock)	2	7	3	3	5	5	0	0	2	2
Trypanosomiasis	2	7	0	0	5	5	0	2	0	0
Camel respiratory problem	2	7	0	0	5	5	0	0	4	4
Calf respiratory problem	2	7	0	0	5	5	0	0	7	7
Tick paralysis	2	7	2	1	5	5	0	3	1	1
Camel chronic respiratory problem	2	7	0	0	5	5	0	5	0	0
Anthrax	2	7	2	2	6	6	0	3	0	0
Mange *cadho*	2	7	2	2	5	5	0	3	4	4

Notes:

Traditional = local strategies of animal treatment and management using herbs and other techniques such as changing the pen or location, or not moving animals because of specific health hazards.

Religious = religious people are called to read verses of the Koran to the animals in the pen, asking God to heal the flock.

Modern medicine = any type of medicine commercially made.

Box 6.10 Paired proportional piling to assess changes in cattle mortality, Oxfam UK/Ireland, Karamoja, Uganda

When using this method informants were asked to name the most important causes of cattle mortality at the time before Oxfam set up a community-based animal health project. The relative importance of these causes of mortality was shown by dividing a pile of 100 stones. The informants were then asked to further subdivide the piles of stones, or add to the piles, to show the situation after the project had been operating. The results are shown below in the two pie charts.

before

after

→

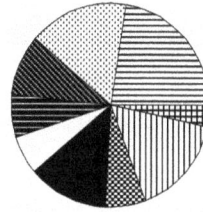

total 30 stones

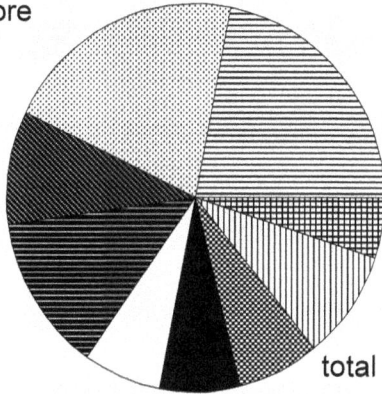

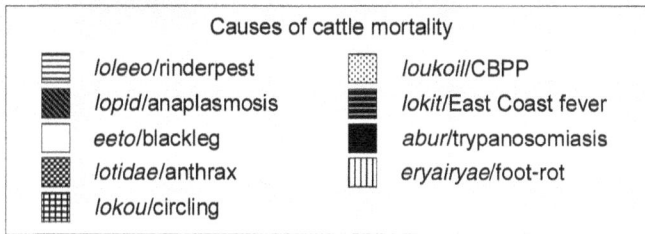

total 100 stones

Causes of cattle mortality	
loleeo/rinderpest	*loukoil*/CBPP
lopid/anaplasmosis	*lokit*/East Coast fever
eeto/blackleg	*abur*/trypanosomiasis
lotidae/anthrax	*eryairyae*/foot-rot
lokou/circling	

The informants were asked to think about and name the various factors that might have influenced the reduction in cattle mortality that had been shown in paired proportional piling. Six factors were named and then scored using 30 stones.

Scoring of factors affecting cattle mortality

Factor	Score
Provision of drugs and vaccines*	7
Construction of cattle crushes*	4
Peace and reduced raiding	3
Good water points	4
CAHW activities*	7
Good grazing	5

* = input from the animal health project.

Again, it is not the precise numbers that are important when using this type of method, but the trends. Some of the information can be cross-checked using CAHW treatment records.

Box 6.11 Paired proportional piling with a Nuer community in southern Sudan

Veterinary staff from VSF-B and VSF-CH projects in southern Sudan tried out a paired proportional piling method with six groups of people in Ganyiel. Seven important diseases of cattle were scored for the period 'before' the project and the period 'now'

Disease names	Informant groups						Totals
	Chiefs	Cattle owners	Community leaders	Community leaders	Non-cattle owners	Traditional healers	
	before/ now	before/ now	before/ now	before/ now	before/ now	before/ now	
Gieng	48/1	34/0	34/0	28/0	32/0	21/0	163/1
Liei	12/42	28/11	14/14	7/6	7/4	16/23	84/77
Rut	7/2	9/1	–	6/4	18/5	–	40/19
Doop	23/2	12/1	17/6	17/3	8/1	10/6	87/19
Dat	8/2	5/1	10/7	6/4	5/3	5/2	39/19
Duny	–	3/7	–	–	–	–	3/7
Yieth Ping	–	–	12/6	11/6	52/20	9/5	84/37

Method: 'before and now' proportional piling of lalop seeds. The figures in the table are the numbers of seeds used by the groups of informants.

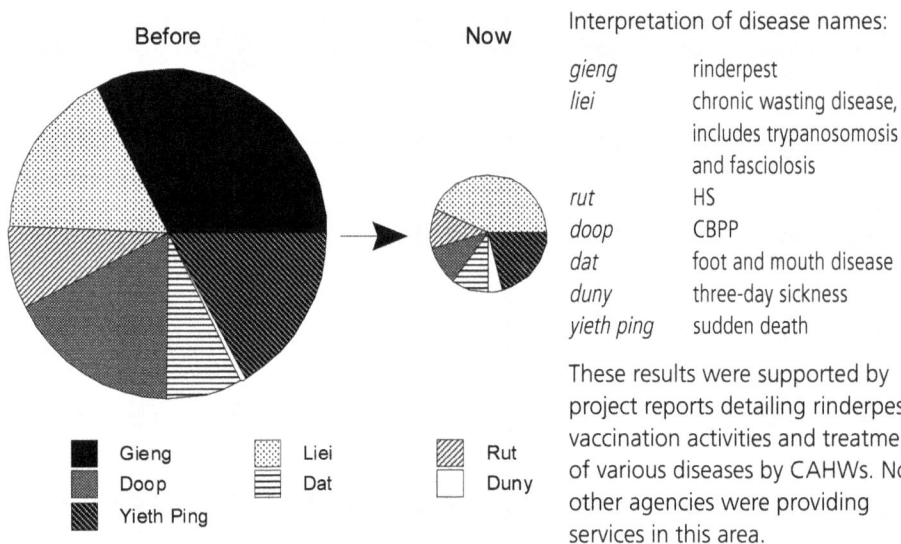

Before   Now

Legend:
■ Gieng   ▦ Liei (dotted)   ▨ Rut
▩ Doop   ▤ Dat   □ Duny
▨ Yieth Ping

Interpretation of disease names:

gieng	rinderpest
liei	chronic wasting disease, includes trypanosomosis and fasciolosis
rut	HS
doop	CBPP
dat	foot and mouth disease
duny	three-day sickness
yieth ping	sudden death

These results were supported by project reports detailing rinderpest vaccination activities and treatment of various diseases by CAHWs. No other agencies were providing services in this area.

Box 6.12 Timeline for a Dinka community in southern Sudan provided by Muorwel-Makiekdit, 1999

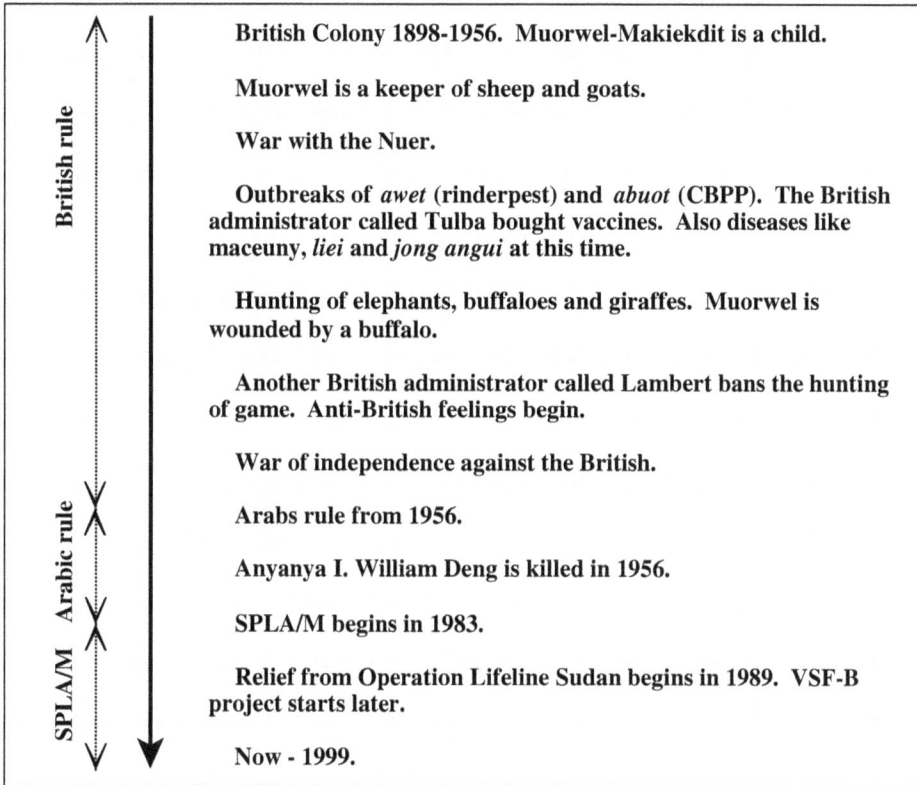

British rule / Arabic rule / SPLA/M

British Colony 1898-1956. Muorwel-Makiekdit is a child.

Muorwel is a keeper of sheep and goats.

War with the Nuer.

Outbreaks of *awet* (rinderpest) and *abuot* (CBPP). The British administrator called Tulba bought vaccines. Also diseases like maceuny, *liei* and *jong angui* at this time.

Hunting of elephants, buffaloes and giraffes. Muorwel is wounded by a buffalo.

Another British administrator called Lambert bans the hunting of game. Anti-British feelings begin.

War of independence against the British.

Arabs rule from 1956.

Anyanya I. William Deng is killed in 1956.

SPLA/M begins in 1983.

Relief from Operation Lifeline Sudan begins in 1989. VSF-B project starts later.

Now - 1999.

Measuring participation

In projects that aim to build the capacity of local players to manage community-based activities, it is useful to assess how the participation of different stakeholders develops or diminishes as the project progresses. One approach to measuring participation in primary human health projects is shown in Box 6.13. At the beginning of a project an arbitrary score of 1 was assigned to five participation criteria that make up the 'spokes' of a radar diagram. As the project developed, different people involved with the project were asked to assess the criteria by reference to a set of questions and issues. People assigned a score of 0 to 5 to each question or issue, and these scores were averaged in order to give an overall score for each of the criteria. Diagrams for year 1, year 3 and year 5 of a project are illustrated.

Box 6.13 Use of radar diagrams to show changes in participation as a project evolves

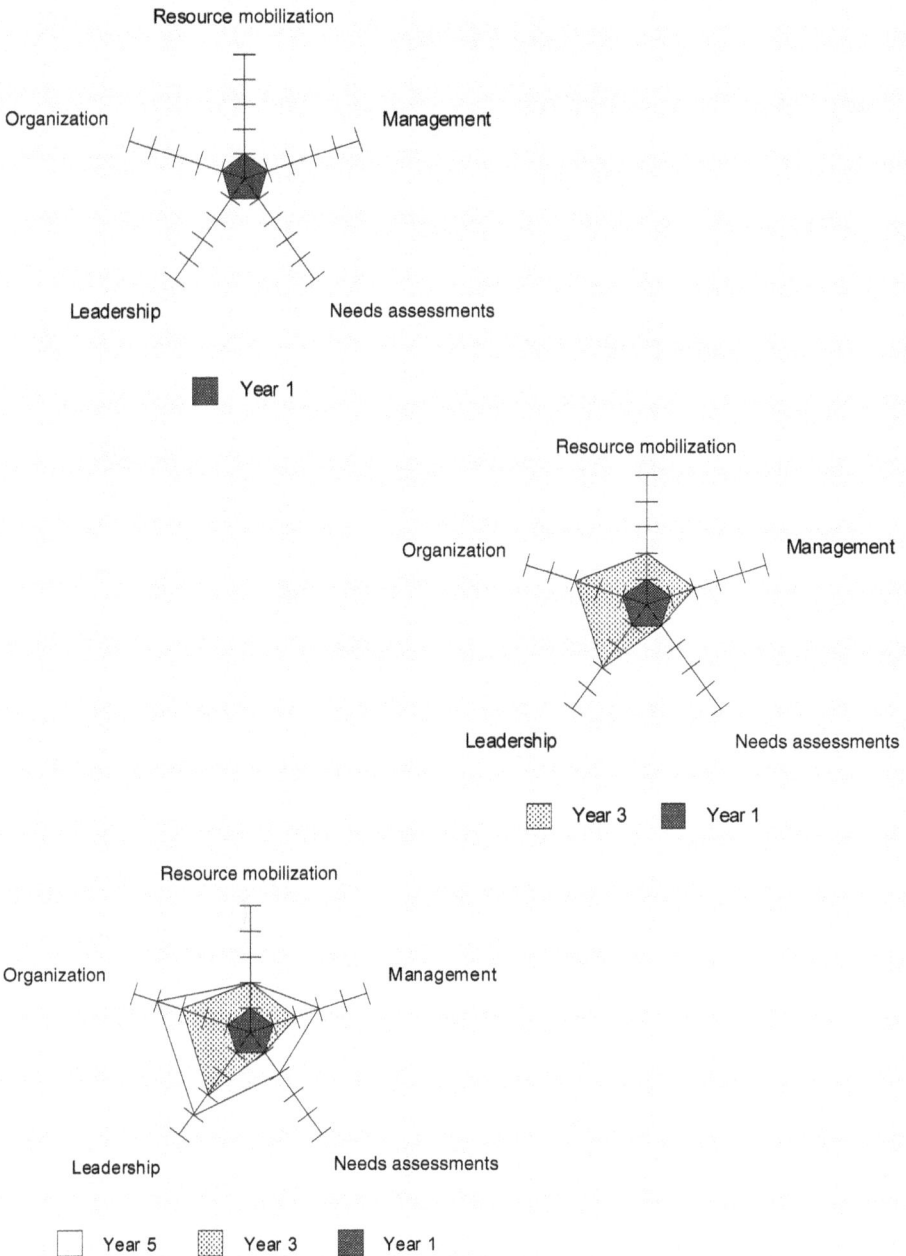

For each criterion of participation (the five spokes of the radar diagrams), scores are developed by reference to sets of questions and issues as follows:

Needs assessment

◆ How were needs identified?
◆ What was the role of the community in analysing needs?
◆ If surveys were used, who designed and conducted the surveys?
◆ Was the assessment used to further involve potential beneficiaries in future plans and programmes?
◆ Was the assessment used to increase beneficiaries' decision-making role in the programme?
◆ Did the survey involve various possible beneficiaries and/or stakeholders?

Leadership

◆ Which groups does the local leadership represent and how does it represent these groups?
◆ How was the leadership chosen and how has it changed?
◆ Is the leadership paternalistic and/or dictatorial, limiting the prospects for wider participation by various groups in the community?
◆ How does the leadership respond to poor or marginalized people in the community?
◆ Have most of the decisions by the leadership resulted in improvements for the majority of the people, for only the elites, for the poor?

Organization

◆ What is the relationship between local organizations and project professional staff? Do local organizations have a decision-making role and, if so, how important is that role?
◆ If new local organizations were created, how do they relate to existing organizations?
◆ Has the representation and the focus of the organization(s) changed since it was created, and, if so, how and to whose benefit?
◆ Who staffs the organization(s) – professionals, beneficiaries and which beneficiaries (elites or the poor)?.
◆ Is the organization flexible and able to respond to change or is it rigid, fearing change?

Resource mobilization

◆ What have beneficiaries contributed to the project?
◆ What proportion of total resource requirements comes from these groups?
◆ Who has decided how indigenous resources should be used?
◆ Do all groups that contribute have a decision-making role?
◆ How are resources mobilized from the community?
◆ Which groups influence mobilization and how do they do it?
◆ Whose interests are being served in both the mobilization and allocation of resources?

Disadvantages of participatory approaches and methods

Although it is widely accepted that participatory approaches to monitoring and assessment have an important role to play in development work, it should be noted that no single approach or set of tools works well in every situation. Some of the pitfalls of participatory monitoring and assessment include:

The use of participatory methods can be time-consuming

Although many participatory methods evolved from 'rapid rural appraisal', this does not mean that participatory monitoring and evaluation is quick to perform. Time is required to work with communities to develop and understand those methods that work well, and identify indicators. Some methods can be very time-consuming and, if people are busy, they may prefer not to be involved. In part, this problem can be reduced by focusing on a limited number of key indicators.

Minority groups can be overlooked

As in all development work, it is easy to overlook the views of people who, due to their gender, wealth or age, are marginalized in a given community. In community-based animal health projects, the users of CAHW services might be wealthy or powerful individuals who make claims on the CAHW for various financial and social reasons. For example, if the CAHW was selected by a committee of male elders, there might be an obligation for the CAHW to treat the animals of the elders first before providing a service to other people. Consequently, participatory assessments should seek out those members of the community who do not use the CAHW and understand the reasons for this. Are these 'non-users' somehow excluded from the service or do they have other options for treating their animals? How do they perceive the CAHW system in terms of its strengths and weaknesses? There are many questions that can be asked, but learning about the animal health service available to poorer livestock keepers or women can assist a project to broaden its impact.

6.5　Ideas for evaluating community-based animal health projects

As mentioned earlier in the chapter, an evaluation is a detailed assessment of a project that focuses on project objectives. Specifically, have objectives been achieved and if not, why not? According to the impact achieved by a project, an evaluation can also pose and attempt to answer questions such as: 'Did the project have the right objectives?', 'What are the wider lessons learnt?' or 'Did the project have unexpected impacts or deficiencies?' Another important aspect of evaluation can be to assess the sustainability of the project and project benefits. Finally, evaluations can look at issues of project efficiency and the effective use of financial, human or other resources.

When monitoring systems are well-designed and properly implemented, evaluation can be a relatively straightforward process because it focuses on project objectives. If a project's monitoring system has successfully identified and measured key indicators of change related to objectives, much of the evaluation process can involve summarizing and analysing the monitoring data and comparing it to the original baseline data. Other evaluation activities can then try to cross-check this information and consider broader issues that affect the project. Conversely, when objectives are poorly expressed in project documents, evaluation can be a very difficult process because it is not clear what the project was trying to achieve.

Evaluations are usually conducted either midway through a project or at the end of a project. Mid-term evaluations are useful if there are concerns that a project is not performing well or if inappropriate objectives have been set. An evaluation at mid-term provides an opportunity to re-orientate a project, reformulate objectives and, if necessary, improve monitoring procedures.

An important but often overlooked task of an evaluation is to relate changes that have taken place during the life of a project to specific project activities. For example, although livestock health might have improved during the lifetime of a project, these improvements could have been due to factors that had nothing to do with the project. Animal health might have improved because there had been good rainfall and plenty of grazing for the animals, rather than a vaccination programme or other veterinary activities.

What is the purpose of the evaluation?

There are many reasons for conducting an evaluation of a CAHW project. When designing the evaluation, it is necessary to define the purpose of the evaluation in terms of the people that the evaluation is aimed at and the use of the evaluation findings. Most of this chapter has been based on the idea that monitoring and evaluation can be learning processes that help a range of stakeholders to improve animal health services. With this idea in mind, the design of an evaluation will depend on the specific stakeholders who are expected to learn from the results. As described earlier (see *Looking at the information needs of different interest groups*), stakeholders can vary from CBOs to central government policy makers to donors. Although an evaluation might be relevant to all stakeholders, it can also focus on a limited number of project objectives that are of particular interest to certain groups. Understanding the information needs of these different groups will help to ensure that the evaluation findings are relevant and acted upon.

Defining the objectives of the evaluation

An evaluation most commonly focuses on project objectives and tries to determine whether objectives have been achieved. In other words, one purpose of an evaluation can be to determine whether the project has achieved its objectives. However, an evaluation can also look at wider issues concerning the relevance, impact, sustainability and efficiency of a project. After analysing these issues, the evaluation can then make recommendations about future work. Typically, the specific areas of assessment that an evaluation tries to cover are described in the terms of reference for the evaluation.

An example of the terms of reference for an evaluation is provided in Box 6.14. In this example, the terms of reference are divided into three main sections that involve collecting data and information about the project and the project area, analysing the information and, finally, formulating recommendations.

Box 6.14 Example of terms of reference for the evaluation of a community-based animal health project

In northern Ethiopia an animal health project was implemented as part of a large agricultural rehabilitation programme. The overall programme aim was to improve the food security of the rural population in the programme area and the programme was implemented by an NGO working in partnership with the Ethiopian Ministry of Agriculture.

The animal health project within the larger programme had three objectives as follows:

Objective 1
Improve the capacity of the zonal Ministry of Agriculture to design, implement, monitor and evaluate a community-based animal health system.

Objective 2
Establish a community-based animal health system in two zones based on 35 community animal health workers serviced by seven Ministry of Agriculture veterinary subclinics.

Objective 3
Support the Ministry of Agriculture veterinary drug revolving fund through technical support on fund management and financial reporting.

Towards the end of the animal health project, an evaluation was designed with the following terms of reference.

Terms of reference

The evaluation will determine:

1. Whether the project has achieved its objectives. If objectives were not achieved, why was this?
2. The impact of the project on the intended beneficiaries. How has the project affected the people in the project area? Who has benefited and why?
3. Whether the project has had any negative effects on people in the target area.
4. How external factors such as political events, other development work or natural disasters affected people during the project.

The evaluation will assess:

5. Whether the aim and objectives of the project are still relevant.
6. Whether project objectives might be achieved via alternative approaches or activities.
7. The efficiency of the project in terms of management, costs and use of human resources.
8. The sustainability of the project, particularly in view of the project's dependence on government veterinary drug supply systems.

Based on the findings of points 1 to 8 above, the evaluation will recommend:

9. How the project could be improved.
10. Modifications or revisions to the project objectives.
11. How to improve monitoring of project impact.
12. How to improve the sustainability of the project.

Who should be involved?

At some stage during the organization of the evaluation it will be necessary to consider whether internal or external evaluators should be used. Internal evaluators are usually project staff who have been closely associated with the project but may lack objectivity when assessing the project. External evaluators may be agency staff from another location, or consultants who are recruited specifically for the purpose of the evaluation. The latter can be relatively costly, but might bring new insights to the project and assist in developing an evaluation that can be regarded as an independent piece of work. The advantages and disadvantages of internal and external evaluators are summarized in Table 6.5. When recruiting external evaluators, many NGOs, private consulting firms and individuals claim to offer an evaluation service. There is considerable variation in the skills and knowledge that external evaluators can bring to projects and two useful rules when choosing external evaluators are:

◆ Ask to see previous evaluation reports that have been produced by the potential evaluator. Do these reports reflect the type of skills and knowledge

Table 6.5 Some advantages and disadvantages of external and internal evaluators

External	Internal
Can take a 'fresh' look at the project.	Knows the project only too well.
Not personally involved, so it is easier to be objective.	Finds it hardest to be objective.
Is not part of the normal power structure.	Is part of the power and authority structure.
Gains nothing from the project, but may gain prestige from the evaluation.	May be motivated by hopes of personal gain.
Trained in evaluation methods. May have experience in other evaluations. Regarded as an 'expert' by the project.	May not be specially trained in evaluation methods. Does not have (or only has a little more) training than others in the project.
An 'outsider' who may not understand the project or the people involved.	Is familiar with and understands the project, and can interpret personal behaviour and attitudes.
May cause anxiety because project staff and participants are not sure of his or her motives.	Known to the project so poses no threat of anxiety or disruption. Final recommendations may appear less threatening

(source: Marie-Therese Feuerstein, *Partners in Evaluation* – see Further reading)

that could be usefully applied to your project? Are the reports well-written, comprehensive, analytical and presented in a professional manner?
◆ Ask other organizations about their experiences with external evaluators. Can they recommend people they have worked with successfully in the past?

In addition to internal and external evaluators, there are other people who can contribute towards, or learn from, an evaluation. Depending on the particular project, an evaluation team might include the following people:

◆ community representatives such as women's group members, community elders;
◆ members of a community-based organization(s);
◆ NGO staff;
◆ private veterinary workers;
◆ government veterinary workers – they can include personnel from central offices if the project is trying to influence policy on veterinary service delivery;
◆ external evaluators;
◆ donor staff.

When CAH projects are implemented by NGOs in partnership with government veterinary services, it is usual to invite local veterinarians to participate in the evaluation. If the project is trying to influence policy, then senior-level staff could also be asked to participate. Depending on funding arrangements, some evaluation teams include donor representatives. There are also many other technical specialists who can offer support to evaluations of CAH projects. These people include social development specialists, gender specialists and economists. The team that conducted the evaluation described in Box 6.14 in Ethiopia comprised a Team Leader (an external consultant veterinarian), the NGO Livestock Project Officer (an animal production specialist and project coordinator), a gender specialist (from another NGO, but working in the same project area) and the Ministry of Agriculture Zonal Veterinary Officer (representing the government partner in the project).

Evaluation design

In general, two types of evaluation are used to assess CAHW projects. One approach is to compare project sites with non-project sites and determine whether there is evidence of different levels of animal health and human well-being in the two locations. Results are then related to project activities in order to find out if and how varying levels of impact are linked to the project. When designed properly, this approach can provide very useful information on CAHW services. However, it is important that the design includes a full description of animal health services in the non-project sites and this exercise in itself can be time-consuming. In addition, there may be limited baseline data in the non-project sites and informants in these areas may exaggerate livestock health problems in the hope of attracting assistance from aid agencies or government. Such exaggeration will tend to heighten apparent differences in animal health status between project areas and non-project areas.

The second approach to evaluation focuses only on project areas, and compares recent animal health information with baseline data. This approach also uses 'before and after' methods to compare two or more points in time, while also looking at the impact of improved animal health (if any) on people's well-being. Within both of the approaches outlined above it is possible to concentrate attention on a particular aspect of a project. For example, some evaluation work looks mainly at the economic issues concerning CAHW activities and the cost–benefit of projects. Other evaluations focus on the service offered by CAHWs and their technical competence. Regardless of which approach is used, two useful lessons are:

◆ Although livestock mortality is a very useful measure of animal health status, in areas with limited veterinary facilities it is often difficult to cross-check information on the number and causes of mortality provided by CAHWs or livestock keepers. When information cannot be cross-checked, this can be stated in the evaluation findings together with the evaluators' assessment of possible sources of bias in the mortality data that is available.

◆ One indirect way to cross-check changing patterns of livestock disease is to link specific uses of veterinary vaccines or medicines to reductions in the presence of diseases that these products are intended to prevent or treat. For example, if a project is providing anthelmintics via CAHWs, it should be possible to comment on the use of anthelmintic in relation to formal or participatory assessments of changes in morbidity or mortality due to worms. Similarly, if ticks are considered to be a problem in an area due to physical damage rather than tick-borne disease, dramatic reductions in livestock mortality attributed to acaricide usage might be questioned.

In the project identified in Box 6.11, CAHWs had been vaccinating cattle against rinderpest (local name, *gieng*). Project reports indicated that the volume of vaccine used by the CAHWS was substantial and that confirmed outbreaks of rinderpest and rumours of rinderpest had decreased during the project period. The results of the paired proportional piling with different informant groups indicated agreement over a dramatic reduction in cattle deaths due to rinderpest.

Some methods for evaluation

Many methods are available for evaluating CAHW projects. Some of these are similar to those that are used during either initial surveys or project monitoring, while others are specific for evaluation purposes. This section summarizes some useful evaluation methods that have been applied in animal health projects and discusses their strengths and weaknesses. Once again, refer to books in the 'Further reading' section for details of more methods that might be applied to CAHW projects.

To a large extent, the choice of methods for an evaluation will depend on the terms of reference for the work, the design of the evaluation and the primary users of the evaluation findings. When a project involves or is trying to influence a diverse group of stakeholders it is likely that different stakeholders will have varying opinions regarding the value of different methods. For example, a government veterinary officer or livestock adviser to a donor might prefer to see quantitative data on livestock mortality rather than read a series of case studies. On the other hand, a social development specialist might prefer to see the findings of focus group discussions with women, men, community leaders, government veterinary staff, CAHWs and project workers.

For projects that are committed to participatory approaches and developing the capacity of local community groups, one objective of an evaluation can be to learn about alternative evaluation methods. In this type of evaluation, the discovery of methods that can be designed and controlled by groups such as CBOs becomes an integral part of the evaluation process. Essentially, the approach prioritizes local perceptions of change above the views of 'outsiders' such as project staff or government workers.

Regardless of which methods are selected for the evaluation and the context of the work, there are some basic guidelines that help to ensure the trustworthiness of the results:

Use a selection of different methods rather than relying on a single method

There is increasing use of combined 'formal/quantitative' and 'informal/participatory' methods in evaluations. It is very unlikely that a single method will produce all the information that is required for an evaluation.

Repeat the same methods with different stakeholders and different locations

This allows results to be compared and the evaluation to describe the perceptions of different interest groups.

Use a multidisciplinary evaluation team of mixed gender

Multiple perspectives and experience are useful during evaluations. A single, technically orientated evaluator can produce results that are biased by personal attitudes or a narrow point of view. This problem is reduced when findings are reached through team discussion and consensus.

Invest in training people in evaluation methods

This is important if the evaluation requires facilitators for participatory methods, enumerators for questionnaire surveys or simply translators for interviews.

Describe the methods in the evaluation report

Many evaluation reports provide very limited information on methods. Although it can be a tedious process to describe methods, this part of a report enables the reader to understand how the information was obtained and, therefore, assess the validity of the report.

a. Reviewing documents

An important activity in any evaluation is a review of project documents and other literature relating to the project or project area. Members of the evaluation team should have access to the original project feasibility study (or equivalent document), the project proposal (with project objectives and activities) and monitoring and progress reports. Other documents such as letters of understanding between implementing partners, minutes of meetings, training manuals and CAHW activity reports should also be made available. Economic assessment of projects will require access to financial reports.

In addition to the above documents, it can be useful for evaluators to view formal, government reports on animal diseases in the project area. Such reports might be obtained at district veterinary offices and they provide an official view of livestock health status in a given area. Indirectly, these reports also reflect the capacity of government veterinary services to monitor livestock diseases and confirm disease diagnosis. Other technical information on animal diseases can be obtained from veterinary journals and a wide range of published and unpublished reports. In recent years, the development of the internet has improved access to literature search facilities that can provide abstracts of papers on key topics.

Although the documents mentioned above are all useful background reading for an evaluation team, in some areas information can be extremely limited. In conflict and post-conflict situations, government facilities and records may have been destroyed. In other areas, it is possible that very little formal veterinary investigation work has been conducted. Despite potential problems and limitations of the secondary data, the review of documents has at least three important functions:

- ◆ It enables the evaluators to determine the extent to which the project is described in writing. Projects with poorly defined objectives, vague activities or limited monitoring data tend to be more difficult to evaluate.
- ◆ It acts as source of information for cross-checking information derived from other sources.
- ◆ It informs the process of developing participatory methods for use during the evaluation, including the formulation of checklists. Whenever possible, the evaluators should also be familiar with local names for the main animal health problems and the extent to which local and western disease names overlap.

A thorough evaluation often makes frequent and accurate reference to the project and secondary literature. For example, direct transcription of project objectives and activities can be useful for organizing the description of the project in the evaluation report.

From a technical perspective, evaluators may also wish to see background information on livestock diseases in the project area. This information may exist in the form of government reports, published papers, participatory surveys or formal veterinary investigations conducted by the project. In those areas where very little background information is available, this in itself can be a useful finding because it reflects veterinary activity in the project area before the project began.

b. Listening to people: interviews, questionnaires and discussions

Interviews and discussions encompass numerous methods varying from informal chats and discussions, to individual case studies, to formal questionnaire surveys. All of these methods are valuable and are commonly used evaluation tools. Techniques for conducting interviews, questionnaires and discussions are well-described in other books but a few points to note are:

- ◆ The skills, attitude and behaviour of the interviewer (and translator) are major determinants of the value of interviews. This aspect of interviewing applies to both informal or semi-structured interviews, and more structured questionnaire surveys. In both cases, the relationship that develops between the interviewer and informant has an important influence on the quality of the information that results. Insensitivity to cultural norms, poorly worded or poorly articulated questions, non-attentive listening behaviour and inexperience with open or probing questions can limit the value of interview methods.

◆ Interview techniques are simple to practise and fine-tune using techniques such as role play before the evaluation proper.

A few specific interviewing and discussion methods are described in more detail below:

Structured interviews

In a structured interview, all of the questions are predetermined and usually listed in the form of a questionnaire. This approach enables information to be collected in a systematic manner and there is less need for interviewers to be experienced in the use of open or probing questions. However, as the questions are formulated in advance by the evaluators, structured interviews tend to be biased towards the perspectives and priorities of outsiders. A questionnaire designed by veterinarians during an evaluation would probably include questions on project impact related to animal production or disease occurrence. However, other forms of impact related to social–cultural uses of livestock may be overlooked. Even when questionnaires contain well-thought-out questions and have been pre-tested, they are still subject to interviewer bias and can easily become 'data driven'.

Semi-structured interviews

In a semi-structured interview a number of key questions are defined but there is scope to follow up interesting lines of enquiry according to responses from the informants. This type of interview requires more skill on the part of the interviewer, confidence to enable discussions to develop and experience with open and probing questions. When used well, semi-structured interviews have the advantage of being both systematic and flexible. The use of key questions enables information from different informants to be collated and compared, while more spontaneous questions provide an opportunity for informants to have a greater influence on how the discussion develops.

Individual case studies

Individual case studies are detailed accounts of a person's history, experiences, livelihood, interaction with a project and hopes for the future. As far as possible, this type of case study is a close transcript of what an informant actually says, with minimum editing. The main strengths of case studies are that they reflect the complexity of people's lives in people's own words. This can help outsiders to understand the diverse and often difficult circumstances in which people live and the relative importance of a particular project compared with other needs and services. When using individual case studies it is important to interview people from different social and wealth groups. Case studies of CAHWs can also be interesting. The method requires good interviewing and translation skills.

Focus group discussions

Focus group discussions are conducted with small groups of people (no more than 15) and are based on a single or narrow range of topics. The composition of the focus group can vary from people with similar interests, social status or identity to mixed groups of people who are likely to hold differing views and opinions. In evaluations of CAHW projects, examples might be the topic of 'Cost recovery and incentives' with a group of CAHWs or 'The qualities of a good CAHW' with a group of women. Good facilitation skills are required during focus group discussions to ensure that people do not digress too far from the main subject and to provide opportunity for each member of the group to contribute.

c. Participatory approaches and methods

Participatory approaches to evaluation are attracting increasing interest from development organizations. The attitudes, behaviour and methods required for participatory evaluation are similar to those used during participatory needs assessments and participatory monitoring. As previously noted, this approach allows scope for innovation and development of new methods according to local conditions and capacity. Also, the approach recognizes that livestock keepers – particularly pastoralists and agropastoralists – tend to have well-developed indigenous knowledge on livestock matters. They have close contact with their animals, observe them on a daily basis and are well-placed to describe changes in disease patterns.

One approach to designing a participatory evaluation is summarized in Box 6.15 and is drawn from ActionAid-Somaliland's work with the Sanaag CBO. In this methodology the principles of soft systems are used to look at ways to define the project as a system, identify the boundaries of the project in time and space, and describe and analyse changes that take place within the system. Various participatory methods are used and these are repeated with different informants in order to compare perspectives in different locations and between men and women.

Box 6.15 A participatory methodology for evaluating a community-based animal health project

There is increasing interest in the use of participatory approaches and methods to evaluate animal health projects. An example of a methodology for a participatory evaluation is presented below and comprises four main stages.

1. What are the geographical (spatial) boundaries of the project?
As part of the evaluation, the location and boundaries of the project need to be confirmed. There is also a need to understand the relationship between the project area and adjacent areas. Using participatory mapping, one or more diagrams of the project areas can be obtained. At least one map should illustrate the locations of different social groups. In community-based animal health work, it can be useful to show the locations of the CAHWs on the map and indicate the areas that they are supposed to service. Also, medicine stores, private pharmacies or government veterinary offices can be illustrated together with routes and modes of transport from the CAHWs' location to these facilities. Participatory maps can be related to more 'official' maps on a district, regional, national or even international scale.

---

2. What are the time (temporal) boundaries of the project?

Once the location of the project is known, the life of a project can be defined using tools such as timelines. In the timeline, it is useful to summarize key events that took place in the community before the onset of the project, and clearly define when the project began. Key stages in project implementation can also be demonstrated.

3. What changes have occurred during the project?

Assess changes that have occurred within the project's spatial and temporal boundaries. In the first instance, this process should focus on the project aims and objectives. An animal health project might have tried 'To improve human nutrition by improving animal health'. In this case, the evaluation should identify local indicators of human nutrition and animal health, and compare the situation at the beginning of the project with the situation at the time of the evaluation. Local perceptions of change can be determined using various 'before and after' ranking or scoring methods. Results can be compared with project activity reports or conventional assessments.

4. How are changes in the community linked to project activities, if at all?

Changes in people's well-being or livestock health and production can be due to many reasons. Participatory methods are useful for understanding how local people relate project work to an improvement or worsening of their situation and the health of their animals. Ultimately, these views should feature prominently in the evaluation because these people are the intended beneficiaries of the project. Scoring, ranking, flow diagrams, Venn diagrams and many other methods can be used to describe and analyse associations between project activities and changes that have taken place during a project.

d. Use of audio-visual methods

Photographs

Good photographs are a useful way to enhance an evaluation and make the evaluation report more interesting. Scanners are not affordable for all projects but the cost of these items is gradually coming down. Photographs can be used in at least two ways. Members of the evaluation team can take photographs and include them in the report, or cameras can be given to local groups for them to record aspects of a project that they consider important. It is easy to leave copies of photographs with local groups as a record of the evaluation process that is accessible to both literate and illiterate people.

Video

In common with photographs, video recordings of project and evaluation activities can be a lively and informative way to capture the evaluation process. Video screenings are also a useful way to refresh memories during report writing, cross-check information and present to community groups for feedback. Video equipment is relatively expensive but, in some areas, cameras and camera operators can be hired on a short-term basis to film specific parts of an evaluation.

e. Situation analysis

A number of analytical tools are available for assisting project evaluators to collate key information and identify areas of further work. These tools can be used at various stages of an evaluation but, if used towards the end of the process, can also analyse evaluation findings. A popular tool is called SWOT analysis, meaning analysis of project strengths (S), weaknesses (W), opportunities (O) and threats (T). A SWOT analysis is usually conducted with a group of people such as key stakeholders in a project. The process involves brainstorming on each of the four features of the SWOT as follows:

Strengths   The good things that have happened during the project. These can be specific activities, events, new or stronger relationships or other positive aspects of a project.

Weaknesses   The shortcomings of the project; those things that were planned but did not happen and mistakes that were made.

Opportunities Given the current situation and what we have learnt about the project, what should we do in the future? How can we build on our strengths and reduce the weaknesses?

Threats   What are the factors that might prevent us achieving our future aims? These constraints can include external political, environmental or economic factors.

The results of a SWOT analysis from a CAHW project in northern Uganda are shown in Box 6.16. These results show some common results and challenges, such as CAHWs trained and working but concerns over incentives and sustainability (see Chapter 3).

Box 6.16 Example of a SWOT analysis of a community-based animal health project in Karamoja, northern Uganda

This example of a Strengths, Weaknesses, Opportunities and Threats (SWOT) analysis was conducted as part of a review of a community-based animal health project implemented by Oxfam UK/Ireland in Karamoja, northern Uganda. This project worked with local communities to select and train CAHWs, and construct cattle crushes to hold cattle for rinderpest vaccination.

The project also established a local development organization called the Dodoth Agropastoral Development Organization (DADO) and, under this organization, a

---

network of smaller Resource Management Committees (RMCs) at cattle crush sites was set up. The SWOT analysis was conducted by members of DADO, local councillors and chiefs, and Oxfam staff.

Strengths	Weaknesses
◆ Oxfam worked closely with community ◆ eight crushes constructed ◆ co-operation with local government administration and vets; including influence on Oxfam's strategic plan ◆ process has happened over five years involving community, administration and local political leadership ◆ selected and trained 16 paravets ◆ formation of DADO and RMCs ◆ involvement of women (i.e. 8 paravets) ◆ promoting peace, for example sponsorship of six peace meetings ◆ community has increased openness and acceptance of new ideas ◆ improved trust and transparency at community and government levels ◆ 316 424 cattle vaccinated for rp and 124 456 cattle vaccinated for CBPP over five years	◆ termites have damaged two crushes (though can be repaired) ◆ poor commitment of some RMC members ◆ some people have broken the peace ◆ mistrust between some CAHWs and some livestock owners ◆ lack of government extension service so programme needs more publicizing ◆ tradition of free government vet service hinders cost recovery ◆ delay in procurement of veterinary drugs ◆ selection of CAHWs trainees needs improving ◆ lack of transport for CAHWs (although bicycles now procured) ◆ not enough time for DADO to talk to livestock keepers ◆ poor record keeping ◆ unreliable livestock statistics such as livestock numbers or disease incidence/ prevalence
Opportunities	**Threats**
◆ DADO/Oxfam/vet department can increase the awareness of the community in Dodoth ◆ DADO to strive for self-reliance ◆ DADO to set up effective system for collecting drug sale revenue ◆ networking with other pastoral organizations ◆ research on traditional livestock practices and production ◆ increase DADO's institutional capacity ◆ identify means of rewarding the paravets ◆ improve paravet skills through more training ◆ use different ways to pass message to the community (e.g. role plays, dramas, etc.)	◆ change in government policies ◆ episode of total breakdown of peace within the region ◆ severe drought ◆ strange disease outbreak (epidemic) for humans or livestock ◆ quality (professionalism) of companies supplying vet drugs ◆ poor supply of vaccine from PARC or vet department ◆ large projects coming in and overriding small projects ◆ lack of funding

Presenting and sharing the information

Evaluations require a great deal of organization and effort, but they are key learning events for CAH projects. However, many of the lessons learnt can easily be lost or forgotten if experiences are not properly documented and shared with relevant stakeholders.

a. The evaluation report

In the long term, the evaluation report will be the main reference document for the evaluation. The way that information from an evaluation is collated and presented is partly dependent on the intended target audience because, as previously discussed, different stakeholders tend to have different information needs and criteria for assessing the value of reports. In common with other aspects of CAH systems, there is no standard style of presenting information. Also, when using participatory approaches and methods, there is scope for flexibility and presentation of information in novel ways.

When producing the evaluation report it is useful to consider the following points:

The report structure

The report should follow a logical structure, in a similar way that a scientific paper is organized according to a summary (or abstract), introduction, methods, results, discussion and references (or bibliography).

Regardless of the quality of the report, some readers will only read the summary and perhaps skim through other sections. Therefore, a good summary of key findings and recommendations is one of the most important sections of a report. It is often useful to organize the summary according to specific terms of reference and even add a note to each main point such as 'This point addresses item xx of the terms of reference'. The summary can also include cross-references to parts of the main body of the report where more detailed information on a particular issue can be found.

An example of an evaluation report structure is provided in Box 6.17. In this case, the report has clearly defined sections for introduction, methods, results, discussion and recommendations. The introduction should provide background information on the project and the project area. This should include notes on the broader political, economic, social and environmental context in which the project operates. The project objectives and terms of reference for the evaluation can also be mentioned in the introduction.

Well-presented methods and results sections enable readers to make an independent analysis of the information and, if necessary, compare their own interpretation of the data with the analysis provided in the discussion section of the report. Sometimes data can be summarized as tables and diagrams in the results section, and the complete data provided in an annexe. However, when summarizing data try to avoid reducing data from numerous sources or stakeholders unless it can

Box 6.17 A structure for an evaluation report

Although many of the things to be included in the report may seem obvious, it is surprising how often useful information is left out of reports, for example a summary or a contents page.

Title page

◆ report title;
◆ authors of the report, named as individuals or organizations;
◆ date.

Acknowledgements

◆ Try to list all the people who contributed towards the evaluation and describe their affiliations to organizations and agencies.

Contents page

◆ Produce a clear and well-spaced contents page with page numbers.

List of abbreviations

◆ List the abbreviations in the report. It can also be useful to provide a brief description, for example MoA, Ministry of Agriculture – the main implementing agency for the project.

Summary

◆ a brief introduction to the evaluation;
◆ main findings;
◆ main recommendations.

Introduction

◆ background to the project area;
◆ background to the project;
◆ objectives of the project;
◆ main agencies and stakeholders involved in the project;
◆ reasons why the project chose to conduct an evaluation;
◆ terms of reference for the evaluation.

Methods

◆ Give clear description of methods used.
◆ Detail different informant groups by type of group and number of informants.
◆ Use annexes to provide copies of questionnaires or checklists used during interviews.
◆ Clearly state use of statistical test, if any.

Findings

◆ Present findings in a logical order according to the terms of reference and the methodology.

◆ Use tables, graphs and other diagrams to summarize and visualize information.
◆ Avoid over-elaborate diagrams.
◆ Use annexes to present raw data (or summaries of raw data).

Discussion

◆ Analyse and discuss the findings. Cross-reference specific discussion points to specific terms of reference and specific findings.
◆ Include discussion on how external factors (political, economic, environmental or others) affected the project.
◆ Comment on methods used – their value, weaknesses and limitations of the information presented.

Recommendations

◆ Recommendations should be succinct and directly supported by information provided in other sections of the report.
◆ Link each recommendation to the terms of reference for the evaluation.
◆ If there are many recommendations, try to prioritize them and group them under subheadings.

Bibliography

◆ Provide a list of the literature that was used by the evaluation team, arranged alphabetically and using a standard and full referencing format.
◆ In theory, readers of the report should be able to locate copies of each reference according to the information provided in the bibliography – incomplete references can be difficult to locate. For grey literature, provide a contact address where the literature can be obtained.

Annexes

◆ Annexes can be used to present information that is too bulky to include in the main body of the report or is of secondary importance.
◆ Common annexes include a detailed annexe on methods (this might contain an itinerary for the evaluation team, a copy of a questionnaire or checklists for interviews) and an annexe with full accounts of interview results and individual case studies. Another annexe might be a draft proposal for future work.

be shown that the results from these different groups are similar. When data is analysed statistically, the statistical test that is used should be clearly stated.

The discussion section of the report should present an analysis of evaluation findings. This part of the report should also relate project events and experiences to the broader setting of the project, such as the general economic situation, political events, the policy environment, donor strategies and so on. This type of analysis is important for placing the project in a given, often complex context and helps to avoid the view that projects exist in isolation of the wider world.

Length of the report

How long should the report be? In most cases, there is a compromise between making a report succinct and likely to be read, and yet comprehensive enough to demonstrate that a thorough evaluation has been conducted. As a general rule, few people will read a long report. Therefore, keep the report concise and to the point, link findings and recommendations to the terms of reference for the evaluation, and avoid digressions away from the terms of reference. Twenty pages is sufficient for the main report and annexes can be used to present additional information such as specific methodological details, examples of CAHW monitoring reports and raw data from surveys.

General presentation

A report that looks professional and well-organized, with clear headings, type and diagrams is more likely to be read than a cramped or cluttered report. Use a type font that is easy to read and avoid fancy borders or other graphics that detract from the main writing and pictures in the report. Carefully check the spelling and grammar in the report and use a good photocopier to make clear, neat copies. The overall presentation and 'look' of the report has a big influence on how the report will be received and the extent to which it is read. Bound reports with strong plastic covers last longer than unbound reports held together by staples.

Writing style

Reports are easier and more interesting to read if they are written in an active style, rather than a formal or scientific style. Try to use short sentences and avoid long words. Technical words can be included but should be explained in a glossary or footnote. For example, some livestock disease names (e.g. trypanosomiasis) can be tricky for non-veterinary readers. Numerous writing and formatting devices can be used to break up large blocks of text and make key points easy to find. These include the use of bullet points and text boxes. Also, direct quotations from interviews can be used to enliven a report.

Use of pictures and diagrams

Pictures and diagrams enliven a report and present information that is cumbersome to describe using text. For example, it is much easier to draw a map rather than describe the positions of villages, roads or other features using words alone. Computer software now enables colourful and sophisticated graphs and other diagrams to be produced relatively easily and added to reports. Graphs are useful for summarizng and visualizing information, but simple black and white graphs that are easy to understand are often a better option than complicated three-dimensional, multicoloured graphs that do not photocopy well. Pie charts are particularly useful for summarizing information in a visual manner.

When presenting the results of participatory mapping or other diagramming exercises, the use of scanners allows diagrams to be inserted into documents and edited. However, for projects without this equipment, good results can be obtained simply by using hand-drawn copies of the original diagrams, gluing these into the top copy of the report, and then photocopying.

Timing
Try to produce the evaluation report within a reasonable timeframe, for example, within one month of the end of the fieldwork. This helps to ensure that reports are acted upon and can build on the momentum and interest for improvement that an evaluation can initiate. Reports that are submitted after many months can easily be out of date.

The draft report: seeking feedback and checking the report's contents
As most evaluations involve multiple players it is useful to distribute a draft copy of the report for feedback and comments. This is particularly important if the report contains information that may be contentious because it provides an opportunity for people to challenge the points in question. If necessary, these comments can be included in the report in order to present two sides of a discussion. Another way to obtain feedback is to organize community workshops in which the main findings and recommendations of the report are presented and discussed.

Distributing the report
The project and evaluation team should formulate a list of agencies and individuals who should receive a copy of the report. A brief letter should be produced to accompany the report.

Producing a special summary report or newsletter for community-based groups
In order to share the evaluation findings and recommendations with the community in general, newsletters can be used. These can summarize the main points of the evaluation, say who was involved and can be made more appealing if photographs, cartoons or direct quotations are included.

b. Presentations at meetings and conferences
In addition to producing a written account of the evaluation, verbal presentations at workshops or conferences can be used to present evaluation findings to a wider audience and seek ideas from others. This topic is discussed in more detail in Chapter 9 on networking.

Summary
Monitoring is one of the most important, but often one of the weakest components of CAHW projects. Difficult terrain, the location of workers in remote areas and the logistical problems of physically reaching CAHWs to check their activities are just some of the constraints to effective monitoring. In addition, there is a tendency for projects to underestimate the time and resources required for effective monitoring, or attempt to use methods that are cumbersome and indicators that are inappropriate or

too numerous. Despite these experiences, a well-designed and properly implemented monitoring system can be a considerable asset to a project. It enables problems to be corrected quickly and allows new opportunities for improving a project to be identified.

Participatory approaches that combine local perspectives and professional judgement are highly appropriate for monitoring and evaluating CAHW projects. These approaches help to overcome some of the difficulties with using conventional quantitative methods in remote areas with limited resources. Crucially, they also enable livestock keepers to have a greater stake in measuring change in their communities and working with veterinary workers to assess and improve animal health services.

CHAPTER

Community-based animal health workers and disease surveillance

7

Jeffrey C. Mariner

CONTENTS

7.1   Introduction

Good animal health surveillance is the key to designing effective national animal health programmes and to participation in international trade. Animal health intelligence is the basis for identifying national programme priorities, newly emerging

Box 7.1 Some terms used in this chapter

Active surveillance – health information gathering systems based on outreach to encourage more complete reporting or uncover more detailed information. An example would be telephoning or visiting clinics in an outbreak area in order to get a more complete listing of cases.

Case definitions – a specific description of the clinical, epidemiological, pathological and/or laboratory test results that are considered characteristic of a disease category and are used as the criteria to classify sick individuals to a particular disease category. Disease categories may be highly specific and definitive such as measles, or very broad and preliminary such as 'fever of unknown origin' depending on the objective of the categorization process. Existing veterinary knowledge disease descriptions based on the clinical, epidemiological or pathological features of a disease are comparable to the clinical case definitions used in western medical and veterinary practice.

Immunohistological diagnosis – a confirmation of the causative agent of disease based on the staining of microscopic tissue slices with specific antibodies linked to dyes and visible under the light microscope.

Polymerase chain reaction (PCR) – a process whereby one or a few copies of an organism's genetic material (DNA or RNA) can be amplified into millions of copies for easy diagnosis, identification and epidemiological characterization.

Passive surveillance – health information gathering systems built up from many routine tasks such as the posting of monthly activity reports by clinics to a central office.

Genetic probe – a sequence of genetic information (DNA) with a dye or radioactive label that is a matching complement to the natural sequence in an organism being tested for in a diagnostic exam. If the probe binds to the test sample, the microbe being searched for is present. The label attached to the probe will stick with the probe and be detectable and confirm that the sample is positive for the agent.

In situ hybridization – this process uses genetic probes on microscopic tissue slices to detect the presence of infectious agents.

Zoonotic disease – a disease that affects both animals and humans and is transmissible from animals to man or vice versa.

---

health threats and effective intervention strategies to enhance the productivity and profitability of animal agriculture. The implementation of the Agreement on the Application of Sanitary and Phytosanitary Measures (SPS Agreement) through the Office International des Epizooties (OIE) and the World Trade Organization (WTO) has established surveillance data as the basis upon which international trade decisions on access to markets will be made.

The initial source of most animal health surveillance data throughout the world is the livestock owner. Unless livestock owners alert society to occurrences of concern, animal health events may go undetected until they reach crisis proportions. In the developed world, where the availability of service and value of stock are both high, livestock owner reports usually take the form of calls for assistance for herd-level problems to public or private professional services.

In the developing world, the availability of animal health service is low in most rural areas. In part, this is due to the non-sustainability of tax-funded colonial-style services in the modern economic environment. A lack of sustainable funding for field operations has resulted in state veterinary services becoming office-bound, and a widening communication and service gap between farmers and tax-funded institutions. The collapse of colonial services is compounded by the slow start of current western models of private veterinary service delivery in the developing world. This is related to the lack of enabling policy environments and the inherent high cost of mobile services relative to the value of individual stock in rural areas. Since livestock owners' primary motivation in making reports is to find a solution to their own problem, farmers are often unlikely to make reports or seek help if they have learned through experience that little help – paid or unpaid – is available. Thus, the lack of animal health services in rural areas goes hand-in-hand with a lack of animal health information.

Beyond the local impact of neglect, nations suffer from biased animal health information and frequently fail to assess animal disease risks accurately. This can have dire consequences for the national herd. For example, in the 1980s and early 1990s, the authorities in Ethiopia received very few reports of rinderpest from the Afar pastoral area due to the paucity of staff in the region and limited contact between the veterinary services and the pastoral community. Numerous reports of epidemic rinderpest were received from more sedentary communities surrounding the Afar, who had more regular access to services. This information bias led authorities to further focus rinderpest control resources around the Afar area but not in the Afar area itself. Control efforts in the sedentary communities had little impact on the occurrence of outbreaks because the source of the problem was never addressed. Subsequently, active surveillance in the Afar region led to the identification of the region as an endemic focus of rinderpest infection resulting from the non-availability of vaccination. The lack of services and surveillance in Afar was the root cause of the recurrent epidemic disease in neighbouring communities. Biased reporting due to a lack of services and contact had resulted in an inappropriate assessment of the epidemiological situation and an ineffective allocation of resources.

Upon realization of the true epidemiology of the rinderpest in the region, authorities quickly dedicated resources to the Afar region and developed community animal health (CAH) programmes that addressed rinderpest. The result of these appropriate surveillance and control efforts was that rinderpest was eradicated from

Afar and the surrounding communities within three years and Ethiopia achieved provisional freedom from rinderpest at the national level.

In general, animal health information arising from indigenous sources is poorly integrated with government veterinary services. Among veterinarians, there is declining familiarity with traditional knowledge systems and lack of exposure to the participatory and qualitative systems of enquiry. Veterinarians trained in 'old school' faculties are following models designed for other societies and economic environments. Sadly, many veterinarians have been steeped in colonial bias that considers traditional knowledge to be a form of ignorance rather than collective wisdom. Modern science, it is said, prefers cool, crisp numbers as measurable and verifiable information. On the other hand, epidemiologists are aware that considerable bias and confounding can be lurking in quantitative data, unless significant time and expense has been invested in controlling for such problems. Good quantitative data is extremely expensive.

Disease reporting and surveillance data is especially prone to bias and often falls within the category of 'numerator data' – observations in the context of an undefined population. 'Was it three cases out of ten, a hundred or ten thousand exposed animals?' Thus, disease reporting and surveillance is often qualitative data in a numeric disguise. It is still extremely valuable information. The strengths and weaknesses of disease intelligence and reporting data is best interpreted in the context of local observations and perceptions. In a sense, these can serve as alternative denominators where conditions preclude the availability of population-based quantitative data. However, in order to effectively recognize, collect and use good-quality qualitative data, veterinary and development professionals need training in appropriate methods.

This guide presents privatized, community-based animal healthcare as one solution to the problem of delivery of animal health services to rural areas that complements the role of publicly funded services. The recommended approach is that livestock owners, community-based animal health workers (CAHWs), consumers, veterinarians and public, private and non-government institutions concerned with animal health are all viewed as stakeholders or beneficiaries in a socio-economic network of mutual interdependence. Each group has legitimate needs and functions. This chapter completes the cycle of service delivery by presenting appropriate methods for gathering animal health intelligence. It will discuss the integration of CAHW networks and community-based veterinary practices into national disease surveillance systems. As such, the chapter defines a role for the CAHWs, not only as service providers in their immediate community, but as service providers to veterinary services and the public at large. But, we should not fall into the altruistic trap. In order for surveillance systems to be sustainable, surveillance must be recognized as *information for action* that results in tangible benefits to the information providers at the local level. The primary motivation for reporting is still the desire for assistance with local problems.

Livestock owners in various cultural and ecological settings know much about their animals. However, local knowledge varies and it is critical that project and veterinary staff understand the strengths and weaknesses of indigenous veterinary knowledge in each community. Chapter 2 describes the process of needs assessment and participatory survey. Chapters 4 and 5 focus on CAHW training and participatory training as an information exchange process. These are essential learning opportunities for surveillance personnel. This chapter provides a brief overview of the characteristics of effective surveillance and highlights aspects of indigenous veterinary knowledge of particular value as epidemiological intelligence. Thereafter the discussion turns to practical matters and suggestions for successful programmes of community-initiated disease reporting and surveillance. The final section describes participatory disease searching, a form of active surveillance. Active surveillance is a term for information collection where epidemiologists initiate or 'reach out' to encourage reporting by going to the field and contacting informants.

Recognition of the pivotal role that community animal health networks can and should play as a resource to all stakeholders in the broader context of national animal health surveillance is key to assuring that public services buy into the concept of community animal health development. Timely and representative disease reporting demands a solid foundation of farmer contact and farmer reporting. In the traditional sector, CAHW programmes are the key to credible and transparent surveillance systems that meet the requirements for national participation in the global livestock economy.

Box 7.2 Can basic-level workers provide useful information for disease surveillance? Testing a CCPP surveillance system in central Somalia

In 1986, Gesellschaft für Technische Zusammenarbeit (GTZ) designed and established the Nomadic Animal Health Auxiliary System (NAHA System) in the pastoral rangelands of central Somalia. The system was part of the German contribution to the multi-component and multi-donor Central Rangelands Development Project (CRDP).

The project used 53 trained Nomadic Animal Health Auxiliaries (NAHAs) who were selected by communities in 14 traditional grazing areas, called *degaans*. The NAHAs received training in basic animal healthcare and were supplied with a kit of equipment and medicines. Veterinary medicines were replenished via a revolving fund system operated under the Ministry of Livestock, Forestry and Range.

Studies on CCPP

One aim of the GTZ project was to investigate the role of NAHAs in epidemiological monitoring and surveillance. Therefore, a study on contagious caprine pleuropneumonia (CCPP) was conducted in which data provided by NAHAs was compared with laboratory sero-diagnosis in selected flocks.

Over a two-year period, a project veterinarian and his Somali counterpart visited and interviewed the NAHAs every two months in order to collect information on the number of clinical CCPP cases seen by the NAHAs, the number of affected flocks and the number of cases treated. The Somali disease name *sambab* ('lung') was used by the NAHAs to describe CCPP cases, as verified by the project in baseline assessments. Treatment figures were cross-checked against the use of oxytetracycline and qualitative information on treatment success, case fatality and traditional practices was also collected.

Serum samples were collected from 1989 goats in 80 flocks and the complement fixation test (CFT) was used to detect antibody to *Mycoplasma* F38. A further 1717 serum samples from 153 goat flocks were tested for antibody to *M. mycoides* subspecies *mycoides*, also using the CFT.

Comparing the two sets of data

In order to correlate NAHA's knowledge about *sambab* cases with CCPP serology results, the number of goats affected with *sambab* per flock was compared with the pooled number of goats tested positive for *M.* F38 and *M.m.m.* antibody. Using Spearman Rank Correlation and Kruskal-Wallis one-way analysis of variance, NAHA disease surveillance information for sambab was found not to be statistically independent from the CCPP serology results. Therefore, it was concluded that NAHAs could play a useful role in a CCPP surveillance system in central Somalia.

The disease intelligence system already established at herd/flock level could have been expanded and stepped up to make a regional livestock health surveillance system. In this way the government veterinary service would have benefited from the potential and the flexibility of the system in a cost-effective way. Although the project in Somalia was interrupted by civil war, these experiences were an indication that community-based systems in other African pastoral areas could also be used for animal disease surveillance.

(contributed by Dr Maximilian P.O. Baumann, Freie Universität Berlin)

7.2 Effective surveillance

Epidemiological surveillance can be defined as the collection, analysis and dissemination of animal health information for the design, implementation and assessment of animal health interventions. Essentially, surveillance should produce information that leads to *action*. It is important to note that most workers distinguish surveillance from epidemiological research or targeted studies. Surveillance is a real-time or ongoing data collection activity. This means that surveillance information reflects the current or near-current situation on the ground. On the other hand, epidemiological research tends to have a broader time horizon and, when an epidemiological question arises, requires lead-time for the design of studies and collection of data. Surveillance can complement and be complemented by research. Surveillance may highlight the need for a study or provide key data to meet part of a study's needs, but the uses of the output, time course and level of rigour differ fundamentally. It is more appropriate to view surveillance data as epidemiological intelligence.

Disease surveillance and reporting are key functions coordinated by public veterinary services that require the participation of all components of the national animal health service: public institutions, agribusiness, private practitioners, community-based programmes and individual livestock owners. Each of these players collects and uses animal health information. Although co-ordinated by government, animal health information systems are more than just information for authorities. Surveillance systems are services to the industry, public and private professionals and

---

Box 7.3 Key requirements of effective animal health surveillance systems

Sensitive

The system must be capable of detecting the majority of disease events of economic or zoonotic significance. The concept of economic significance includes both commercial and subsistence benefits.

Specific

The system must be able to correctly identify the cause or nature of disease events.

Timely

Information must be made available within a time-frame that permits an appropriate response or intervention to be put in place, if one is warranted. Information is a perishable commodity that looses value with the passage of time.

Representative

The system should generate information that accurately depicts the spectrum and relative importance of animal health events in all regions, societies, livestock keeping systems and segments of the population.

Acceptable

The results of the system should be of sufficient interest and value to all participants to justify the workload and other opportunity costs created by the activity.

Flexible

The system should be capable of adapting to new, unforeseen events or needs.

Cost-effective

The cost of the system both in terms of direct costs and hidden costs such as human labour should be reasonable relative to the benefits derived from the surveillance information.

Simplicity

The system should be no more complex than necessary with the aim of encouraging participation.

---

sub-professionals, as well as livestock owners. Thus, timely information dissemination is an integral part of surveillance systems. In fact, feedback to the original suppliers or sources of information is essential to assuring their continued participation. Animal health surveillance systems must meet several basic requirements in order to be effective as outlined in Box 7.3.

Only a surveillance system made up of a combination of different surveillance activities can fully meet all of the requirements detailed in Box 7.3. In an effective surveillance system, different activities will focus on different system requirements and the whole will constitute a series of integrated checks and balances. As an example, general disease reporting based on livestock owner reports and clinical diagnosis made in the field is essential for the detection of health events. The capacity of the system to detect and report health events is the sensitivity of the system. However, reports and clinical diagnosis often lack a specific, confirmed diagnosis. It is the job of disease investigations and laboratory-based surveillance to confirm or refute some or all of the field reports. The capacity of a system to confirm disease diagnoses using scientifically recognized methods is the specificity of the system. If either the sensitivity or specificity of the system is lacking, health surveillance is inadequate (see Box 7.4).

Box 7.4 Sensitivity, specificity and action in surveillance systems

Sensitivity	Specificity	Characteristics of surveillance system
Low	Low	Poor capacity to detect disease in the field. When disease is detected, poor capacity to confirm disease diagnosis. Low ability to inform appropriate action.
High	Low	Good field-level detection of disease events and reporting but capacity to confirm clinical or traditional diagnoses is limited: 'We know diseases are present but we cannot easily give western names to these diseases.' Ability to inform appropriate action related to quality of local knowledge.
Low	High	Poor detection of disease events in the field. Should samples be collected, good capacity to confirm diagnosis: 'We can diagnose disease but we do not receive information or samples from the field.' Ability to inform appropriate action jeopardized by lack of samples or intelligence.
High	High	Good capacity to both detect disease events and confirm diagnoses. High ability to inform appropriate action.

The actual content of surveillance programmes varies with the objectives of the system, but some common components can be identified. The following activities are representative of components of a comprehensive surveillance system:

◆ general disease reporting – a component for the routine collection of clinical, slaughter and/or laboratory data on animal diseases, poisonings or other health-related events from public, commercial, private and community sources;

◆ outbreak detection and investigation – an activity for the recognition and investigation of significant or emerging animal health events;

◆ laboratory diagnosis – the activity of confirmation of clinical and epidemiological diagnoses of significant or emerging animal health events;

◆ targeted surveillance – an activity focused on the detection or measurement of specific diseases identified for control or eradication:

  – active surveillance – the process of searching for specific disease(s) where information collection is initiated by the veterinary services or their authorized representative;

  – sero-surveillance – objective, statistically driven, laboratory test-based surveillance for evidence of disease exposure.

A significant health event is an occurrence or incident that represents a major risk to livestock production or human health. Some significant health events, such as outbreaks of contagious bovine pleuropneumonia (CBPP), are internationally defined by the OIE. Such diseases are identified on the OIE List A as diseases of international significance to trade due to their economic impact and highly infectious nature. Other significant health events are defined nationally based on the priorities and problems of local production systems and economies. Not all of the activities mentioned above are directly relevant to community-based animal health projects, but the participation of livestock owners is the foundation and a prerequisite for all effective surveillance.

7.3   The community's role in disease surveillance

Indigenous veterinary knowledge as epidemiological intelligence

Livestock owners who are dependent on livestock for a major component of their income or subsistence place a high value on livestock information. Consequently, in many pastoral and agropastoral groups regular, even daily meetings are held to discuss the health of the livestock and decide how they should be managed. In part, decisions on livestock management are based on a constant reassessment of the animal health situation, including exposure to parasites on pasture, or proximity to diseased herds or wildlife. Livestock topics, including animal health, form a substantial part of everyday conversation in such communities.

Indigenous surveillance systems already exist and people already act on the information arising from within these systems.

Many pastoral and agropastoral groups have evolved efficient management strategies that take into account the basic epidemiology of disease and they

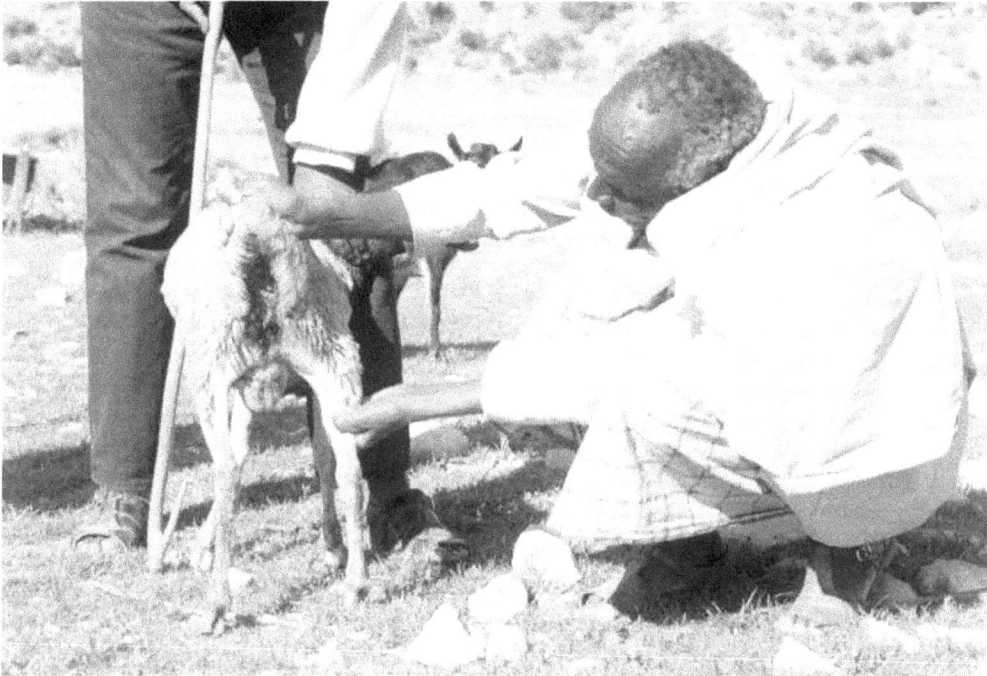

Plate 7.1 In many communities which rear livestock, animals are checked regularly for signs of disease and infestation with parasites. This herder in Somaliland is inspecting his sheep for ticks. (*Andy Catley*)

successfully reduce morbidity and mortality to tolerable levels without the use of modern pharmaceuticals. Such approaches warrant study as environmentally friendly and cost-effective methods for preventing disease. Examples are herding patterns that limit the exposure of livestock to tsetse flies and the muzzling of sheep as they pass natural water sources combined with the watering of sheep from vessels rather than at stream banks to prevent liver fluke.

Pastoralists and agropastoralists have a rich and detailed knowledge about significant health problems affecting their animals. This indigenous veterinary knowledge is based on oral tradition, shared information and the life experience of the individual. The core of this knowledge is clinical, pathological and epidemiological observations that serve to organize disease information into recognizable entities described by a traditional terminology. Although traditional disease entities and terminology often correspond to western systems, indigenous veterinary knowledge may be uniquely structured and care is required in interpreting traditional diagnosis.

Documented examples of the significance and extent of indigenous veterinary knowledge are worth considering. In some cases, modern epidemiology recognizes the importance of this traditional knowledge as hypotheses for more formal enquiries; other cases are 'missed opportunities'. In regard to reservoirs of disease, the Maasai of East Africa were the first people to recognize the association of malignant catarrhal fever (MCF) with wildebeest and, specifically, the wildebeest calving season. In fact, the Maa word for wildebeest and MCF are the same. Recognition of the importance of this observation by veterinarians led to formal experimentation that confirmed the role of the wildebeest as the reservoir for MCF. Livestock owners can be credited with the hypothesis that led to the first demonstration of an arthropod vector of disease. The famous experiments conducted by Kilbourne, a veterinarian, demonstrated that ticks were responsible for the transmission of Texas fever (babesiosis due to *Babesia bigemina*). These experiments were designed to test the cattle owner's view that ticks were the cause of the disease. In fact, cattle workers called the disease 'tick fever'. It is interesting to note that these experiments were undertaken despite the medical and veterinary professions' view that the parasite was harmless.

In addition to general knowledge on disease, livestock owners make diagnoses on a day-to-day basis and take note of trends in disease occurrence. Table 7.1 provides examples of diseases routinely recognized by pastoralists in Africa and Asia. This information is valuable intelligence for surveillance systems. Each term has a consensus definition that can be elucidated during participatory enquiry. From an epidemiological perspective, these definitions can serve as 'case definitions'.

Hence, detailed local knowledge about livestock and a well-developed diagnostic ability have evolved in pastoral and agropastoral communities. These skills and interest can provide the entry point for CAHW-based service delivery programmes to the community and within the programme; the CAHW training process builds on this local knowledge. CAHWs are key resource people for surveillance systems in remote, and not so remote areas.

Just as with animal health service delivery, rural societies are often marginalized communities that are poorly served by animal health information systems. This is unfortunate due to the high value livestock owners place on livestock information exchange. Their flexible and opportunistic systems of production in inherently risk-prone and unstable environments make accurate livestock-related intelligence a necessity.

Table 7.1 Examples of traditionally recognized disease syndromes and their equivalents in modern veterinary terminology

Culture, country	Indigenous disease name	Western equivalent
Afar, Ethiopia	*dugahabe*	rinderpest
Somali, Somalia	*sambab*	contagious bovine pleuropneumonia
Pathan, Afghanistan	*mach*	trypanosomiasis in camels due to *T. evansi*
Fulani, Cameroon	*mboru*	foot and mouth disease
Pokot, Kenya	*lokiit*	East Coast fever
Pathan, Afghanistan	*panni, garg*	fasciolosis
Caprivians, Namibia	*kankotwe*	Newcastle disease
Kavango, Namibia	*ombindu*	botulism

Integration of indigenous veterinary knowledge into surveillance systems

In order for surveillance systems to function, regular contact is required with livestock owners. In the current economic climate, this has been a constraint for a number of national veterinary services. Veterinary services' operational budgets and transport availability have been contracting over the last decades and this trend is unlikely to change. These constraints have reinforced the trend towards the development of alternative systems of delivery such as private veterinary practice and CAHWs. Just as these approaches are being integrated into service delivery systems, they need to become a core component of the information collection system.

A prerequisite for the integration of indigenous veterinary knowledge into surveillance systems is effective participatory practice. An attitude of respect for people and appreciation for the value of the farmers' knowledge are required on the part of professionals if they desire the full and open sharing of information. Thus, participatory training for veterinary staff is essential for the success of surveillance systems (see Chapters 2 and 4).

In order for a surveillance system to be sustainable, it must have a perceived benefit to the providers of data. Historically, many surveillance systems have withered due to a data 'mining' design that did not have relevance to the stakeholders who provided the data. Ultimately, district-level staff, monitors, CAHWs and livestock owners must derive benefit from the output of the surveillance system that they directly recognize as a return on the surveillance activity and workload.

For professional and subprofessional participants one benefit can take the form of written feedback reports provided on a timely basis. For CAHWs and livestock owners, oral or participatory information exchanges during the data collection process and specific activities in refresher training workshops would be effective. For the livestock owners, benefits might include appropriate rural radio programmes on diseases they have identified. One aspect of participatory research is that participants learn from the data collection process. Data collection exercises that have elements of 'participant discovery' could be valuable for ensuring the sustained interest of information providers. Emphasis should be placed on making the data collection process a benefit in itself.

The overall objectives of the surveillance system must encompass the needs of the productive sector. The specific needs may include but are not limited to:

◆ timely advice on current animal health problems through appropriate media;
◆ timely availability of correct inputs, vaccines and drugs against appropriate payment;
◆ effective treatment strategies adapted to local conditions;
◆ management innovations based on traditional approaches that minimize the impact of disease and environmental degradation.

As in any other type of community development, the experts on needs are the participants themselves. This fact suggests that focus group discussions and community dialogue with CAHWs and livestock owners are probably the best route to identifying desirable output from the surveillance system at the community level.

Community-based animal health workers and surveillance systems

Most CAHW networks provide for monthly monitoring contacts by a subprofessional – either an assistant veterinarian or production specialist under the supervision of a veterinarian – to review the activities of the CAHW and provide guidance. Ideally, each of these CAHW monitors is responsible for 12 to 15 CAHWs. Regrettably, effective monitoring is often one of the weakest aspects of CAHW networks (see Chapter 6). This is unfortunate because monitoring events are data collection opportunities for the formal veterinary sector both in terms of general disease reporting and active surveillance. The challenges CAHW programmes face in establishing effective monitoring programmes result in part from the gap between the formal and informally trained sector discussed earlier. A further constraint has been the lack of effective policy environments and the general recognition that CAHW network supervision must operate through market-based incentive programmes that reward both the CAHWs and their monitoring and support system for the activities of the network. The economic rewards must be structured so that both active CAHWs and monitors who promote and support their activity receive quantity and quality-based incentives. Feedback of accurate activity reports and surveillance data from CAHWs to monitors and the monitors to higher levels in the network should be viewed as a quality-of-service issue. Incentives for activity are usually achieved through mark-ups on the resupply of drugs (which in itself has problems with over-prescribing and diagnosis based on what treatments are available rather than on disease). Quality can be maintained by establishing certain standards as a prerequisite for continued participation in resupply of medicines, participation in refresher training activities, or provision of 'advanced' benefits at cost such as bicycles. Reporting standards can and should be a part of the explicitly defined programme standards.

In the better monitoring systems, the CAHW monitors prepare monthly or quarterly summaries of CAHW activities in their area together with comments on trends to be fed into the project reporting system. In most projects, annual summary reports and end-of-phase reports summarize global statistics. In addition to animal health information, these reports are often informative in terms of animal health economics. It should be a rewarding process to integrate these reports into a general disease reporting system.

A disease reporting system using CAHWs can also have limitations. For example, health worker activity reports may be a reflection of the availability or non-availability of selected drugs. The renewed availability of a drug after a period of absence frequently results in a flurry of treatments that may mimic an outbreak. Ideally, CAHW reporting should include a section for debriefing by the monitor where descriptive and explanatory information can be appended. As with much passive

Box 7.5 Community-based surveillance systems in action: experiences from southern Sudan

In southern Sudan, NGOs and UNICEF have worked with local administrations and communities to establish an extensive network of some 700 CAHWs, under the Operation Lifeline Sudan (OLS) Livestock Programme. In this programme, CAHWs are supported by CAHW supervisors, who are workers who receive more training than CAHWs. Also, the CAHW supervisors have usually received some formal education and are more literate than the CAHWs.

Southern Sudan is in the midst of a chronic civil war and much of the region is under rebel control. In the rebel-held areas there are no veterinary laboratories and it is not possible to transport samples to government veterinary laboratories in areas under government control. Save the Children (UK) and UNICEF have therefore set up a very basic veterinary laboratory in Lokichokio, Kenya, close to the Sudan border. This laboratory receives samples from southern Sudan by air and road, carries out examination of blood and lymph node smears, faecal samples and skin scrapings and conducts serology for brucellosis. Samples are also forwarded to laboratories in Nairobi, Kenya. This obviously presents logistical constraints, limits the type of samples that can be collected and delays reporting of results.

Based on the experience of field vets, CAHWs and CAHW supervisors, the OLS programme has been using and developing a disease monitoring and surveillance system since 1993. The system continues to evolve as the programme develops and new requirements emerge. The system uses eight types of information, as summarized in Table 7.2.

Reporting and responding to disease outbreaks

The eradication of rinderpest in southern Sudan requires comprehensive surveillance in order to detect outbreaks, define endemic foci and investigate stomatitis/enteritis cases. A system for responding to disease outbreaks has been developed and uses:

◆ standard formats for documenting radio messages from the field;
◆ standard 'outbreak forms' for documenting epidemiological information;
◆ field sampling kits;
◆ protocols for carrying out disease investigation.

Although the impetus to develop the system was rinderpest eradication, the system can cater for many other diseases and the sampling kits enable field workers to collect a range of samples. The system is aimed primarily at CAHW supervisors who conduct the preliminary investigation and complete the various written forms. However, CAHWs are not only the crucial link in the disease outbreak and response chain but they are the point of contact with livestock keepers. Therefore, it is often the CAHWs who are the first trained workers to hear about a disease problem, collect information about the problem and pass the news to their supervisor. CAHWs also assist with disease investigation because they know the local community's movements and terrain, and they can collect samples such as blood and faeces.

Procedures for responding to disease outbreaks are being institutionalized in the programme through CAHW supervisor training and refresher training. Submission of outbreak information is encouraged by ensuring that action is taken as a result of the outbreak report. This action can take the form of:

◆ a full field-level investigation by a team of vets and other workers;
◆ provision of appropriate medicines or vaccines to deal with the outbreak;
◆ in some cases, advice by programme vets on how to deal with the outbreak.

The last confirmed outbreak of rinderpest in southern Sudan was in Torit County in 1998 and was reported initially by a livestock keeper to a CAHW, who reported it to his CAHW supervisor, Quinto Asaye. Quinto followed up the report, sent a radio message to his supporting NGO, German Agro-Action, and to UNICEF, and initiated rinderpest vaccination in the affected and neighbouring villages. His radio message was acted upon by vets from GAA and UNICEF who visited the area, examined animals and collected samples. The outbreak was subsequently confirmed as rinderpest in Kenyan and UK laboratories. Additional advice and support were provided for outbreak control, but the CAHWs and the CAHW supervisors were crucial in controlling the outbreak through a systematic vaccination campaign, covering areas that were too insecure to be accessed except by local people.

Assessing vaccination efficiency

Sero-monitoring is carried out to monitor the efficiency of vaccination. Approximately 40 serum samples are collected from each cattle camp or village in order to check the rate of sero-conversion to vaccination. Samples are collected by CAHW supervisors and CAHWs, under the supervision of vets. More recently, a filter paper serum collection system has been used to ease the collection and storage of samples in the field, and transportation of samples to the laboratory. Due to operational constraints in southern Sudan, sero-monitoring is not comprehensive or based on random sampling. However, the procedure is useful for identifying major problems with vaccination or cold chain. Furthermore, developing local capacity to conduct sero-surveillance activities will assist future assessments of disease freedom.

Completing the information loop: feedback to field-level players

Feedback of information to the CAHWs and CAHW supervisors is considered to be a key aspect of the system. It helps to ensure that field-level staff know that their work is valued and that action is taken when serious problems arise. Despite this, feedback has not always been timely or comprehensive. Constraints to effective feedback have been:

- the system collects large volumes of data and the entry of data into the database is slow;
- database reporting formats have taken time to develop;
- lack of communication channels into southern Sudan;
- delayed reports from laboratories.

However, the OLS livestock co-ordination meetings that are held three times a year for UNICEF and NGO field staff and CAHW supervisors provide a good forum for presenting data collected since the last meeting. Feedback of this information from the supervisors to the CAHWs in the field is variable.

Developing an active surveillance system

The active surveillance system is still being developed, but will comprise methods for use by CAHWs and CAHW supervisors for active stomatitis/enteritis searching, part of the rinderpest eradication campaign. In the course of their normal activities, CAHWs will be asked to carry out some basic interviews and exercises to detect the presence of possible stomatitis/enteritis cases. They will report information to their supervisor who will then carry out a basic stomatitis/enteritis investigation, including sample collection. Suspicious cases will be followed up with a detailed field investigation by UNICEF/NGO vets. The CAHWs and the follow-up by CAHW supervisors will form a comprehensive network of surveillance throughout southern Sudan. This will provide an effective early warning system to detect the last cases of rinderpest and, eventually, help to demonstrate that southern Sudan has eradicated the disease.

The experience in southern Sudan demonstrates that CAHWs can play very important roles in a disease monitoring and surveillance system. In the system, CAHWs acquire information because they examine and observe livestock, interact with livestock keepers, and treat and vaccinate animals. CAHWs also:

- act as key informants in the system by providing background information on livestock populations and locations;
- assist with disease investigations and sero-monitoring.

(contributed by Bryony Jones)

disease reporting information, CAHW reports will be largely numerator data. The treatment reports will reflect the cases whose owners requested and accepted to pay for treatment, but not all cases observed. Further, unless some effort is made to build population size into the reporting system, the data will not be suitable for estimating epidemiological rates or proportions such as attack rates, incidence or prevalence. Efforts could be made to define the population size served by the CAHW and use this figure as a denominator in rate estimation. This approach would probably be feasible

Table 7.2 Components of Operation Lifeline Sudan Livestock Programme community-based surveillance system, southern Sudan

Type of data/activity	Method for field-level data collection	Method for documenting information at field level	Management of information at central, programme level and feedback	Remarks
Background information				
Maps, livestock populations, seasonal movements, trade routes, raiding routes	Participatory mapping by NGO vets and supervisors with key informants including CAHWs	One-off events and maps documented. Updates as situations alter (e.g. displacement of communities)	UNICEF transfers data into mapping software. Reports and copies of maps provided on demand	Transfer to mapping programme in early stages
Livestock population figures	Estimates by geographical area and community structure by supervisors and NGO vets, with key informants including CAHWs	Livestock census forms used by NGOs, annually	UNICEF transfers data to spreadsheet. Disseminated at quarterly livestock coordination meetings (LCM) and to NGOs	Quality of estimates variable, system still being improved
Routine CAHW activities and rinderpest control				
Livestock treatment figures	Monthly pictorial monitoring forms completed by CAHWs	Data from CAHW forms summarized by CAHW supervisors each month	UNICEF transfers data to database. Reports provided at LCM and to NGOs on demand	
Vaccination figures	Punchcards used by CAHWs	Summarized each month by CAHW supervisors	UNICEF transfers data to database. Reports provided at LCM and to NGOs on demand	
Sero-monitoring	Serum collection (vacutainers or filter papers) by teams of NGO vets, CAHW supervisors and CAHWs	Sero-monitoring forms completed by NGO vets or CAHW supervisors	Laboratory report (Kenya or overseas) copied to NGO vets/CAHW supervisors; results summarized and presented to LCM	Slow reporting from labs – negative effect on future sample collection
Disease outbreaks				
Disease outbreak reporting	Verbal reports by CAHWs and livestock owners	Outbreak report forms used to document information for radio message to CAHW supervisors, NGO vets	Information recorded in Outbreak Report Register. Advice, field investigation, appropriate medicine/vaccine, summary report to LCMs	Details passed to PACE, Nairobi
Disease outbreak investigation	Field-level veterinary investigation conducted by UNICEF/NGO vets assisted by CAHW supervisors and CAHWs	Investigation report and laboratory submission form completed by UNICEF/NGO vet	Results entered into Outbreak Report Register with laboratory results. Summary report to LCMs; laboratory report to CAHW supervisor	Details passed to PACE, Nairobi
Active surveillance	Disease searching in cattle camps and villages; PRA methods used by vets with CAHWs and CAHW supervisors	Active surveillance forms for use by CAHW supervisors, NGO vets	UNICEF vets collect and react to information. Summarized reports for LCMs, with mapping of information	This system is in the planning stage

256

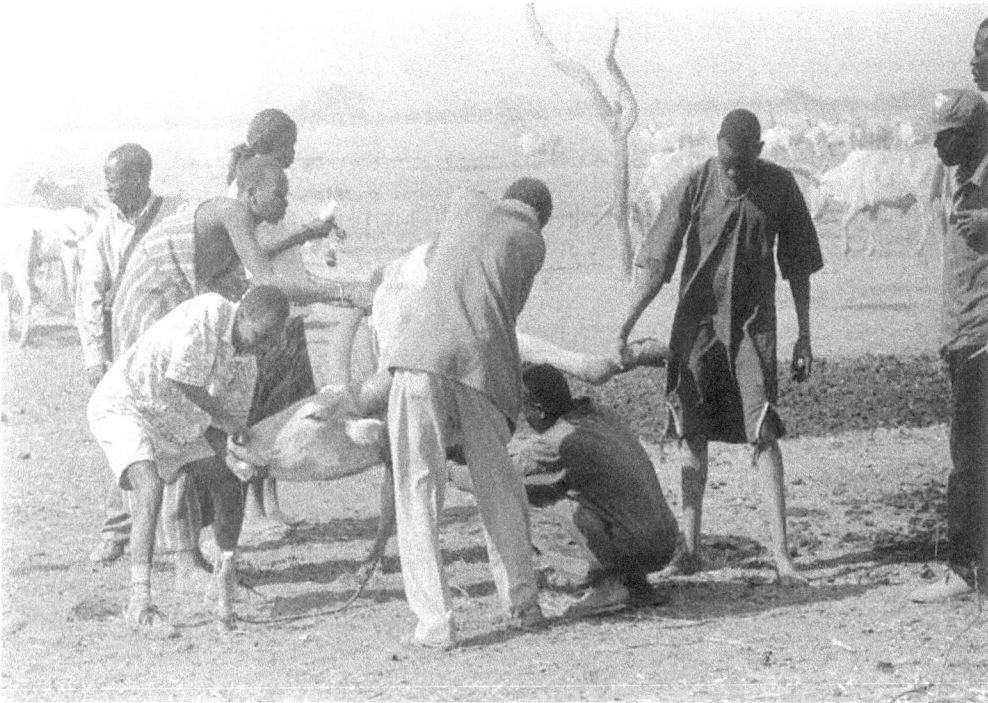

Plate 7.2 CAHWs can be useful for sample collection. They may need extra training to collect blood or faeces samples. These workers in southern Sudan are collecting samples under the supervision of a veterinarian. (*Andy Catley*)

in sedentary systems, but might have applicability in pastoral systems with more rigid social structures.

These concerns regarding use of CAHW record keeping systems in surveillance are not fundamentally different from disease reporting systems based on the clinical activities of private and public veterinarians. What these systems lack in specificity and representativeness, they make up for in their sensitivity and timeliness. Just as was described for overall national surveillance systems, CAHW reporting is only one piece of an effective surveillance system. It is key epidemiological intelligence that must be interpreted in the context of the overall picture.

Where CAHW networks with record systems are in place, this information is not routinely reaching the national surveillance framework. There are various possible reasons for this.

◆ In many cases, CAHW networks are implemented by separate lines within the government, projects or non-government organizations (NGOs). Even with the best efforts on all sides, institutional barriers can be difficult to bridge. One approach to promoting effective communication and collaboration is participatory leadership forums where representatives of the various government, project and NGO-based programmes come together to establish common goals and approaches through dialogue. In addition, field visits to expose decision makers and surveillance workers to the benefits of community-based work that include surveillance activities would be an appropriate approach as well.

◆ Even when CAHWs are identifying serious disease outbreaks, their reports may not be heard, or may get lost within other more routine monitoring information.

In the case of disease outbreaks, a typical CAHW training course includes training in history taking and basic clinical examination of sick livestock. Therefore, CAHWs should be able to obtain useful information on disease outbreaks that can be passed on to formal veterinary workers. Such information does not necessarily have to be written down by the CAHW, who might be illiterate, but can be passed verbally to the monitor.

◆ When a CAHW reports the occurrence of a serious disease outbreak, the monitor should report this event separately from the routine monitoring mentioned above. It is usually advisable for the monitor to investigate the event using a combination of participatory techniques and conventional disease investigation and sampling procedures (see later in this chapter). Such an approach requires the monitor to collect the testimony of several livestock owners and, if possible, inspect some cases. If the disease reported is subject to an official eradication or control programme, such as rinderpest or CBPP, the monitor should comply with any special reporting requirements. In some countries, special report registries exist for rinderpest and all livestock owner

---

Box 7.6 Community animal health workers as reporters of disease outbreaks

There are examples of field-level reports from CAHWs providing the first indication of important disease outbreaks. In some cases, the diseases in question were of major international importance. For example:

◆ In Karamoja, Uganda, in 1994 and Eastern Equatoria, southern Sudan, in 1998, CAHWs provided the first news of rinderpest outbreaks to their supervisors. This information was then transmitted to programme veterinarians who were able to visit the areas in question, collect samples and confirm the presence of rinderpest. This unsolicited action of CAHWs in remote areas could play a crucial role in identifying the remaining foci of rinderpest in the final stages of eradication programmes.

◆ In the Afar region of Ethiopia, a CAHW provided the first indication that a mysterious respiratory disease was affecting camels in the area. This disease was later to spread through Ethiopia, Somalia and northern Kenya.

and CAHW reports should be recorded in these registries with the results of follow-up. If triangulation supports the nature of the report, the monitor, or the concerned CAHWs, should immediately inform district authorities and request a disease investigation.

As examples, CAHWs have made key unsolicited reports that led to the detection of rinderpest in Uganda and southern Sudan on different occasions. They also made an early report of an emerging epidemic of respiratory disease in camels that subsequently swept East Africa. This information was beyond value, but someone had to be listening in order for the benefit of the information to be captured.

◆ Even where CAHWs and livestock keepers are active in reporting outbreaks of disease, they do not always receive the attention they merit. This is an unfortunate state of affairs, but highlights the communication gap between formally trained service providers – whether public or private – and traditional livestock owners. In addition to the attitudinal issues stressed above, the long-term solution includes increased empowerment of the consumers of services through fee-for-service approaches that minimize the employment entitlement and lack of accountability of tax-funded services.

In countries that have extensive CAHW networks, it would be useful for a representative of the national surveillance staff to become involved in the training and monitoring of CAHWs, at least on a part-time basis. This will give headquarters staff direct experience with the programme and make them better able to take advantage of the information derived from CAHWs.

◆ Disease reports from the field may be misinterpreted through misunderstanding of local usage of disease terms. CAHW programmes normally construct a lexicon of disease terms and these documents should be made generally available. National surveillance staff should have an inventory of documents covering the ethnoveterinary knowledge (EVK) of all communities in the country. They actually serve as the case definitions for reporting purposes in the specific communities where they were constructed. In the event that lexicons are not available from all major livestock owning cultures, surveillance staff should conduct participatory surveys to complete the gaps and, when necessary, use conventional veterinary investigation methods to relate local disease terminology to western terminology.

One point where data quality may become compromised is in the translation process. In one example, subgroups in one ethnic community used terms from a traditionally defined category referring to clostridial disease in contrary senses. The result was that farmers sometimes reported anthrax and the veterinary services turned up with blackleg vaccine, or vice versa. Asking a few questions on symptoms would have cleared up the discrepancy. Another example of this type of confusion occurs when animal health staff translate a broad category of disease as due to only one specific agent contained in that class. An example from the Fulße of Burkina Faso is *wilseré*. This disease concept includes, but is not limited to, trypanosomiasis. Animal health personnel frequently misunderstand the term and automatically dispense trypanocidal drugs in response to a report. Misinterpretations could lead to substantial errors or over-reporting in a surveillance system. In order for data auditing to be possible, it is important that the reporting process retain the EVK diagnosis and the ethnic origin of the report.

a. Developing forms for disease reporting

Most CAHW training programmes incorporate some form of record keeping system. These systems are generally designed to provide a programme-monitoring tool, a means of professional supervision of CAHWs and to help CAHWs keep track of their finances. Record books usually tally the types of treatments provided and moneys received. Record books often serve a useful training function as a memory aid by summarizing disease, species, drug and dosage in simple charts. Examples of recording formats are provided in Chapter 6.

Record keeping systems can be designed for literate or non-literate programmes, as appropriate to local conditions. Beware of building a literacy requirement into the programme. As already mentioned in Chapters 2 and 4, literate candidates can be overqualified 'job seekers' with little long-term commitment or interest in being a CAHW. Non-literate systems are largely pictographic and symbol-based. Simple symbols such as clouds and moons that represent years (rainy seasons) and months, respectively, are effective for indicating age, time of year and treatment intervals. Sketches of animals can depict the species and class of animals treated, and drawings of syringes with levels indicated, boluses or tablets are used to record dosages. Finally, specific symbols can be developed for various amounts of money. When project resources are limited, a great deal can be achieved using simple but clear black and white pictures. In most communities there are local artists who can draw pictures that illustrate local conditions, types of animals and diseases.

For projects with access to modern computer equipment, image scanners have greatly eased the production of high-quality, illustrated reporting forms. For example, very accurate images of medicine labels can be added to forms. In addition, low-cost libraries of copyright-free livestock and animal health images are now available which contain pictures of livestock types, disease signs, basic veterinary equipment and veterinary medicines (see Chapter 4).

Regardless of how the disease reporting forms are produced, it is important to try to develop and test the forms with the CAHWs who will use them. For example, during CAHW refresher training the trainees could be provided with draft forms and asked to comment on the clarity and ease of use of the forms.

b. Incentives for disease reporting

Some people have suggested that incentives for CAHWs may be necessary to ensure successful routine data and sample collection. This is not an entirely new concept – physicians in Britain are paid a minimal fee for the completion of measles and pertussis reporting forms to cover the time and effort required. It is recognized that both

CAHWs and monitors require incentives in order for community-based programmes to be sustainable and that incentives related to the quantity and quality of work are the most effective.

In regard to treatment, it has been found that sustainable incentives can only come from the beneficiaries themselves. However, in regard to surveillance, it is unlikely that livestock owners will pay to provide information or allow sampling. Government could pay an incentive to CAHWs, but this is unlikely to be sustainable on a routine basis and could lead to confusion about who is the CAHW's real employer and reinforce the psychology of dependence. It may be sustainable for government to pay an incentive to the monitor for routine, good-quality reporting. It is challenging to envision how the incentive could be linked to the quality and quantity of reporting. One method already suggested is to establish a minimum standard of reporting for continued participation in the resupply network. A second possibility would be a quarterly bonus for individuals who meet their reporting standard consistently. Ideally, the bonus would be a percentage multiplier times the cash volume for the month – thus linking quantity and quality intimately.

Experience from the field

In northern Karamoja, Uganda, a national epidemiological project paid CAHWs to assist in the collection of about 4000 serum samples with great detriment to the long-term sustainability of the programme. After the experience, the CAHWs in question felt entitled to payments in regard to any request. Another serological study in Karamoja that was more directly associated with the CAHW programme collected approximately 3000 samples during the same time period without provision of any payment. This second study team invested time in discussing the purpose and benefits of the study with participants and collected a significant amount of ancillary information to support the serological study using participatory techniques – a process that enhances the participants' self-awareness. Both studies met their immediate objectives. The first study disrupted the main focus and long-term sustainability of the programme by reinforcing the psychology of dependency by paying people to do what was essentially a personal responsibility to the community. The rumour quickly spread that CAHWs were on the government payroll and 'double-dipping' when they requested payment from their clients for medicines. The second study reinforced the concepts of community employment and self-reliance by asking for and obtaining the time and energy of the participants in support of community objectives. Ultimately, the results of the second study were used to restructure and strengthen the sustainability of the CAHW programme through better targeting of activities, fostering a sense of self-reliance and tailoring incentives to local needs.

It would be unreasonable to expect individuals to sustain work on targeted studies without incentives. However, the issue of paid incentives needs to be approached with caution. The risks are great. With sufficient community dialogue and depending on the society, the role and purpose of specific incentives paid by institutions can be satisfactorily defined so as not to endanger the sustainability of the programme. However, it would be better to identify non-cash incentives for routine sampling and reporting. The best incentive would be a prompt diagnostic report and the availability of an appropriate intervention when warranted. Confidence in the public services to respond is probably what is really lacking.

The CAHW is working within the context of the community where peer pressure as well as peer recognition are key driving forces. A rinderpest report once began through a letter from a CAHW's father calling his son home to help with the outbreak. The CAHW clearly took great pride in being asked and able to mobilize assistance for his community on such a significant problem. The CAHW had to persist in his reporting efforts for several weeks before he was heard and only highly emotive forces could have enabled him to overcome the disbelief, inertia and complacency he encountered along the way.

Private, community-based veterinary practice

The concept of community-based veterinary practice – the implementation of a veterinary practice through a CAHW network – has been identified and tested as a solution to the challenge of animal health service delivery in remote areas. In this approach, a private veterinarian together with an institution experienced in the establishment of CAHW networks team up to build the system, maintained and supervised by the private veterinarian. Commercially, the CAHW network functions as a service pyramid with the community workers forming the base, subprofessional monitors facilitating hands-on training and day-to-day supervision and a veterinary professional responsible for the overall management and supervision. Inputs are passed down the pyramid and cash to cover costs plus incentives or service fees flow up. The overall activity of the community-based practice is determined in the same manner as a CAHW programme. It is arrived at through the participatory appraisal (PA) and community dialogue process and is based upon community needs tempered by economical feasibility. When this model was tested in Salamat, Chad, a veterinarian who was previously unknown to the community was able to rapidly integrate his practice into local society and build a strong rapport with livestock owners. By investing in the CAHW network, the veterinarian communicated to the community that he was seeking to build a mutually beneficial relationship. This veterinary practice also benefited from a state vaccination contract to provide rinderpest vaccination with heat-stable vaccine delivered by the CAHWs. The practice rapidly generated good vaccination coverage and was highly successful at collecting a cost-sharing fee of CFAfr50 per vaccination from the livestock owners. A predefined portion of this fee was retained by the CAHW and his monitor with the balance paid to the veterinarian. Thus, all levels received incentives (also see Chapter 3).

An extension of this community practice can be envisioned where the veterinarian is contracted to provide additional services for the remote area. Certainly, collection of surveillance information could be remunerated through a contractual arrangement. The contract would need to define the standards of surveillance and reporting methods, and also specify the rewards and penalties for non-compliance. In the case of the community-based practice, the managing veterinarian could pay out bonuses for good-quality reporting by CAHWs and monitors. In addition, the system could reward the early detection of epizootic disease targeted for national or regional control.

Biological sample collection methods for use by CAHWs

Remote communities provide additional challenges in terms of the confirmation of diagnoses because travel to the outbreak site may be difficult and many common diagnostic processes routinely use samples collected and stored on ice. As a result, disease reports from remote areas are often unconfirmed and dismissed as non-specific rumours. It is important to bear in mind that achieving specificity in surveillance in remote areas is not always feasible and that animal health authorities must accept less specificity in data from such areas or risk a severely biased assessment of the national health situation.

There are, however, a variety of robust sampling methods for the collection of diagnostic material in remote areas that do not require refrigeration or coolant. Use of 'Appropriate Technology' in sample collection and diagnoses can greatly enhance the specificity of surveillance information from remote areas, although it will never fully eliminate the constraint of remoteness. Use of these techniques requires diagnosticians and surveillance experts to 'think outside the box' and place themselves in the shoes of remote farmers and the animal workers of all descriptions that serve livestock owners in such areas. As we shall see, the techniques that use appropriate sampling technology are either 'state of the art' or classic scientific standbys. In both cases, they are high-quality science. Examples of various sample collection methods are provided in Box 7.7.

Box 7.7 Robust sampling methods for use by CAHWs

Collection in formalin

Collection of tissues or faeces in formalin is a robust method of sample collection that allows specific diagnoses to be made:

◆ Tissues can be processed histologically and examined by a pathologist. Small pieces of diseased tissue 1 cm square should be placed in 10 per cent buffered formalin; use at least 20 times the volume of formalin for each sample. Malignant catarrhal fever can be diagnosed using this method.

◆ Formalin-fixed tissues can be used for immunohistological diagnosis or in situ hybridization with genetic probes. These techniques can be performed on fixed samples collected months or even years previously. Research has shown that even moderately autolysed samples can be diagnostic. It is of value to collect tissues from carcasses up to 24 hours old. This technique is most useful when a particular disease

---

or set of diseases is targeted for study and confirmation. Prior to implementing a sampling scheme, laboratories need to be identified that are both willing and capable to carry out the desired testing. Although the testing is relatively simple, basic histological preparation capabilities (sectioning and staining) are not always present at the national level. After seven days in 10 per cent buffered formalin, samples can and should be transferred to phosphate-buffered saline or normal saline. Provided the host and destination countries agree, samples can be mailed to appropriate laboratories for testing – formalin-fixed tissues are stable and non-infectious. The samples should be small in quantity and well-sealed in unbreakable laboratory-grade containers obtained from a scientific supply source. A wide range of viral, bacterial and parasitic diseases such as rinderpest, peste des petits ruminants, or hog cholera or heartwater can be diagnosed using this method provided the laboratory has a specific antibody for the disease of interest.

◆ It is also possible to extract genetic material from formalin-fixed tissues for polymerase chain reaction (PCR) analysis. In PCR, small quantities of genetic material are amplified enzymatically for identification by genetic probes or sequencing. Techniques for the diagnosis of most major animal disease have been described in the literature and PCR-based diagnosis is rapidly becoming the diagnostic standard. This technique can be readily applied to viral, bacterial and parasitic diseases such as bluetongue, foot and mouth disease, CBPP or East Coast fever.

◆ Faeces that have been fixed in formalin can be used for worm eggs counts and detection of fluke eggs. Approximately 3 g of faeces is placed in around 20 ml of 10 per cent formalin and thoroughly mixed. The formalin prevents the parasite eggs hatching.

Collection of samples in alcohol (70 per cent ethanol)

◆ Parasites such as ticks, flies, lice, gut worms and flukes can be preserved in 70 per cent alcohol.

◆ Lice can be detected from hair samples plucked from infected animals.

◆ Tissue samples in 70 per cent ethanol are also suitable for PCR diagnosis.

Collection of dried samples

◆ CAHWs can prepare blood smears that are air-dried and wrapped in tissue paper. Care must be taken to protect the slides from flies during drying or the entire sample can 'disappear' in a matter of minutes. These samples are useful for the diagnosis of various haemoparasitic and some bacterial infections.

◆ Sera can be blotted and dried on filter paper and then placed in plastic bags. Once in the lab, the samples can be eluted with buffers and tested serologically for the presence of infectious agents. Although the drying process undoubtedly reduces the sensitivity of the isolation process, isolation or antigen detection is diagnostic. Diseases that can be diagnosed using this method include Newcastle disease.

Sample collection activities can be incorporated in CAHW programmes as supporting evidence for reports or as part of targeted surveillance programmes. The materials can be distributed and incorporated in the training process. Prior to introduction of sample collection, the programme implementers should be sure to identify a reasonable level of laboratory support that will actually be willing to test samples in a timely fashion. Placing emphasis on sample collection will create an expectation of results. Failure to provide feedback on collected samples may disillusion participants at a critical juncture and endanger more basic network activities.

Guidance should also be given on what and how frequently to sample. Some diseases are easily diagnosed from specific tissues or types of samples collected at specific times. If a CAHW programme identifies clinical problems that merit laboratory back-up, appropriate materials to be collected should be described in the training. Also, it is usually the case that only a few representative cases at a particular stage in the disease process need to be sampled. This again varies by disease. For viral diseases, it is often early or acute cases that are the best candidates for sampling. For some haemoparasitic diseases, advanced chronic cases are probably more usefully sampled.

CAHWs should also be trained in what not to sample. Sampling certain zoonotic diseases (diseases transmitted from animals to humans) requires special precautions. Rabies and anthrax are two good examples. In some areas these diseases

Using to CAHWs to prepare samples

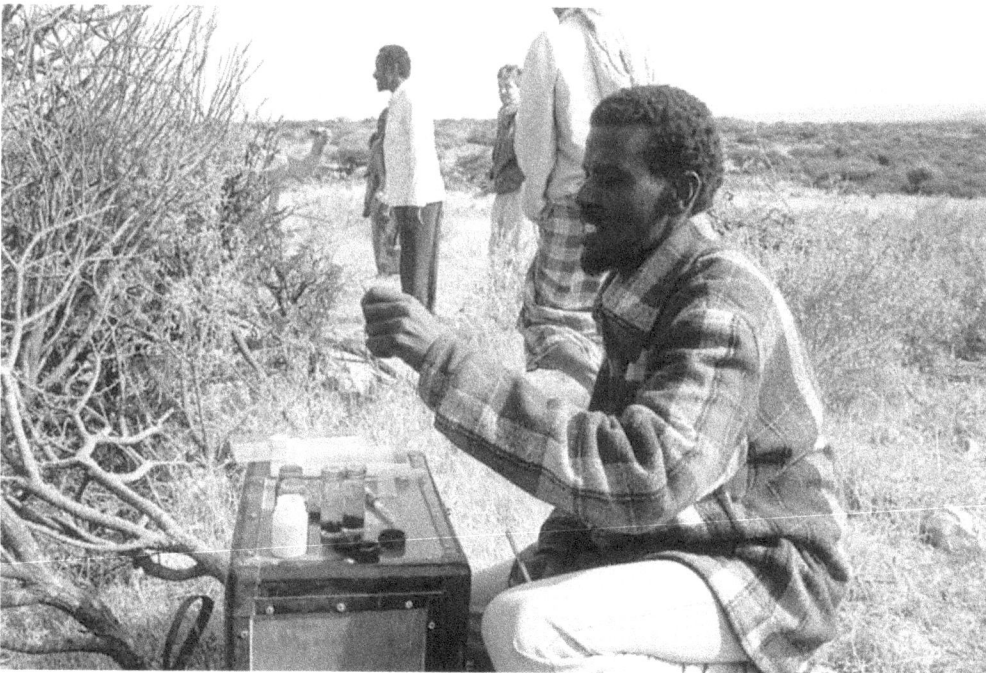

Plate 7.3 A CAHW in Somaliland assists with an investigation into trypanosomiasis in camels by collecting blood samples and preparing smears. (*Andy Catley*)

265

are well-known and the risks a matter of common knowledge, whereas in other areas the risks of handling carcasses are not understood. Training courses should, however, explicitly state that, if these diseases are suspected, professional assistance should be sought.

The availability and adoption of cold chain independent sampling techniques should enhance epidemiological surveillance in remote areas. One note of caution is perhaps necessary. Inappropriate dependence on laboratory data can lead to the failure to respond to obvious disease situations. As has been mentioned, epidemiological surveillance is an intelligence-gathering activity designed to generate best-bet scenarios upon which to base animal health interventions. The absence of laboratory confirmation does not justify the failure to recognize or respond to significant animal health events in remote areas detected by prudent participatory, clinical or epidemiological investigations.

7.4   Active surveillance and participatory disease searching

Definitions, roles and approaches

Active surveillance implies that the surveillance system initiates the data collection activity rather than passively waiting for reporters to send in a form and so on. There is no strict dividing line between active and passive surveillance. Many activities have both active and passive elements. Disease searching is a surveillance activity where trained personnel undertake investigations to try to locate cases or outbreaks of a specific disease. Disease searches are usually performed as part of an eradication programme. Disease searching methodologies include clinical searches, questionnaire surveys and participatory methods. In eradication campaigns, disease searches can be used to delineate the extent of endemic and epidemic areas or to assist in the verification of eradication of the disease from an area. Participatory disease investigations are responses to outbreaks or outbreak reports that rely on participatory methods to collect information on an outbreak, identify sources and trace outbreaks forward for sample collection.

Participatory disease searches (PDS) are probably the most powerful tool available for active surveillance. Participatory search is a sensitive and rapid intelligence-gathering activity for the detection and investigation of animal health events. Clinical surveys or questionnaire surveys, on the other hand, can be based on random sampling and can be analysed statistically. In reality, however, animal health questionnaire surveys in remote areas often use non-random sampling such as convenience sampling because of limited household or population data, or logistical constraints and are analysed statistically regardless of these limitations. Although statistical significance is a useful trait, the real function of disease searching in the surveillance system is to enhance sensitivity. It is the function of other components of the system, such as serosurveillance, to make statistically valid inferences about the population.

Participatory disease searches are an appropriate response to livestock owner reports of epidemic disease or the results of CAHW surveillance programmes. As such, disease searches are an important non-monetary reward to communities and CAHWs for participation in disease reporting and surveillance systems. It demonstrates that their information and investment in surveillance result in action. It is also appropriate to view government veterinary services and private veterinarians as stakeholders and customers in community animal health programmes, in addition to their other roles. The newly emerging veterinary services will be geared towards surveillance and coordination of animal health programmes. Community animal health programmes are standing networks of key informants ready for more formal epidemiological enquiry. It is important that professional services, whether public or private, perceive the power of such a resource and encourage and support its development.

How to conduct participatory disease searches

A PDS usually begins from a report or suspicion of an outbreak in an area. The first step is to identify what community or communities live in the area, either permanently or temporarily. Next, in common with other types of participatory systems of enquiry, consult secondary sources, if any are available, regarding the community and its livestock. This secondary data might include any significant reports, literature or maps related to the local community's structure, decision-making processes, livestock keeping and agricultural practices, or animal health situation. For epidemiological issues, mobility, trade and interactions with other communities can be valuable background information for assessment of risks. These will be explored in greater detail with the livestock owners themselves and the unavailability of background information should not prohibit the undertaking of participatory work. In fact, it highlights the need to get to work, so do not worry. It is also useful to seek out livestock or other workers who have been involved in projects or other activities in the area of interest. Often these people will have the required secondary sources readily available.

The next step is to use participatory methods in order to understand local perceptions of the animal health situation in the area. These methods include semi-structured interviews (SSIs), focus group discussions and visualization methods such as mapping. Clinical and post-mortem examinations are also an excellent opportunity for probing knowledge, issues and terminology. In order to use these methods effectively, training in PA will be helpful if courses are available (see Chapter 2). Such training helps to ensure that investigators develop skills such as active listening and pay attention to appropriate, respectful behaviour when interacting with livestock keepers. In addition, participatory enquiry requires the use of both open questions (non-directed questions using words such as 'why', 'who', 'what', 'where', 'when', 'how') and probing questions (which may need to be directed). The fluent and creative use of these types of questions is central to PDS, but requires practice and is greatly helped by familiarity with the secondary data.

Participatory disease searches rely on key informants and CAHWs are probably the most critical key informants available on local animal health issues. Active CAHWs are seeing cases on a daily basis and keeping abreast of the local news. Depending on community interactions, CAHWs may travel substantial distances to observe or assist at important outbreaks within the greater society.

Community animal health workers can also act as guides or entry points to the community. They can assist in organizing focus group discussions and SSIs with livestock keepers in order to identify the diseases of interest in the area, and to gather the local history of the disease under investigation. It is important that the subject of the investigation, if it is a specific disease, is not communicated to the community or the CAHW before completion of the basic data collection process. This is to avoid bias in the responses. An example of a PDS checklist is provided in Box 7.8. This process can be adapted to several diseases, as long as the diseases are identified by livestock keepers and outbreaks are perceived as significant events.

In PDS, CAHWs can be interviewed and probed for details on the occurrence of disease, epidemiological factors and the symptoms or severity of outbreaks. Their basic training in western concepts provides a slightly different perspective that can

---

Box 7.8 A checklist for a participatory rinderpest disease search

Avoid mentioning rinderpest before the cattle owners do.

1. Introduce the appraisal team as an animal health appraisal.
2. Identify the respondents and establish if they own cattle.
3. Establish their main herding locations (mapping).
4. What are the current cattle disease problems in their herd? If tearing or diarrhoea are mentioned, explore these syndromes in detail.
5. What are the current cattle disease problems in the area?
6. Historically, what are the most important disease problems of cattle? Invariably rinderpest is mentioned in the response to this question if the cattle owners have experienced outbreaks in the last two decades. Frequently it will be the first disease mentioned.
7. Have they personally seen rinderpest in their lifetimes? What does it look like?
8. When was the last time their cattle were affected by rinderpest? Where? Where did it come from?

As warranted, further probing questions can be added to cross-check reports made in other interviews, further define cattle movements which may affect the epidemiology of the disease, or to contrast current outbreaks with previous outbreaks in regard to the severity of disease.

both add and detract from the information communicated. In some cases, their training assists them to recognize the details of interest, however the risk is that they will communicate their 'book learning' rather than what they actually observed.

Experience from the field

A CAHW in Gedo region, Somalia, was probed in 1996 about a mild disease that was characterized by tearing and occasional oral erosions and diarrhoea. His responses reflected careful observation of the syndrome and consideration of the diagnosis. The real value of the interview was in identifying subtle characteristics of the field syndrome that either fit or did not fit with a diagnosis of rinderpest. The CAHW declined to voluntarily categorize the disease. When pressed at the end of the interview, he stated that the balance of information suggested the disease was not shifow *(rinderpest) since it did not kill. This response reflected the fact that high mortality was part of the traditional case definitions of rinderpest used in the area. This interview demonstrated the importance of understanding local disease terminology as case definitions and the need to understand traditional diagnostic criteria in order to interpret reports.*

Participatory analysis is another component of participatory disease searches where the CAHWs play a major part. Participatory analysis occurs after the team has identified and refined hypotheses. A focus group can be asked to consider the hypotheses and discuss/debate their relevance to their perceptions of the community situation. This is a further tool to refine and test the accuracy of hypotheses. The training, accessibility, local knowledge and confidence of CAHWs make them useful sounding boards.

Assessing cases: ante- and post-mortem examination of animals and sample collection

In PDS and participatory epidemiology in general, ante- and post-mortem examinations as well as biological sampling serve as an additional tool available for triangulation of participant information. The approach is somewhat different from other epidemiological sampling procedures in that the sampling is purposively directed; it is 'key sampling' to support or refute hypotheses derived from participant-provided data.

In the case of PDS, the investigation should continue until current cases are detected for clinical or post-mortem examination and sampling. Although SSIs are best conducted before examination, the participatory process should continue during examination. If the main SSI is conducted at the same time as examination of animals, it is difficult to compare the oral information with the physical evidence as two separate forms of information in the triangulation process. The examination and the actions of the investigator will influence participants' responses and could potentially be highly leading. The best process, should time permit, is to collect the knowledge, views and opinions of the livestock owners prior to physical investigations and then to continue

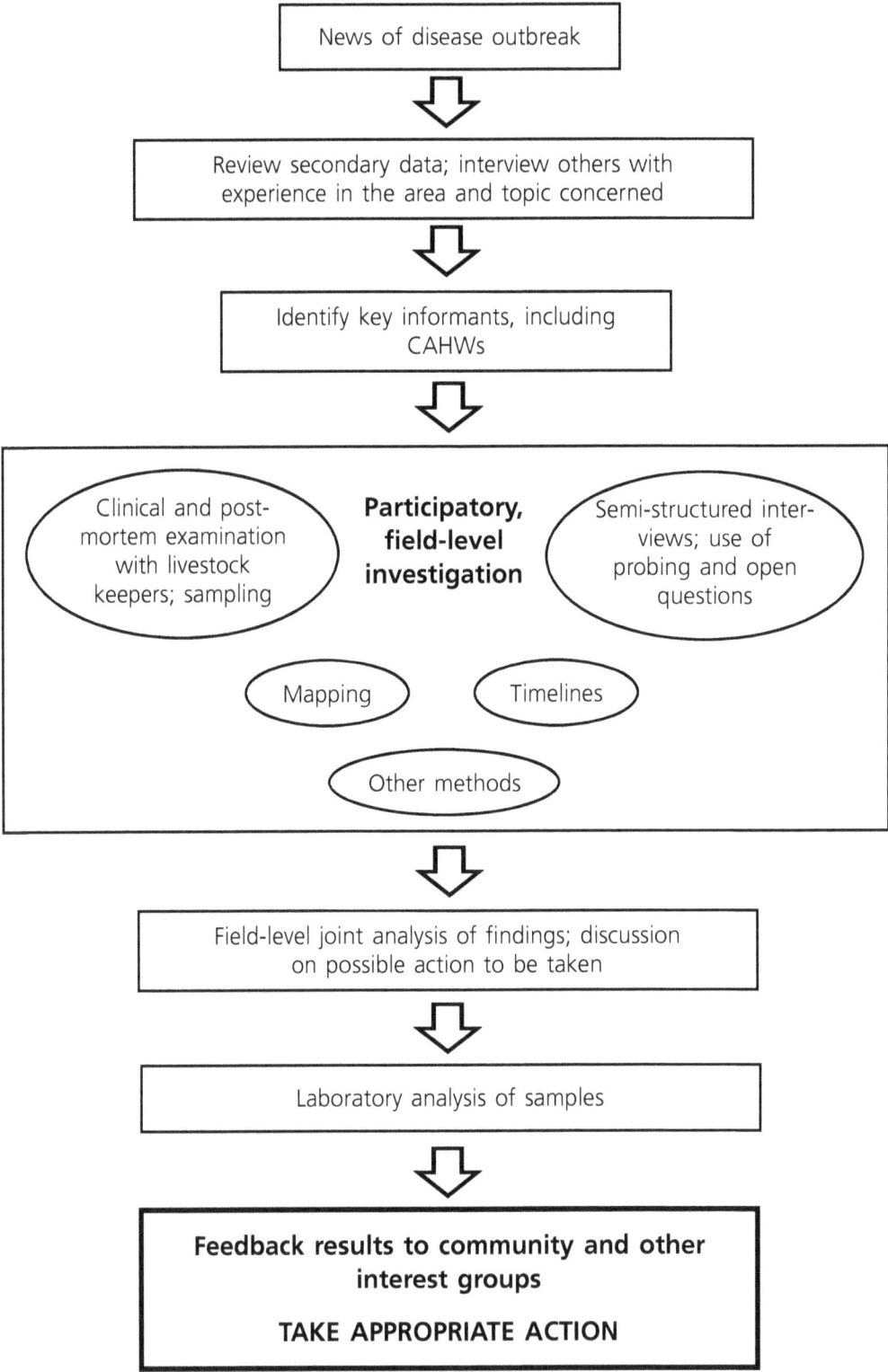

Figure 7.1 Key activities in participatory disease searching

probing the participants as physical and post-mortem exams are ongoing. It may be that examinations are not possible due to time or local security constraints. In these instances, CAHWs can be provided with suitable sampling materials with arrangements for submission of samples through monitors. As discussed above, appropriate sampling materials include filter paper for sera, formalin for tissues, or ethyl alcohol. As these investigations often take place in remote areas, the investigating team should also consider using these methods as back-up systems for sampling. Most field epidemiologists working in remote areas can identify with the frustration of finding cases just as the ice ran out or watching their samples deteriorate while searching for car parts.

Incentives for CAHWs in active surveillance and PDS

An approach that warrants further experimentation is the payment of rewards for reports leading to the identification of cases of a disease subject to control or eradication. This approach was successfully applied in the eradication of smallpox and, in fact, a reward is still in place for a report of a smallpox case leading to a confirmed diagnosis. This approach has the advantage that it is linked to the quality and quantity of information. It was tested in an animal health context as part of the Pan African Rinderpest Campaign to verify the eradication of rinderpest from the Afar region of Ethiopia. A reward of Birr100 was offered to any CAHW who could locate a case of rinderpest. Despite substantial interest on the part of CAHWs, no reports were made. This contributed to the verification of rinderpest eradication from the area and reinforced the decision to cease vaccination.

Rewards should be paid only for reports that lead to confirmed diagnosis. In order for rewards to work in all situations, all parts of the reporting chain probably require an incentive. The reward should be split between the reporting CAHW or livestock owner, the field staff responsible for transmitting the report and carrying out

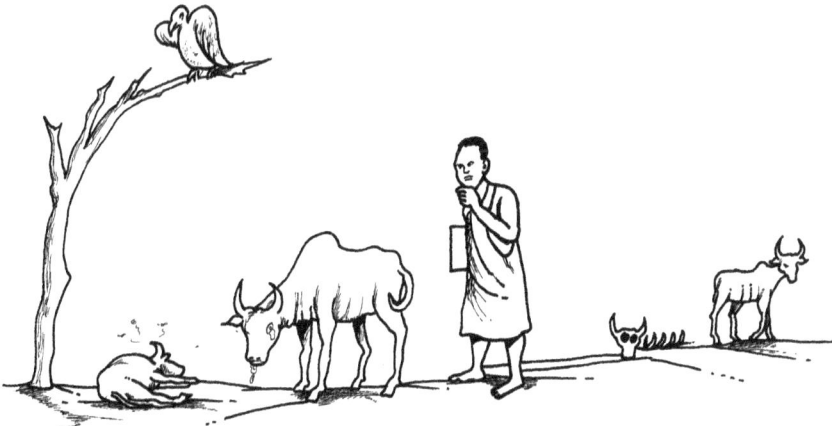

'This looks like rinderpest. I'll take some samples and carry them to the doctor in town – perhaps I'll get a reward!

the initial investigation, as well as the team responsible for confirmation of diagnosis. This is due to the fact that local disincentives to report and investigate selected diseases occur. Simple jealousy or fear can derail a professional investigation. Thus, do not assume that any level of the reporting and investigation chain can be left out. Some have suggested that unscrupulous professionals that have access to infectious material could abuse rewards. Involving several levels in the reward process would help to ensure honesty. Further, with the advent of routine molecular epidemiology, trace-back of isolates can be so precise that identification of such acts would be straightforward.

7.5 Summary

This section has suggested some roles for CAHWs in surveillance and reporting systems. The main concepts to bear in mind are as follows:

- Livestock-owning communities often have very well-developed existing veterinary knowledge and these knowledge systems are the basis of the case definitions used by livestock keepers for reporting purposes. Surveillance systems require an adequate understanding of existing veterinary knowledge in order to interpret reports.
- Animal health surveillance is one of the primary functions co-ordinated by public animal health services and one that requires the collaboration of all stakeholders in animal health services – livestock keepers, community-based animal healthcare networks, all levels of animal health workers including vets, and industry.
- The livestock keeper is the primary source for all surveillance information. Effective interaction and communication with livestock keepers is essential to the sensitivity of surveillance.
- CAHWs are ideal intermediaries for the collection of surveillance information in remote and not so remote areas. This includes both routine reporting and key intelligence in regard to outbreak investigations.
- Veterinarians and other animal health workers have the important role of translating local knowledge into a definite diagnosis, then facilitating an appropriate course of action.
- Inexpensive, cold chain independent sample collection and transport methods are available for use in biological sampling of sera, blood and tissues in remote areas.
- Community animal health programmes that incorporate disease reporting and surveillance functions should insure that the system provides real benefits to the participating communities and CAHWs. Incentives need to be identified to sustain activities. They should be linked to the quantity and quality of information provided.

The rules of the game and how to influence policy

8

John Young and John Woodford

CONTENTS

8.1 Introduction

Brexy Roring is a licensed Tonkeswan (CAHW) working in Minahasa District in Indonesia. Although he dropped out of his studies in the Faculty of Animal Husbandry, University of Sam Ratulangi in Manado in 1985 after the fifth semester because he could not afford to continue, his neighbours in Kauditan sub-district immediately started asking his help for any problems they faced with their livestock.

Brexy admits that most of his knowledge was learnt 'on the job', and, although illegal, he was able to earn enough from this work to buy some livestock of his own. Then, in December 1998, the Decentralized Livestock Services in Eastern Indonesia (DELIVERI) Project working with Dinas Peternakan (the District Livestock Services) in Minahasa invited him to attend CAHW training, and he became a 'licensed' Tonkeswan. Since then he has expanded his business and has bought a motorcycle to enable him to serve a larger area. He now serves between ten and 15 clients each day. He was delighted with the training: 'It provided the opportunity to share knowledge and skills with my fellow Tonkeswan in Minahasa, and having a permit has boosted my career.'

The service provided by Brexy and his colleagues is popular, and since he and his colleagues started work the percentage of farmers who think that animal health services are good in Minahasa has increased from 22 to 78 per cent. But legally they can work only under the direct supervision of a government veterinarian; their licences, only valid for a year at a time anyway, could be revoked at any time. That is one of the rules governing animal health services in Indonesia, and, by working carefully within and around these rules, DELIVERI's Community Animal Health Worker programme was a great success.

Much earlier, in 1980, Voluntary Service Overseas (VSO) was asked by a small NGO in Sri Lanka to send a vet to help train CAHWs to serve members of a small milk producers' association. VSO placed an advertisement in the *Veterinary Record*, the British Veterinary Association's professional journal, for a vet to 'train paravets in Sri Lanka', and a young British vet duly applied and got the job. But before he could set off for Sri Lanka, VSO received a letter from the Chairman of the Sri Lankan Veterinary Board. The letter pointed out that, before being allowed to practise veterinary medicine in Sri Lanka, the successful candidate would need to pass the Sri Lanka Veterinary Board's professional examination, *and* that, since paravets could not legally practise veterinary medicine in Sri Lanka, VSO might like to rethink the job description. By failing to understand and start work within the rules, the project never got off the ground.

The laws governing veterinary practice form part of a broader set of institutional factors, or 'rules of the game' for animal health services. In many countries, these rules do not favour the establishment of CAHWs, and it is vital to understand them thoroughly, work with them, and then work to change them so that CAHW projects can improve access to animal health services, especially for poor livestock keepers. This chapter describes some of these rules and provides ideas, based on practical experience, about how to help to change them.

8.2   The rules of the game

The rules of the game governing animal health services in most countries are deep-rooted, complex, confused and constantly changing. Some – for example the demand for, supply and control of medicines – may change very rapidly due to economic or political situations, such as natural, economic or political disasters or conflict. Others – for example structural and institutional changes to government and private livestock service organizations – change very slowly and lag far behind changes to national policy, such as structural adjustment programmes, decentralization or privatization. Changes to the legal framework often take decades. The 'rules' therefore rarely fit the 'game' very well.

Legislation inherited from colonial systems prohibiting non-veterinarians from providing clinical veterinary services makes little sense in countries where the few qualified veterinarians are usually willing only to live in the more urban areas. Entrenched attitudes among both civil servants and farmers developed over decades of free public veterinary services may make it difficult to establish private or community-based services. The absence, or inexperience of, private-sector veterinary associations makes it very difficult to develop veterinary codes of conduct, or systems for professional development to promote private veterinary practice.

The 'rules' include laws and regulations, government and donor policies and strategies, operational systems within government, private- and third-sector livestock service organizations, veterinary education systems, and the attitudes they engender among service providers and recipients.

Historical perspective

Professional veterinary services emerged in many countries during the colonial era – primarily to protect cavalry and pack horses against disease – then gradually expanded to meet the needs of colonial farmers. Civilian veterinary services copied veterinary services in colonizing countries and sought to protect emerging livestock industries through disease control programmes, mainly involving quarantine, movement restriction and the slaughter of infected animals. Rapid increases in the understanding of tropical diseases, expansion of colonial government capacity, and the extension of clinical services to local farmers left an elite group of overseas-trained veterinary professionals seeking to emulate services in developed countries. However, with few trained staff at their disposal they often relied on a cadre of committed, practical animal health auxiliaries working at field level.

Following the establishment of veterinary schools in national universities with funding from rapidly expanding government budgets, university or technical school graduates quickly replaced the animal health auxiliaries. Although better trained, these graduates usually expected cleaner work and higher incomes, and were reluctant to live in rural areas. Increasing populations, the high cost of rapid infrastructural development and the collapse of commodity prices left veterinary departments with high professional expectations but little money for operational activities. Consequently, government veterinary services in many countries entered a period of serious decline; veterinarians with a western-style university education were unable to find new ways to deliver services. Until recently, few senior government veterinarians were enthusiastic about CAHWs. A survey among chief veterinary officers at the Office International des Epizooties in 1995 found many did not support CAHWs, fearing increased drug resistance due to uncontrolled drug use and malpractice.

Policies

There is a general trend throughout the developed world away from large government departments providing free services towards smaller, streamlined departments whose job is to set standards and create an enabling environment for the private sector to provide services. This trend has been promoted in developing countries, particularly in Africa, through structural adjustment programmes built into World Bank and IMF loan agreements. Many governments are now pursuing policies to reduce the size and increase the efficiency of bureaucracies through decentralization, privatization and public participation.

Government livestock departments in many countries are therefore rethinking the roles and responsibilities of the public and private sectors to ensure livestock services and productivity are enhanced. Public sector roles in developed countries focus on setting priorities and policies, establishing standards and systems for certification and quality control, and developing control programmes for economically and socially important diseases and research. Increasingly, clinical services are being provided by the private sector, sometimes under contract to the government. Developing countries are also moving in this direction (see Box 8.1).

Box 8.1 Public and private sector roles in animal health services

Most countries in Africa are currently sharing the responsibility for animal health service delivery between the public and private sectors:

Public sector

Public sector roles are generally considered to be the following:

◆ setting sector-wide development priorities;
◆ formulation of policy guidelines and execution of policy;
◆ licensing and certification, for example:
   – quality certification of livestock sector inputs such as drugs and vaccines;
   – restricting the use of drugs and chemicals to qualified providers;
   – licensing of sectoral workers.
◆ provision of quality control of, for example:
   – hides and skins;
   – pharmaco-surveillance of the efficacy of drugs and vaccines.
◆ enforcement of quality control and certification regulations;

- enforcement of quarantine and livestock movement controls;
- epidemiology and surveillance of livestock diseases;
- control of epizootic (notifiable) diseases;
- provision of legal services;
- establishment of information networks;
- provision of extension services;
- research.

Private sector

Private sector roles are generally considered to be the following:

- provision of veterinary clinical services;
- provision of artificial insemination services;
- production of animal vaccines and veterinary drugs;
- supply and distribution of veterinary drugs and other animal health inputs;
- management of dips and crushes;
- research and diagnostic support services.

Joint services

The joint services could be as follows:

- provision of meat inspection and inspection of slaughter houses;
- vaccination against notifiable diseases;
- collection of samples for disease surveillance and monitoring;
- provision of research and veterinary laboratory services for selected diseases.

(source: Dr Walter Masiga, opening address at Conference on the Delivery of Animal Health Services in Eastern Africa, December 1998)

Legislation

Most countries have legislation defining the responsibilities and rights of veterinarians, and providing mechanisms for their regulation. In ex-colonial countries, this legislation was usually copied from the colonial country and, therefore, was designed according to veterinary services in Europe. The legislation usually sought to protect animals from malpractice and protect the right of veterinary professionals to charge a fee for services. It often restricted the right to practise veterinary medicine to fully qualified veterinarians, and usually invested authority to provide and revoke a license to practise in a government or non-government body. This persistence of this regulatory set-up means that, in many countries, it is technically illegal for CAHWs either to practise veterinary medicine, or to charge for their services. Supplementary regulations may define more precisely what treatments or practices may be provided, and charged for, by non-veterinarians.

Animals may also be protected from potentially cruel procedures under legislation covering animal welfare, wildlife or endangered species. Statutory provisions for the control of economically important diseases or zoonoses are usually defined in specific legislation about animal diseases. These diseases include foot and mouth disease, Newcastle disease, anthrax and rabies. The legislation usually charges government with responsibility for disease control and such diseases are commonly termed 'notifiable'. Livestock keepers and veterinarians are responsible for informing government in the event of a suspected disease outbreak. The legislation can also force livestock owners to comply with control measures such as slaughter policies. CAHW programmes must also comply with these provisions.

The provision and sale of medicines is also regulated, often by laws aimed at ensuring that drugs can only be provided or sold by suitably qualified pharmacists or other professionals. These laws restrict access to potentially harmful drugs, including 'prescription-only' medicines and 'class-1 poisons', to medically qualified personnel. This legislation is also based on legislation in colonial countries and assumes good infrastructure and plenty of qualified pharmacists and vets. However, if fully implemented in developing countries, it would probably make essential drugs more or less unavailable in many areas.

In addition to the problem of inappropriate legislation, supplementary regulations governing animal health services are often issued piecemeal by government

---

Box 8.2 Laws governing veterinary services in Kenya

The Animal Diseases Act, Cap. 364

The Animal Diseases Act provides for the control of animal diseases with special emphasis on notifiable diseases. One of the major and important provisions in the Act is the conferment of sufficient powers to the Director of Veterinary Services (DVS) to control diseases. The Act also makes adequate provision for the minister responsible for veterinary services to make rules necessary for better carrying out of the Act. Similarly, the inspectors appointed by the DVS have sufficient legal powers to institute appropriate measures for the enhancement of disease control.

The Veterinary Surgeons Act, Cap. 366

The Act provides for the registration of veterinarians and the manner in which a veterinary practice should be conducted. The Kenya Veterinary Board (KVB) is established under this Act and the mandate of the Board is to ensure that the Veterinary practices are conducted by qualified and registered veterinarians.

The Pharmacy and Poisons Act, Cap. 244

The Act provides for restoration of health of both animals and humans through control of the profession of pharmacy and the trade in drugs and poisons.

The Prevention of Cruelty to Animals Act, Cap. 360

The Act plays a unique role in the delivery of animal health services. Under the Act, it is an offence for anybody to neglect his or her animals generally or specifically when the animal is in need of veterinary treatment. Similarly, it is an offence for anybody to cause an act of negligence to an animal.

The Meat Control Act, Cap. 356

The Act aims at providing wholesome meat and meat products for human consumption through inspection and licensing. The Act defines the inspector as any veterinary officer, health inspector or any other person duly authorized in writing by the Director of Veterinary Services.

The Cattle Cleansing Act, Cap. 358

The Act primarily aims at controlling East Coast Fever and other tick-borne diseases in the scheduled areas (mainly dairy farming areas). Under the Act the Government provides dipping facilities and enforces compulsory dipping in scheduled areas.

The Rabies Act

The Act provides for the control and suppression of rabies, which is a zoonotic disease. The provisions in the Act are sufficient for the intended purpose.

The Dairy Industry Act, Cap. 336

The Act provides for improvement and control of the dairy industry and its products. The Kenya Dairy Board (KDB) is the implementing agency.

There are many other laws related to the delivery of animal health services in one way or another but which have no direct significance on the delivery of animal health services.

(source: Dr Julius K. Kajume, Conference on the Delivery of Animal Health Services in Eastern Africa, December 1998)

departments in the face of new situations. As this can occur without repealing earlier, contradictory regulations, it can be very difficult to interpret the exact legal position for CAHW programmes. These problems are illustrated in Box 8.2, which outlines the basic laws governing the delivery of veterinary services in Kenya. An example of how legal frameworks can be difficult to interpret is provided in Box 8.3.

Box 8.3 The legal framework for CAHWs in Indonesia

Under the existing legislation veterinary surgeons have the sole right to provide clinical veterinary services and use veterinary pharmaceuticals. However, non-veterinarians are entitled to perform certain clinical procedures and use drugs as long as they are supervised by a veterinarian. 'The use of drugs which include vaccines, sera, antibiotics and chemotherapy to prevent and eliminate livestock contagious diseases should be done or supervised by veterinary surgeons.'

Existing regulations specifically define a non-veterinarian technician position which assists veterinarians in the clinical services that they provide (*Paramedis Kesehatan Hewan*). These are graduates of secondary-level education to whom veterinary surgeons can delegate their authority to perform some procedures but always under the veterinarian's control and responsibility. Although *paramedis* normally work in the public sector the regulations also allow for this position to exist in the private sector. This can include members of the community who provide animal health services for a fee so long as they are supervised by a veterinary surgeon.

According to the legislation, the minimum academic requirement for *paramedis* is to have completed secondary education in a high school of livestock. Alternatively, they need to have undergone special training on animal health. Although this training has traditionally been provided by the Agriculture Training Centre of the Ministry of Agriculture at central level and has never included non-government workers, the legislation allows Regional Government Livestock Services to implement this training in the district and make it accessible to non-government persons.

◆ Although these regulations appear to permit Regional Livestock Services to train farmers or other members of the community to provide clinical services in the districts, this has never happened.
◆ Although the regulations stipulate that the training has to be approved by the National Directorate General of Livestock Services, no standards exist for its specific contents.

The existing regulations do not delimit clearly the range of clinical procedures that non-government *paramedis* are authorized to perform, but a draft attempt to do this, based on authorities and permissions for equivalent government staff, has recently been presented for discussion to the Ministry of Agriculture.

The procedures that community-based animal health workers could be entitled to perform are even less clear. Drawing from the existing regulations it could be argued that their activities should be similar to the responsibilities proposed for the government animal health workers. However, they also fall within the activities that private veterinarians are entitled to undertake. They do not include any activities related to control and eradication of infectious diseases. It is ultimately up to the veterinarian to delimit the range of procedures that non-veterinarians are entitled to perform by delegating his or her authority.

In conclusion, the existing regulations do allow Regional Livestock Services to train and authorize farmers or other members of the community to provide clinical services, and for the government veterinarian to define the permissible procedures provided they operate under his or her supervision and responsibility. However, there needs to be legal clarification on the standards of training and the limitation of clinical procedures.

Statutory bodies and veterinary associations

Most countries have a veterinary board or veterinary council to regulate the veterinary profession. The veterinary board is usually responsible for establishing the educational and practical standards required for vets, for registration and licensing, and for establishing codes of conduct and disciplinary procedures. In some countries, the veterinary board also provides practical support for practising vets through information and continuing education, although these are more commonly organized by non-statutory veterinary associations. An example of a statutory body with responsibility for governing a veterinary profession is given in Box 8.4 and the broader aims of a veterinary association are described in Box 8.5.

Box 8.4 The Royal College of Veterinary Surgeons, United Kingdom

History

The Royal College of Veterinary Surgeons (RCVS) was formed in 1844 after the Royal Charter was granted. Veterinary practice became a profession distinguished by the title 'veterinary surgeon'. The first Veterinary Surgeons Act in 1881 confirmed the Charters and authorized the establishment of a Register and imposed certain restrictions on unauthorized people. An amendment in 1920 allowed the Royal College to charge an annual fee for all members practising in the UK. A new Act in 1948 recognized the veterinary degrees awarded by the Universities of Bristol, Cambridge, Edinburgh, Glasgow, Liverpool and London, and in 1949 'unqualified' veterinary practice became illegal, except for certain minor treatments and operations, although a Supplementary Veterinary Register was created for people allowed to undertake these minor procedures. A new Veterinary Surgeons Act in 1966 replaced all previous legislation, re-enacting some of the provisions of the 1948 Act, and additional powers were granted to the RCVS for temporary registration, disciplinary proceedings and a number of other areas. In 1999, the Council voted to allow non-veterinarians to sit on its Preliminary Investigation Committee.

Purpose

The RCVS safeguards the interests of the public and animals by ensuring that only those registered with it can carry out acts of veterinary surgery through three main statutory functions:

◆ deal with issues of veterinary professional conduct;
◆ monitor standards of veterinary education;
◆ maintain a Register of Veterinary Surgeons who are eligible to practise in the UK.

Box 8.5 The role of the Veterinary Association in Zambia

The full participation of the Veterinary Association of Zambia (VAZ) is recognized as crucial for the success of any sound livestock prevention and control programmes. The VAZ exists to:

◆ promote, within Zambia, the interests of its members and those of the veterinary profession, allied sciences and animal welfare;
◆ maintain the status and traditional ethics of the profession;
◆ facilitate dissemination of professional knowledge and information and encourage the interchange of ideas on and discussion of subjects of common interest;
◆ encourage and assist persons in Zambia desirous of acquiring a veterinary professional qualification;
◆ encourage and assist the government in preparation of legislation on matters relating to the veterinary profession;
◆ ascertain and declare the corporate opinion of members in such quarters as it is deemed from time to time to be desirable and to make or support representation to Government and other appropriate bodies on questions affecting the profession;
◆ encourage good relations and understanding between members and the public;
◆ suggest and if deemed expedient from time to time adjust the scale of charges for the use of members.

The current paid-up membership is fewer than 50 from a possible number of 150.

Institutional structures, systems and attitudes

Institutions and organizations are partly defined by their management and administrative and financial systems. In addition, policies, legislation and structures influence informal relationships, operational norms and attitudes that evolve gradually over time. These informal features of institutions are often the most entrenched rules of the game. When thinking about how to change these rules, experience tells us that new systems are always influenced by old ones. People tend to carry on doing what they know how to do. In many large bureaucracies – including governments, large NGOs, donors and international agencies – employees tend to be rewarded for following procedures rather than proposing innovative improvements to an organization's vision or style of work.

There may be no better example than Indonesia, where government structures and systems and civil servant and farmer attitudes evolved gradually throughout the 32-year 'New Order' of President Suharto. In 1996, government planning, budgeting and resource management systems were highly centralized and hierarchical. All budgets were set in the capital Jakarta, often with little attention to different needs in diverse locations throughout the country, and with little flexibility. For example, if a budget existed for a three-day training course for ten field workers in disease control, the same budget could not be used for general animal health training. Nor could the money support disease control training for different staff or pay for a longer or shorter course for more or fewer fieldworkers. Furthermore, the budget planning process started over a year before the period for which the budget was required. Basic government salaries were low, and were only made viable through a complex system of bonuses for special project activities and responsibilities that made it difficult and disadvantageous for staff to create time for other activities. Salary increments and promotion prospects were linked to the acquisition of 'points' through in-service training, which encouraged managers to spread out training opportunities among their staff evenly rather than to provide specific training to help individual members of staff do their existing jobs more effectively, or to do new jobs. Resources for non-specific field activities, travel outside the district or province, and general training, were particularly difficult to access. As a result, most civil servants thought their job was to 'serve the state' rather than 'serve the community'. They were used to implementing programmes designed in Jakarta, following detailed instructions, and being told what to do by their immediate boss. Farmers simply waited for government projects to happen to them. Similar bureaucratic structures and procedures have led to inefficiencies in many state veterinary services. This problem is also described in Chapter 3, particularly in relation to government-managed revolving funds for veterinary drugs and the substantial hidden administrative costs that can prevent full cost recovery and sustainability.

On top of this general institutional inertia and bureaucracy, veterinarians who control animal health service development are often extremely cautious of supporting alternative approaches. Some feel that community-based or ethnoveterinary systems do not fit comfortably with the scientific basis for veterinary medicine, while others assume that such approaches will weaken the service's professional competence or undermine the quality of the service. Related to these beliefs is the widely held view that livestock keepers who are poor, illiterate or from different cultural backgrounds to a professional elite cannot know much about animal diseases or be trained to use veterinary medicines. In general, the knowledge and skills of livestock keepers are not respected by vets or regarded as valuable resources for improving basic veterinary services. Such attitudes among vets contrast markedly with the principles of participatory development.

Where there is no government

Much of the above is less relevant in countries at war or suffering extreme poverty or natural disaster. In these areas, government can be non-existent or have very limited meaningful influence. The normal rules of government and civil society do not apply and are replaced with 'local rules' set by indigenous social institutions, rebel movements, militias, warlords or even aid organizations. In many areas affected by conflict and lack of governance, livestock are crucial livelihood assets. For example, livestock rearing is the main economic activity in much of the Horn of Africa and CAHW programmes can be enormously important in these areas.

As noted in Chapter 3, the challenge under these circumstances is to build programmes that look to the future and a time when peace will come. This involves working as closely as possible with any civil structures that emerge during the conflict period (and these might change over time). It also means working with representatives of previous veterinary structures who are likely to re-emerge into positions of influence and authority when the conflict eventually abates. In some cases, rebel authorities who have supported effective community-level initiatives during a conflict have changed radically once in power and reverted to top-down, bureaucratic systems. Boxes 8.6 and 8.7 describe experiences in two conflict-affected areas where close partnerships between CAHW programmes and local administrations have enabled a future perspective to be developed.

Box 8.6 Promoting CAHW services in Afghanistan

The Dutch Committee for Afghanistan (DCA) and other NGOs had been training CAHWs (called paravets in Afghanistan) for many years. In March 1999, a workshop was organized to address the following issues:

◆ What is the future for the paravets in Afghanistan?
◆ How can we upgrade them to a level that will be recognized by the Government?
◆ Can an 'educational board' or 'steering committee' be established to guide this process?

Workshop participants included NGOs and representatives for the Ministry of Agriculture, Ministry of Planning, Ministry of Education, the Veterinary Faculty, Veterinary Institute and Food and Agriculture Organization (FAO).

The workshop allowed all participants to air their opinions and experiences. From this has come a greater feeling of cooperation and common purpose, better working relationships on the ground, and a better climate for taking forward discussions on the future of Afghanistan's animal health services. After two days of meetings, the General Recommendations of the workshop on the role of paravets in the veterinary infrastructure of Afghanistan were as follows:

1. The Group recognizes the critical role that has emerged for paravets in the delivery of animal health services at the local level for livestock owners in Afghanistan under the *extreme conditions* the country has witnessed in recent years.
2. In recognition of that valuable service, the Group recommends that paravets should continue to work in Afghanistan.
3. The Group identified numerous advantages to government and the people of Afghanistan by having paravets work on a fee for service basis. The Group

---

recommends that paravets continue to work in the private sector and not become government employees. However, the Group also recognizes the need of governmental oversight and regulation of paravet activities.

4. The Group recommends an addition to the Afghan law governing veterinary practice to specifically define the qualifications and responsibilities of a paravet and to legalize the paravet as a legitimate provider of local veterinary services.

5. In support of legalizing the future function of paravets, the Group recognizes the need for a licensing mechanism for working paravets, as well as a system to certify the credentials and evaluate the competence of paravets prior to licensing.

6. The Group recognizes the need to continue to produce new paravets to meet future staffing needs, as well as to upgrade or broaden the skills of some existing paravets.

7. The Group recommends the use of the existing educational facilities to a maximum, thereby avoiding duplication, and encourages the cooperation of the existing training institutions, both government and NGO-supported. The Group recognizes also that certain definite positive elements in the ongoing paravet training should be incorporated in future intermediate-level training.

8. The Group recommends the identification of specific requirements for upgrading a selection of the present paravets, also in relation to the specific tasks they are asked to fulfil.

9. The Group recognizes the authority of the existing Educational Board/Attestation Committee to deal with the issues regarding training, certification and upgrading of paravets, but recommends that other interested parties be offered ex officio status to participate in discussion on issues related to paravets. The following institutions or organizations are proposed for this ex officio status: FAO and DCA.

10. The Group also recommends the establishment of a Paraveterinary Steering Committee, comprised of representatives of relevant ministries, FAO, DCA, other relevant NGOs and interested donors. This Committee can serve in an advisory capacity to Government as it continues to develop and refine policies relative to the role of paravets in Afghanistan.

Box 8.7 Developing a future perspective in southern Sudan

In areas affected by severe and long-term conflict, the rules of the game are often unwritten and controlled by unofficial bodies. The conflict in Sudan is the longest-running civil war in Africa and yet, in the south of the country, a large-scale CAHW programme has been delivering veterinary services since 1993. Bryony Jones and colleagues describe the situation and approach of the Operation Lifeline Sudan (OLS) Livestock Programme as follows:

Southern Sudan has a long history of underdevelopment and conflict. Since independence was granted to Sudan in 1956, there has been civil war between north and south apart from a period of peace between 1972 and 1983. The current conflict continues with no immediate end in sight. Millions of civilians have been killed, displaced or are refugees. Southern Sudan is controlled partly by the government and partly by several rebel groups, some of whom have signed a peace agreement with the Government of Sudan. The prolonged conflict has created what is described as a chronic, complex emergency. Development has been prevented, infrastructure has been destroyed, trade and transport routes have been disrupted, schools and health facilities are almost non-existent, and administrative structures are minimal and have few resources. A series of droughts have been exacerbated by the conflict, causing periodic famines.

The OLS Livestock Programme aims to facilitate the development of an animal health service that uses a network of CAHWs. As the war continues this structure can provide basic animal health services to all areas. When peace eventually comes, this network will provide a basis on which any new government in power can build its animal health services. The programme interacts with potential future decision makers in the north and south. It is creating awareness of the advantages of a community-based system, linked to private vets and pharmacists. In the absence of adequate technical support in rebel-held areas OLS has been taking the role of coordinator of animal health services, but is working closely with counterparts to build their capacity to fill that role in future.

(source: Jones *et al.*, 1998)

8.3   Changing the rules of the game

Reducing government budgets, collapsing services and increasing pressure from strengthened civil society have put many government livestock departments under intense pressure to reform. Most are already committed to privatizing clinical veterinary services, and are working on mechanisms to put privatization policy into practice. As explained in Chapter 3, CAHWs afford opportunities to strengthen rural, private veterinary businesses by increasing service coverage and, therefore, profitability and sustainability. When such businesses include veterinary supervision of CAHWs and are contracted by government to conduct vaccination programmes or disease surveillance (see Chapter 7), the prospects for sustained improvements in veterinary services look promising. However, we have also seen that in many countries CAHWs are not supported by helpful policy and legislation. Therefore, influencing the institutional environment or 'changing the rules of the game' is becoming one of the most important elements of CAHW projects. For this process to be effective, it is essential to:

♦ develop a good understanding of the situation at local, national and even international levels;
♦ identify the key stakeholders and work closely with them to:
  – develop a clear strategy using appropriate participatory approaches and methods;
  – plan and run the project open-mindedly with careful monitoring and evaluation;
  – use information derived from the project to influence the key policy makers.

This section discusses how ways to influence policy can be built into the different stages of a project from 'getting the big picture', through project planning and evaluation to effective use of information derived from the project.

Getting the big picture

Knowledge is the key. Without a holistic understanding of all aspects of the situation, the rules of the game, and the practical situation in the field it is difficult to develop an effective strategy to promote the CAHW approach. Some participatory field approaches have already been described in Chapter 2, and using these can help to provide a good understanding of the situation at field level. Tracking down and reading the relevant legislation, using professional help for interpretation and application if necessary, and open discussions with a wide range of government and non-government veterinary staff, representatives of farmers' organizations, pharmacists and drug companies are also essential.

In addition to fully understanding the situation 'now', it can also be very useful to work with policy makers or their representatives to conduct a more historical review and analysis. This process can help to people to answer questions such as 'How did we reach the current situation?' and describe the strengths and weaknesses of different policies at different stages in a country's development. Commonly, this work will also highlight how policy is not static but changes according to numerous political, economic and other factors. Other opportunities include learning from policy reform in other sectors such as human health, education or natural resource management.

Developing a strategy

Chapter 2, *Getting started*, describes how to ensure that all immediate stakeholders are involved in project design and development. Careful study of the policy and legal context can help to identify high-level stakeholders, including senior livestock service managers and policy makers. The next step is to develop a clear strategy for improving the policy environment. Detailed information is included in the three case–studies later in the chapter, but in summary there are two main strategies:

In countries with limited field experience of CAHW services

In these countries, pilot CAHW projects can be established. The strategy is to work with government partners to expose them to participatory ways of working, and then design, implement and evaluate the CAHW service. Lessons learnt then feed a debate about policy reform. When pilot projects produce convincing results, information is carefully targeted at senior livestock service staff, leading to a series of policy and organizational reforms to promote widespread replication. This type of approach has worked well in Indonesia (see case study 1), Tanzania (case study 2) and parts of Ethiopia (see Box 3.4, Chapter 3).

In countries with long experience of CAHW services, but inappropriate policy

In this situation, there are often weak linkages between field-level players and central-level policy makers. For example, non-government organizations (NGOs) can be the main source of CAHW experience in the field but do not disseminate experiences to policy makers. In some areas, relationships between NGOs and government are characterized by mutual mistrust and avoidance. While NGOs can view government as bureaucratic and corrupt, governments sometimes consider NGOs as 'loose cannons' that seek to undermine government services, and resist coordination or regulation by the state. In this situation, the key strategy is dialogue. Bringing different stakeholders together in well-designed and well-facilitated meetings can help build trust in the relationship. This approach has worked in Kenya, as described in case study 3.

Effective planning as a tool towards changing the rules

Effective planning can ensure that a project identifies policies that may present barriers to success, achieves measurable results, and develops effective strategies to influence, challenge and change policies as necessary. There are various planning models, but one of the most commonly used is the logical framework ('logframe'). Although

---

Box 8.8 Logical frameworks

A logical framework ('logframe') is really just a way of describing a project as succinctly as possible. It shows:

◆ how the expected outcome of the project, its 'purpose', will contribute to the achievement of the ultimate higher-level 'goal';
◆ what the project must produce in order to achieve the purpose, its 'outputs';
◆ any 'assumptions' that must be met;
◆ the 'objectively verifiable indicators' that will be used to show whether the project has succeeded;
◆ and finally what activities and inputs are necessary to achieve the outputs.

To be most effective, logframes should be developed through a participatory process of discussion with all potential project stakeholders to:

1. decide the ultimate goal of the project. This is usually a high-level aim, often related to the quality of life, to which all project stakeholders should aspire, to which the project will contribute, but will not achieve by itself. For example: 'Increased incomes from livestock keeping for poor households'.

2. decide whether it is actually possible, within the prevailing context, to change anything to bring that particular goal closer. If it is, achieving that change becomes the purpose of the project. For example, the above goal could be achieved through 'Increased productivity of indigenous livestock breeds, using locally available resources'.

3. identify as clearly as possible the main obstacles or constraints to achieving this purpose, and what the project must put in place to overcome them. These become the project outputs. They should be practical and measurable. For example:
   – 'Losses from disease reduced from x per cent to y per cent per annum by the end of project year 3';
   – 'Calving interval reduced from 30 to 24 months by the end of project year 4'.

4 identify the activities that will be needed to achieve each of these outputs, and the inputs needed for each of the activities.

At each step it is also important to find out if there are any external factors that could obstruct progress. For example, increased productivity of livestock will only result in improved incomes for poor households if people have good access to markets and can get a good price. Similarly, reduced losses from disease will only result in increased production if there is enough fodder for the increased number of animals to eat. These are assumptions that need to be met for the project to succeed. Any assumptions that can be addressed practically should be addressed within the project. For example, it might be possible to include a fodder production component in the project to make sure there is enough fodder for the livestock, but it might be difficult for a small livestock project to do much about the market infrastructure.

It is also important to identify clear indicators which can be observed during the life of the project to ensure that the project is on track. These become the objectively verifiable indicators in the logframe, and they should be SMART, i.e. Specific, Measurable, Appropriate, Realistic and Time-bound.

A good logframe should be very clear and succinct. Ideally it should fit on one side of a page, so that it is possible to get an overview of the whole project at a glance. But it should be regarded as a working document – more or less everything except the purpose can change in response to changing circumstances. It is common to review and amend logframes every six months or annually.

An example of a logframe is provided in Box 8.12.

logframes can be difficult to work with if used too rigidly, when used as a flexible aid to planning they can be effective.

Assessing impact

Demonstrating the impact and benefits of a project is one of the most powerful tools for influencing policy. To do this requires effective monitoring and evaluation throughout the life of the project. Most livestock services are managed by veterinarians who are accustomed to empirical data on disease morbidity or mortality, or statistical data about improved livestock productivity. However, collecting this kind of data is often beyond the scope of CAHW projects. Chapter 6 describes how it is possible to use a combination of approaches to collect some convincing evidence relatively easily.

Box 8.9 Using impact to influence policy: the case of rinderpest control in Afar

In the Afar region of Ethiopia, 20 CAHWs were trained in 1994. Project impact was assessed by the Pan African Rinderpest Campaign (PARC) by comparing vaccination efficiency and cost of vaccination as performed by CAHWs and government vaccination teams.

In Afar, the CAHWs achieved 84 per cent vaccination efficiency using heat-stable vaccine. This figure exceeded the 72 per cent vaccination efficiency of Ethiopian government vaccination teams and compared favourably with conventional rinderpest vaccination campaigns in Africa generally (which achieved a vaccination efficiency of 60 to 85 per cent). It was also noted that CAHWs in Afar were able to stop rinderpest virus circulation in their communities after only a single vaccination campaign, whereas rinderpest outbreaks continued in adjacent areas where government vaccinating teams were working. The wider application of CAHWs in the Afar region resulted in no reports of rinderpest outbreaks in Afar after November 1995. In less than two years, the community-based approach had controlled rinderpest in Afar, and Ethiopia was able to declare provisional freedom from rinderpest according to the OIE pathway. Prior to PARC, the Joint Project 15 (JP15) rinderpest eradication programme had failed to control rinderpest in Afar using conventional vaccination programmes implemented over a 15-year period.

When comparing vaccination costs, 20 CAHWs moving on foot vaccinated 73 000 cattle in one season. These CAHWs were supervised by two veterinary staff supported by one vehicle. In the same period, government vaccination teams comprising 64 staff in 14 vehicles only vaccinated 140 000 cattle in an adjacent area of Afar. In May 1998, 14 out of 20 CAHWs were still operating in Afar.

(source: Mariner, 1996 – see Further reading)

A quite small amount of empirical data about changes in livestock disease incidence, productivity or economic benefit can make a very convincing case if supported by – or 'triangulated' with – qualitative data, especially if the results are presented in the right format for each audience.

Impact can also be assessed by a comparison of CAHW services with other types of service provision. This is most easily achieved by focusing on a limited number of disease problems and comparing common measures of coverage, efficiency and impact in the two services. An example from the Afar region of Ethiopia is provided in Box 8.9.

Using information effectively

Although many CAHW projects generate useful experiences and information, very few use this information effectively to influence the policy environment. Providing the right information at the right time to the right people in the right format can make all the difference between success and failure. For example:

- ◆ Vets and livestock professionals tend to be convinced by reports that look scientific.
- ◆ Donors and NGOs tend to be convinced by reports that demonstrate, preferably with pictures, that the information has been collected in a participatory way with, or preferably by, the beneficiaries.
- ◆ Field staff and farmers are often more convinced by talking to other field staff and farmers who have been involved in a project than by written reports.

Photographs, electronic presentations and video clips can provide the same practical feel if it is not possible to take people to the field. One technique used with great success by the DELIVERI Project was to take farmers to make verbal presentations at high-level meetings, as described in case study 1.

Workshops: bringing people together

The concept of CAHWs (called 'barefoot vets') first emerged in a series of work-shops organized by the Commonwealth Secretariat in the early 1980s, and workshops and seminars remain one of the most potent mechanisms for sharing ideas, formulating policies and influencing decision makers. The effectiveness of workshops depends on factors such as the selection of participants, the relevance of the topics under discussion and the type of facilitation provided. The workshop should have clearly defined objectives, and activities should be designed specifically to meet these objectives. When topics for discussion might be sensitive, an external and neutral facilitator is useful for ensuring that all points of view are heard and discussed.

Many of the principles of organizing and running CAHW training courses (see Chapters 4 and 5) also apply to running effective workshops. Workshop participants can soon become bored if they are subjected to lengthy presentations with little time for discussion. Rather than being a series of lectures, workshops should use working groups in which people jointly analyse an issue and then present their findings back to the other participants for discussion. Much time needs to be allocated for this kind of process. A workshop should end with sessions on recommendations and action plans and, again, sufficient time is required to ensure that draft recommendations are prepared, discussed with participants and reworked as necessary. The impact of workshops is demonstrated by experiences from Tanzania (case study 2), Kenya (case study 3) and Afghanistan (Box 8.6). In Nepal, workshops were also used to good effect and led to the development of a national skills test for CAHWs (Box 8.10).

It can be seen from these examples that, to a large extent, workshops on policy issues have been dominated by professional or government stakeholders. Although

---

Box 8.10 Using workshops in Nepal to develop the community-based approach

When dwindling budgets and organizational changes in the Department of Agriculture and Livestock Services in Nepal threatened the Village Animal Health Worker (VAHW) programme, the Rural Development Centre of the United Mission to Nepal organized a national workshop bringing all the key stakeholders together to discuss the future. The workshop, in September 1997, was a great success with presentations from a wide range of participants including the Director General of Livestock Services, interviews with a VAHW and a Village Development Committee Chairman, and group work focusing on three critical questions:

◆ The first group's task was to define the proper role for the VAHW in Nepal.
◆ The second group developed a list of minimum skills needed by a VAHW.
◆ The third looked at how best to develop support systems to ensure sustainablility.

The workshop concluded that VAHWs were a vital component of Nepal's animal healthcare systems, but that better mechanisms were needed to integrate VAHW programmes with government services. Participants agreed that all VAHWs should pass some sort of skill test, and should be registered and licensed by the District Livestock Services office. A networking and skill-test subgroup was established to look at these issues in more detail.

The networking and skill-test subgroup completed its primary task, and submitted a proposed VAHW skill test to the Council for Technical Education and Vocational Training. This was approved by the Council and then subsequently endorsed by the National Skill Testing Board and the Animal Health Technical Training Subcommittee.

(contributed by Dr Bob Hott, Christian Veterinary Mission)

CAHWs and livestock keepers might be represented, they tend to be present in small numbers. Considering that community-based approaches to animal healthcare rely heavily on local priorities, skills and knowledge, there are clear opportunities to improve the involvement of communities directly in the policy reform process. Creating activities where policy makers come into direct 'face-to-face' contact with communities can be a powerful way to influence policy. One approach is to use workshops in which livestock keepers and veterinarians work together to analyse constraints and opportunities facing animal health services. This idea was applied in eastern Ethiopia where two stakeholder workshops were conducted, with an emphasis on participation by livestock keepers (see Box 8.11).

'Seeing is believing': the power of field visits

In the early 1990s, the Pan African Rinderpest Campaign (PARC) was facing major problems accessing some remote and hostile areas of Ethiopia and Sudan. In order to solve this problem, CAHW projects were established with an initial emphasis on rinderpest vaccination with a heat-stable vaccine that could be used by CAHWs. Although senior PARC staff gave permission for this approach to be tried, there was

Giving livestock keepers a voice

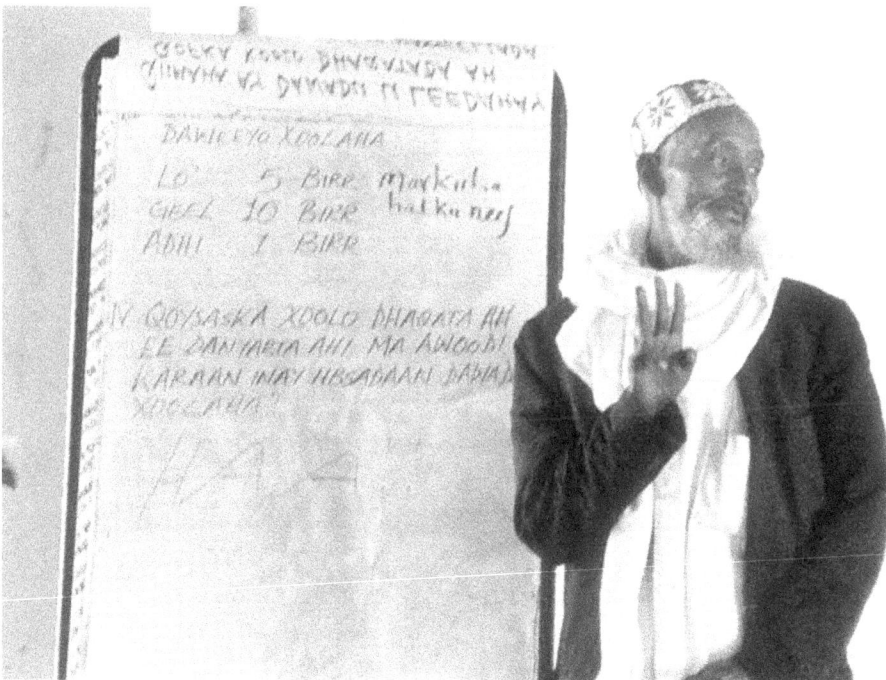

Plate 8.1 Stakeholder workshops on animal health service delivery can be an opportunity for livestock keepers to 'take the floor' and present their opinions to policy makers. (*Andy Catley*)

Box 8.11 Stakeholder workshops to inform policy on animal health service delivery: an example from Ethiopia

In the administrative region of eastern Ethiopia called the Somali National Regional State (SNRS or 'Region S'), stakeholder analysis was used in the design of animal health services at a time when veterinary privatization was being advocated by the Ethiopian Government. The SNRS supports Somali pastoralists and agropastoralists and is a large, sparsely populated dryland area. The stakeholder analysis involved two workshops with livestock owners, community elders, religious leaders, women, traditional livestock healers, private veterinary drug traders, livestock traders and government veterinary personnel.

The workshops were opened in a traditional manner using a well-known Somali poet to introduce the theme of the workshop and describe the various options for treating sick livestock that were available at that time. Workshop participants were divided into groups to discuss topics such as:

◆ the main benefits and diseases of livestock;
◆ the role of women in animal healthcare and options for treating sick livestock;
◆ the role of traditional medicine versus modern medicine for treating livestock diseases;
◆ livestock disease, veterinary services and livestock trade as perceived by livestock traders;
◆ strengths and weaknesses of the existing veterinary services;
◆ ability and willingness to pay for veterinary services;
◆ opportunities for improvement and risks.

During the discussions, participatory appraisal tools such as proportional piling, ranking and scoring were used to identify and prioritize issues, problems and solutions. For example, ranking was used to understand how different stakeholder groups were treating their animals. Representatives from each stakeholder group then presented the findings of their discussion to the rest of the workshop participants and the whole workshop voted on key issues and ideas for improving veterinary services.

The stakeholder analysis workshop was successful because each stakeholder group was able to voice its opinions and needs. More powerful stakeholders such as government veterinarians had to explain the weaknesses of the existing veterinary service to the end-users and work with them to identify a way forward. The stakeholder approach also helped to ensure that less powerful groups were not misrepresented.

In this case, all stakeholder groups gave their support to basic, clinical veterinary services which could be delivered by community animal health workers (CAHWs) linked to private veterinary pharmacies. Government vets agreed to consult regional government officials and produce a 'policy statement' to support private veterinary activities and CAHWs.

SOMALI NATIONAL REGIONAL STATE

POLICY STATEMENT ON VETERINARY SERVICE DELIVERY
September 1997

Livestock production is crucial to the economy and well-being of the people in the Somali National Regional State. In order to protect and enhance the region's livestock assets, the regional government is committed to the development of effective and sustainable animal health services.

The current economic policy of the Federal Democratic Republic of Ethiopia aims to stimulate private sector activities in a range of sectors. The policy reflects growing support to privatization throughout both the developed and the developing world.

Regarding veterinary services, the executive agency responsible for animal disease control in Ethiopia is the Ministry of Agriculture. On a national level, the Ministry of Agriculture is supporting private sector veterinary activities through a joint project with the Pan African Rinderpest Campaign. Criteria and regulations for private veterinary practice, the handling of veterinary drugs and the importation of veterinary drugs have been formulated.

Regarding the development of veterinary services in this region,

1. The Somali National Regional State Government fully supports the development of the private veterinary sector in the region and is committed to creating an appropriate economic and legal environment for private sector veterinary activities.

2. The Somali National Regional State Government will retain control of public sector animal health activities, those activities being disease surveillance (regional and international), veterinary investigation, regulation of veterinary drugs and private facilities, veterinary public health and research on livestock disease.

3. The Somali National Regional State Government supports a gradual transfer of curative veterinary service responsibilities (meaning clinical examination and treatment of livestock) from the public sector to the private sector. The regional government will continue to deliver curative services in those areas where the private sector does not operate.

4. The Somali National Regional State Government will investigate options for joint public–private sector vaccination campaigns in order to increase the coverage of present vaccination activities.

5. The Somali National Regional State Government fully supports the development of trained community-based animal health workers who in partnership with private veterinarians can provide basic animal healthcare to communities in remote parts of the region.

(contributed by the Veterinary Services Support Project, Save the Children, UK)

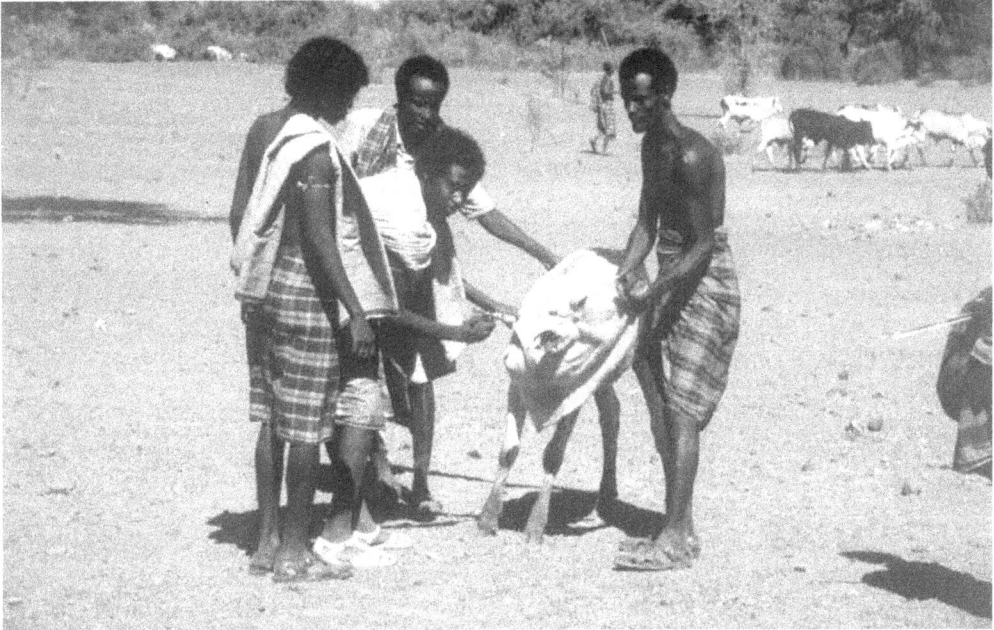

Plate 8.2 When senior staff from the Pan African Rinderpest Campaign went to the field to see CAHWs in action in Afar, Ethiopia, they were soon convinced that CAHWs had a major role to play in rinderpest eradication. (*PARC Communications Unit*)

much scepticism regarding the capacity of illiterate livestock herders to handle the vaccine properly and cover sufficient numbers of cattle. The turning point came when senior PARC staff agreed to visit Afar and see for themselves what was happening on the ground. The change in attitude among the PARC staff was dramatic. They were able to observe the CAHWs in action – mobilizing communities, organizing cattle crushes and using the automatic vaccination syringes and vaccine correctly (also see Box 8.9).

8.4 Evidence of success: Case studies in policy reform for CAHW services

Case study 1: the DELIVERI Project in Indonesia

Background

The Department for International Development of the United Kingdom (DFID) has been supporting the livestock sector in Indonesia for nearly 20 years. Initial support focused on veterinary research, but over the years the focus shifted through human resource development and tertiary training to epidemiology. By

1989, DFID was supporting national animal health planning, and national and local animal health reporting systems. This project soon discovered that local animal health services were dominated by national programmes. The design of these programmes was flawed due to poor information and, because they were implemented in exactly the same way throughout Indonesia, important local needs were often overlooked.

This experience led the project into a number of small pilot projects using 'bottom-up planning' to develop local animal health services in response to local needs. This worked surprisingly well. It also brought DFID into contact with a number of other projects working on services at field level with positive results. However, central government policy makers and planners remained unaware of these initiatives and just continued implementing the same large-scale national programmes. The challenge was how to influence national policy in favour of small-scale local solutions, then how to introduce and establish new participatory planning and implementation systems in the department that would allow them to adopt the new approaches.

The DELIVERI approach

The purpose of the DELIVERI was to 'make livestock-related institutions more responsive to the need of small-scale farmers, including the resource-poor, through the adoption and replication of more client-orientated and participatory approaches'. The strategy to achieve this was to implement a series of pilot projects, use the results to convince senior government managers of their value, then work with them to establish the necessary systems and human capacity so they could replicate them more widely. To achieve this, the project had five distinct outputs, each with a specific set of activities. The DELIVERI Project developed a logical framework with project partners. The logframe details specific policy-related outputs and activities, as shown in Box 8.12.

This was a novel approach in the agricultural sector in Indonesia because it involved an iterative 'process' rather than a blueprint approach. Also, the project did different things in different places, rather than the same thing everywhere, and did not provide any physical or financial resources for farmers or for government staff, except for training and information.

Use of action-research and information

With an explicit focus on making government livestock institutions more responsive to the needs of poor livestock farmers, producing and using information to influence policy makers was a key component of the DELIVERI Project. The project used an action-research approach. Early training courses provided farmers and government livestock service staff with the new information and skills they needed to set up pilot projects to test new approaches. The results of these pilot projects, and the results of other project components – for example the institutional studies – were synthesized into information to influence key decision makers to establish a policy framework for the further dissemination of successful approaches.

Box 8.12 The DELIVERI logframe

Narrative Summary	Verifiable Indicators (OVI)	Means of Verification (MOV)	Important Assumptions
Goal: 1. Sustainable increases in wealth and self reliance of small-scale and resource-poor farmers. 2. Improved institutional arrangements for the delivery of sustainable and accessible rural services in place throughout Indonesia.	1.1 Sustained increases in net incomes attributable to livestock production over 5–10 years	1.1 Bureau of Statistics data	(Goal to Supergoal)
Purpose: 1. Livestock-related institutions more responsive to the need of small-scale farmers, including the resource-poor, through the adoption and replication of more client-orientated and participatory approaches.	1. One or more new systems evaluated and adopted by GoI livestock-related institutions by the end of project year 4. 2. Customer satisfaction level increased from (a) in 1996 to (b) in 2000.*	1.1 Institutional base-line and follow-up surveys. 1.2 GoI plans and proposals. 2.1 Institutional base-line and follow-up surveys. 2.2 Results of customer survey. 2.3 Agreed plan for strategic withdrawal.	(Purpose to goal) 1. Improvements to service delivery replicated throughout Indonesia.
Outputs: 1. Client-focused approaches to the planning and delivery of livestock services to small-scale and resource-poor farmers piloted in Programme locales	1.1 Twelve pilot schemes using new approaches developed, implemented and evaluated with stakeholders over 2 year period, by March 2000.	1.1 Project M&E reports. 1.2 PSC reports and minutes. 1.3 Reports of participatory evaluations of pilot schemes.	(Output to purpose) 1.1 GoI supports testing and replication of innovative approaches to service delivery 1.2 One or more of the approaches tested is successful; target farmers are able to assess constraints and take advantage of opportunities through public and/or private sector services.
2. Participatory, managerial, technical and extension skills of Programme-related livestock service staff improved.	2.1 Participatory, management technical and extension skills appropriate for decentralized livestock services amongst relevant staff and target institutions** doubled by March 2000.	2.1.1 1996 training needs assessment questionnaire scores, and follow-up survey in 2000. 2.1.2 Pre and post training evaluations. 2.1.3 Project training records.	2.1 Dinas staff willing, able and empowered to work with poor farmers, have support of management and have resources to do so.
3. Recommendations produced on improving the institutional framework for more decentralized and responsive livestock services and support provided in implementing them.	3.1 Intermediate Institutional Development Plans agreed/owned with/by Target Institutions. 3.2 Final Institutional Development Plan approved by DELIVERI PSC with a commitment to further action by March 2000.	3.1.1 Institutional study reports. 3.1.2 Intermediate Plans Produced. 3.1.3 PSC Meeting minutes. 3.2.1 Plan Produced. 3.2.2 PSC Meeting Minutes. 3.2.3 Peer Review by International Centre of excellence.	3.1 GoI introduces recommended institutional reforms, at least in programme areas.
4. Methods of assuring quality of service introduced to the Programme and evaluated for use by government livestock services.	4.1 Quality-focused internal project team management system incorporating continuous internal review installed and running by February 1997, and evaluated for use by DGLS/DP by July 1997. 4.2 Strategy for the development of quality systems for Target Institutions produced by February 1997. 4.3 Quality systems operating throughout the programme by March 2000.	4.1.1 Internal project documentation. 4.1.2 Internal review reports. 4.2.1 Quality Assurance Plan produced. 4.3.1 PSC Meeting minutes. 4.3.2 Customer satisfaction survey results.	4.1 Commitment to quality systems throughout programme and livestock services in programme areas.
5. Programme experience and recommendations understood by GoI policy planners.	5.1 Measurable improvement in knowledge of and attitudes to Decentralized Livestock Services amongst policy and decision makers in Target Institutions by mid-term review and at end of project.	5.1.1 Attitude surveys pre/post and with/without project activities. 5.1.2 Pre and post training evaluations.	5.1 Programme produces useful lessons and experience. 5.2 Programme recommendations adopted by GoI

*Figures to be inserted after completion of customer satisfaction surveys in mid 1997.
**Target Institutions includes the Department General of Livestock Services and Dinas Peternakan.

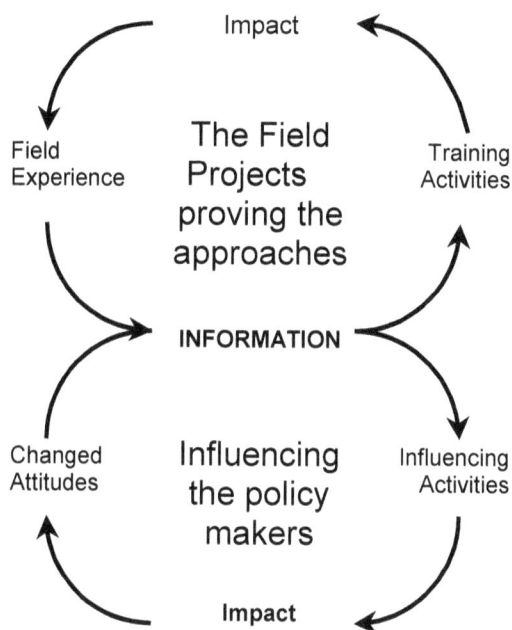

Figure 8.1 DELIVERI's information-influence cycle

Towards the end of the first year, the project conducted a study of information needs by all the different people who needed information about the project, the different kinds of information they needed, and the way they would like the information to be presented:

Policy makers

Senior Jakarta livestock policy makers felt that they had more than enough general information about the project both from the documents produced by DELIVERI and documents produced by the government. They regarded the project Newsletter as 'one-way', and not responsive to the particular information needs of the policy makers. They needed more 'real' information about project impact to help them determine the value of the project in the national development framework. They needed to be convinced of the value of the DELIVERI approaches, in particular what were the benefits. They wanted to see real evidence of impact at output level using indicators that they were comfortable with. They cared more about the value of the information than how the information was presented. They did not want to read long documents. They preferred to meet with project staff face to face to discuss progress. Specialists within technical departments wanted information specifically focused around their areas of interest.

Middle managers

Livestock service staff at regional level wanted a wider range of information than they had received until then. They were also interested in information materials that could help them to communicate better with Jakarta. Staff interviewed specifically mentioned discussion papers, 'progress-in-brief' papers and articles in journals. They stressed the value of personal meetings and discussions with project staff and colleagues involved in the project in different districts, and wanted to collaborate with the press to help to socialize the activities with farmers.

Field staff and farmers

Livestock field staff wanted more informal, practical and motivating information for use in the field. This included information about the project's philosophy and approaches and PRA techniques, as well as technical material on animal health and so on. They liked the idea of technical bulletins, wall posters and photo-albums. They asked for more information to help them explain the principles and benefits of the project more clearly.

Using these results, the DELIVERI Project developed an information strategy based primarily on personal meetings with the different stakeholders, supported with a wide variety of information materials using different media (see Box 8.13).

Presentations at conferences and seminars often combined verbal reports by farmers and field staff with sophisticated electronic multimedia presentations and video clips, supported with brochures and leaflets. The project presented scientific papers at conferences, often co-authoring them with government counterparts, and encouraged local journalists to visit project sites and publish articles in the local press. Attractive annual planners, desk calendars and diaries became very popular with staff throughout the Department of Agriculture, and helped to publicize the project. Within two years, the project had become better known and more popular throughout the Department of Agriculture than many other much older and larger projects, and this contributed substantially to the project's ability to influence policy makers.

Case study 2: the Animal Health Services Project in Tanzania

Background

During the last ten to fifteen years there has been a steady decline in public expenditure in the agriculture and livestock sectors in Tanzania. Furthermore, structural adjustment and a national Agricultural Sector Management Programme resulted in significant reductions in manpower, especially at the field level of the service delivery chain. Therefore, much of rural Tanzania has been left to fend for itself as far as livestock health services are concerned. In some areas, NGOs have introduced CAHWs as primary animal health service providers. However, in many areas the service vacuum has been filled by a variety of untrained and illegal drug vendors.

In response to increasing concerns over improper veterinary drug distribution and drug misuse, and in pursuance of a policy of market liberalization, the Division of Livestock Development (DLD) identified the need to investigate options for the privatization and regulation of animal health services and the drug supply chain, particularly in underserved parts of the country. In September 1998, the former

Box 8.13 DELIVERI's information materials

Key information objectives	Senior managers	Middle managers	Field level	Others
Creating general awareness				
◆ basic information about DELIVERI	A4 brochure	A4 brochure	wall poster	A4 brochure
◆ background to project	PowerPoint presentation	PowerPoint presentation	leaflets	3-fold leaflets
◆ policy issues	world wide web		exhibition	PowerPoint presentation
				world wide web
Building understanding				
◆ goal – purpose – outputs – activities	project description	project description	leaflets	project description
◆ stakeholders – farmers and livestock service staff	newsletter	newsletter	newsletter	newsletter
◆ institutional development	world wide web	world wide web	booklet	exhibition
			wall poster	world wide web
Developing conviction				
◆ demonstrating progress	newsletter	newsletter	newsletter	newsletter
◆ demonstrating potential impact	annual report	annual report	world wide web	annual report
◆ participatory planning of activities	discussion papers	discussion papers		world wide web
	world wide web	world wide web		
Motivating active participation				
◆ close alignment with GoI policy	newsletter	newsletter	newsletter	newsletter
◆ communicating senior support	personal contacts	personal contacts	personal contacts	personal contacts
◆ positive reinforcement of success	workshops	workshops	workshops	workshops
◆ demonstrating impact	feel-good materials	feel-good materials	feel-good materials	PowerPoint presentation
	PowerPoint presentation	PowerPoint presentation		
Reinforcing political will to continue				
◆ proof of advantage of new approaches	personal contacts	personal contacts	personal contacts	workshops
◆ support of external agencies	workshops	workshops	feel-good materials	media/press
	media/press	media/press		
Information for replication				
◆ clear, attractive recommendations	guideline books	guideline books	training manual	guideline books
◆ complete historical information	CD-ROM	CD-ROM	booklets	booklet
◆ approach 'toolkits'	world wide web	world wide web		CD-ROM
				world wide web
Feel-good materials	annual planner, calendar, diary, greeting card, engraved pen, T-shirt, hat, pins			

Ministry of Agriculture and Co-operatives signed a memorandum of agreement with the Department for International Development, United Kingdom (DFID) to provide Technical Assistance and funding to support the Animal Health Services Project (AHSP). This project was located in the Lake Zone of Tanzania and designed as a pilot project to test alternative systems for the delivery of animal health services in the wake of sectoral and ongoing local government reforms. It was intended that the lessons learnt might be used to replicate the process in other areas of Tanzania and influence policy reform and the revision of legislation governing the delivery of animal health services.

Project resources

The project team consisted of four senior Tanzanian nationals, a project manager, a sociologist known as a Community Link Adviser and two field veterinarians. These people worked closely with Regional and District Veterinary Officers (DVOs), private veterinarians, Livestock Field Officers (LFOs) and livestock keepers in the four districts where the project was carrying out its pilot study. The whole team was supported by one technical adviser and a series of short-term inputs from a sociologist, an institutional development adviser and a human resource adviser. A laboratory technology adviser assisted with the rehabilitation of the Veterinary Investigation Centre and training laboratory management and technicians. The project was funded by DFID under a bilateral agreement with the Government of Tanzania for an initial phase of two and a half years from September 1998 to March 2001.

Project approach towards change management

The project team relied heavily on establishing a close rapport with a series of distinct stakeholder groups using a range of participatory techniques. Stakeholders were

Strategic Planning Cycle

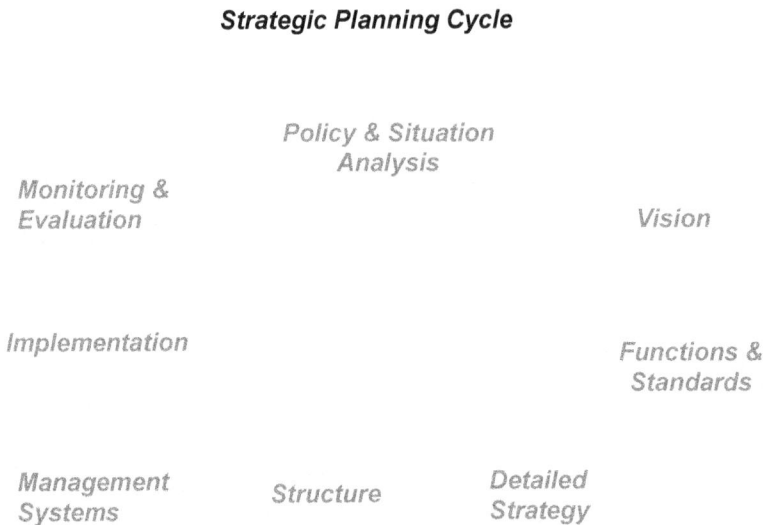

Policy & Situation Analysis

Monitoring & Evaluation

Vision

Implementation

Functions & Standards

Management Systems

Structure

Detailed Strategy

Figure 8.2 The Strategic Planning Cycle of the Animal Health Services Project, Mwanza.

grouped into tiers starting at the farm level and working up to national institutions and policy makers. A strategic planning cycle was used to steer each tier through the process of change. The project saw its role as one of supporting and facilitating change and not driving it.

At half-yearly intervals representatives of all the stakeholder tiers were brought together as a change management team. Change management team meetings allowed the individual stakeholder tiers to become aware of and understand the changes that were taking place at each level. It was important that each tier knew what the others were doing in order to bring about changes.

Initial meetings were held with district veterinary authorities in order to explain the aims of the project. It was made clear that the project was put in place to assist them to effect changes that would result in farmers gaining access to an improved animal health service. Subsequent meetings focused on a situation analysis, identifying problems within the current system for the delivery of animal health services, identifying and ranking objectives to overcome the problems and developing a 'vision'. Similarly, the first approach with livestock keepers was to use group meetings as a means of allowing farmers to express their feelings about livestock issues. Livestock diseases ranked highly as did access to services and input supplies. Action–research, individual, group and team interactions and survey feedback were the main participatory tools used in this process. DVOs redefined their roles and responsibilities in line with the new policy direction and started to develop a new vision with respect to a partnership between the public and private sectors.

Some key issues and concerns

As the strategy for the establishment of a CAHW delivery system emerged so too did a number of issues that required resolution at the highest levels, for example concern over the quality control and regulation of the provision of animal health services and drug supplies. Each tier had a different perspective on these issues. Livestock keepers were mainly concerned about access to and quality of affordable services and drug supplies. Community-based animal health workers were particularly concerned about 'unfair' competition from 'illegal' vendors and state veterinary employees. State veterinarians at the District level were concerned about the use of 'Part 1' poisons by CAHWs with little training and about their own future livelihood. As a private sector service becomes available, government veterinarians will be obliged to withdraw from the commercial side of service delivery and restrict their activities to the provision of advice, regulation and disease surveillance, none of which can be regarded as sources of financial gain. At the national level, state veterinarians and veterinary academics were worried about competition from lay practitioners and lowering of standards of practice.

There was widespread acknowledgement of the problems surrounding the delivery of animal health services at all levels of government and in the private sector. Not least was the need to revise legislation governing the delivery of animal health services and the supply and use of veterinary drugs, particularly in relation to services provided by para-professionals operating in the private sector. The project's role was to help the stakeholders in each sector find solutions to these problems.

Collecting information to inform policy revision

In order to overcome the concerns expressed by stakeholder groups, the project collected evidence to support the need for change from a variety of sources. This evidence was presented to stakeholders at workshops, seminars and meetings organized by the project and at the Tanzania Veterinary Association Annual Scientific Conference, which can attract as many as 150 veterinarians from all over the country. The project team was aware that senior government officers and veterinary academics were especially interested in evidence collected in Tanzania rather than from elsewhere. Each livestock production system and environment was considered to possess unique characteristics that would determine appropriate solutions. The modalities of managing animal health delivery systems will vary according to local needs.

Therefore, the main source of evidence was a pilot study undertaken by the project in four districts of the Lake Zone in Tanzania. This study involved the design and testing of animal health service delivery models. Other evidence was derived from published literature and from a number of ongoing NGO initiatives in Tanzania. The project strived to ensure that the models tested in the pilot districts were both sustainable and replicable.

The project facilitated the state veterinary service in creating an environment that allows the private sector to become established as the provider of clinical services and drug supplies at the farm gate. In order to test the models many activities were implemented using project-derived resources. Increasingly, these activities are now being financed through locally derived resources. As the project withdrew from financing so the sustainability of each intervention was tested as an explicit exit strategy.

Workshops and networking

During the process of collecting evidence from NGOs and other projects concerned with establishing private para-professional animal health service providers, it became apparent that there was a need to develop a network of collaborating partners within Tanzania. It was felt that such a network would help to combine the efforts of each of the partners in championing their collective cause and would help to harmonize an approach towards gaining legal recognition for para-professional animal health service providers. Networking thus provided the project with an opportunity to convene a national workshop to formulate a legal framework for the provision of animal health services by community-based and other para-veterinary service providers.

The workshop brought together a wide variety of opinions and stakeholders representing the main institutions concerned with the delivery of animal health services in Tanzania. Three participants from other countries were also invited. The workshop produced two significant landmarks that are helping to overcome the problem of legal recognition of non-professional animal health service providers in Tanzania:

- First, the workshop participants unanimously agreed that paravets and CAHWs have a vital and essential role to play in delivering animal healthcare services to the people of Tanzania' and that 'the legal framework governing the delivery of veterinary services in Tanzania be changed so as to legally recognize, define, sanction and regulate the status and activities of paraveterinarians and CAHWs, who will work under the supervision of the veterinary surgeons of Tanzania'.

- Second, the workshop participants selected a representative from each of the main stakeholder groupings to form a task force to take the process of developing the legal framework forward. This Legal Framework Working Group (LFWG) includes the Assistant Director of the Tanzania Veterinary Board, a legal adviser to the Ministry of Agriculture and Food Security and other senior government representatives. The LFWG is scheduled to meet at regular intervals over a period of a year and a half. The goal of the LFWG is: 'Policy and legislation governing the delivery of animal health services reviewed and revised to make provision for non-professional service providers'. The LFWG has agreed upon detailed terms of reference and has developed a logical framework matrix and work plan. At intermediate stages in the process of developing recommendations, the LFWG will circulate drafts of its findings to as wide an audience as possible. In this way it hopes to obtain feedback from all the stakeholders involved prior to submission of final recommendations. Once all stakeholders have been given an opportunity to contribute to the debate, the AHSP will assist the DLD to hold a second national workshop in order to allow all stakeholder groups to meet and contribute to the formulation and ownership of final recommendations. Final recommendations will then be presented to the Permanent Secretary of the Ministry of Water and Livestock Development. It is expected that the LFWG will be in a position to make all the necessary recommendations for policy and legal revisions within one year.

The project found that carefully planned national workshops, although expensive, provided one of the best opportunities to gain a wide audience where issues can be brought into the open. It is however important to recognize that, while some individuals appear to concur with resolutions made collectively, they may continue to harbour their firmly held reservations, privately. Peer group pressure can inhibit minority groups airing their feelings in public. A skilful facilitator should be able to recognize when this is happening and provide the right opportunity for such opinions to be expressed openly and without reservation.

The AHSP has now entered a second phase (April 2001 to March 2002) during which it will continue to test the models of animal health service delivery it has established in the Lake Zone. The DLD recognized the value of the project and the process it initiated. It sees the need for an institution within headquarters to take this process forward in the medium and long term. In response to this need, during the final phase of project implementation, the project team will assist the DLD with the establishment of a new 'Animal Health Services Sub-Unit' (AHSSU). The main aim of the AHSSU will be to ensure that sustainable animal health service delivery systems become established, regulated and monitored throughout Tanzania. The AHSSU will be directly responsible to the Assistant Director for Animal Health and will be responsible for:

◆ Liaison between the Ministry of Water and Livestock Development and the Ministry of Regional Administration and Local Government (the two ministries responsible for the delivery of public livestock services) on all matters concerning the delivery of animal health services through both the public and private sectors.

◆ In close collaboration with the Tanzania Veterinary Board, advising on and facilitating the establishment and regulation of the delivery of animal health services through the public and private sectors.

◆ Advising on the quality control of animal health service delivery systems.

◆ Monitoring and evaluation of the delivery of animal health services in Tanzania.

It is expected that the AHSSU will be able to attract funding from a wide range of sources since policy makers are becoming increasingly aware that livestock play an important role in the livelihoods of most of Tanzania's rural poor.

Case study 3: livestock policy and legislative change in Kenya

In the mid-1990s, the Kenyan Department of Veterinary Services and the prime statutory body concerned with veterinary service delivery, the Kenyan Veterinary Board (KVB), were opposed to the development of community-based animal health delivery systems. At the same time the demand for veterinary services in the pastoral areas of the country was not met by the state, while NGOs were rapidly learning that they could get funds to train CAHWs and provide a basic service to livestock keepers, albeit with limited geographical coverage. At this time, the private veterinary sector in Kenya was still immature.

During the implementation of their CAHW projects, NGOs commonly engaged the services of district-level veterinary staff for training CAHWs, without necessarily informing the statutory bodies of their activities. This led to friction and misunderstanding that culminated in the publication by the KVB of a warning to veterinarians in the national press (Box 8.14).

This low point in relations did not last long. Indeed, it actually stimulated a group of stakeholders to formulate a workshop to discuss 'Practice, Policy and the Law in the Delivery of Animal Health Services' in May 1999. This workshop was carefully planned to ensure that the Department of Veterinary Services, the KVB, the Kenya Veterinary Association, the Kenya Association for Livestock Technicians, the private sector and the NGOs all felt involved in the process of coming together to discuss the issues.

> **Box 8.14** Notice in Kenya national press, January 1998
>
> ### KENYA VETERINARY BOARD
> #### STATEMENT ON THE TRAINING OF PARAVETS ON PRIMARY VETERINARY HEALTHCARE ASSISTANTS AND THE DISTRIBUTION/HANDLING OF VETERINARY ETHICALS
>
> The Kenya Veterinary Board under the Veterinary Surgeons Act, Cap. 366 is charged with the responsibilities of ensuring that the practice of veterinary medicine is done within the legal framework in Kenya. It is the legislative body for the veterinary profession in this country.
>
> In the recent past the Board has observed with great concern an escalation of activities of some Non-Governmental Organizations (NGOs), donor agencies, development groups and individuals in matters affecting the animal industry. Special reference is made to *Wasaidizi wa Mifugo* (paraveterinary or primary veterinary healthcare assistants) training programmes and the distribution and handling of veterinary ethical drugs.
>
> The Board's stand on the matter is as follows:
>
> 1. The general public and specifically those involved closely with livestock and animal health should be aware that under the Veterinary Surgeons Act, Cap. 366 it is illegal to treat an animal for reward, whether monetary or in kind unless it is done by a registered veterinary surgeon.
> 2. For the purpose of this Act, the practice of veterinary surgery shall be deemed to include the performance of any such operation and the giving of any such treatment, advice, diagnosis or attendance as is usually performed or given by veterinary surgeons in respect of any domestic or wild animal.
> 3. Any person who subjects any animal to any veterinary surgery in contravention of the Veterinary Surgeons Act, Cap. 366 shall be guilty of an offence under the Cruelty to Animals Act, Cap. 360, Section 3 (1) h.
> 4. It is illegal and unethical for a veterinary surgeon to encourage or cause lay persons to breach the law. The Board takes great exception and will deal with such errant veterinary surgeons in accordance with the law.
> 5. It is illegal to handle veterinary ethical drugs unless one is expressly allowed under the Pharmacy and Poisons Act, Cap. 244, Section 23(e), Sections 26, 28, 29 and 31.
> 6. All persons and organizations involved in training of any aspect of vet practice and equipping primary veterinary healthcare assistants by whatever title are advised to desist contravening the law and, if in doubt, contact the Chairman, Kenya Veterinary Board.

The workshop, hosted by ITDG, proved to be a remarkable success because it allowed both sides – those 'for CAHWs' and those 'against CAHWs' – to see the viewpoint of the other. After initial friction, it was agreed that everyone had the common objective of putting in place viable and credible veterinary services. The workshop brought in legal council to advise on how the current laws might be adapted. As a result of this stakeholders' workshop, practical sets of recommendations were prepared and a task force established to see that they were implemented.

The workshop was followed by others that again allowed NGOs, the veterinary department and the KVB to interact. These workshops occurred in pastoral areas and therefore brought city-based policy makers face to face with some of the constraints to veterinary service delivery in remote areas. By 2000, the task force was at an advanced stage in preparing a standardized curriculum for training CAHWs across Kenya, and the KVB was admitting that it could be possible for it to both approve the curriculum and register trained trainers of CAHWs.

The KVB also began working with other key stakeholders to decided how to consolidate, realign and redraft the 29 statutes affecting the practice of veterinary medicine in Kenya. The aim was to produce four 'pinnacle' statutes for the livestock industry that would serve the best interests of Kenyans and be responsive to the needs of the majority of the stakeholders in a liberalized economy. There was a strong desire to keep the new statutes flexible so that, in future, they could absorb and reflect policy change.

A series of workshops began that were used to formulate livestock sector policy. This process reached an advanced stage in 2001 with the preparation of a draft policy paper. The next stage was to share this document with the field-level livestock service providers through a series of local workshops. Simultaneously, a firm of advocates was employed to prepare the legislative texts of the pinnacle statutes and follow them through the various legal stages until they are made law.

Once this process is completed, it should be possible to legally develop privatized and community-based animal health delivery systems in the drier, extensive grazing areas of Kenya. The chaperone to these legal and policy changes is the proposed expansion of the Kenya Veterinary Association Privatization Scheme to meet the special challenges of privatizing networks of vets, animal health technicians and CAHWs in the arid areas of Kenya. Although this process is ongoing, in just three years there has been a significant and major change in opinions and policy accompanied by the constructive engagement of the most relevant parties. There are still problems to solve but the process of engaging in constructive dialogue accompanied with professional legal advice has now been seen to work and has increasing support at the grassroots level.

8.5 Summary

Although there is much evidence of success with changing attitudes and practices within veterinary services, and a much greater acceptance of the value and validity of CAHW services, few of these experiences have become established in legal or structural changes. Therefore, much work remains to be done to ensure these gains are not lost. Important international bodies such as the OIE are now taking an active interest in community-based services and OIE meetings are important forums for chief veterinary officers to share opinions and learn about progress in other countries and regions. The fourteenth Conference of the Regional Commission for Africa in the Office International des Epizooties resulted in the release of a positive though rather guarded statement.

Box 8.15 The role of paraveterinarians in veterinary services in Africa

OFFICE INTERNATIONAL DES EPIZOOTIES

Organisation mondiale de la santé animale
World organisation for animal health
Organización mundial de sanidad animal

Press Release of 26th January 2001
The role of paraveterinarians in the delivery of veterinary services in Africa

Veterinary services in many countries in Africa are in general traditionally provided by the State. Structural adjustment combined with new thinking on the role of the State has led to a decrease in funding to many public veterinary services. The quality and availability of public veterinary services have subsequently declined in many countries in Africa. Para-professionals in the form of paraveterinarians and community-based animal health workers (CBAHWs) have long been recognized as a means of increasing the availability and affordability of private animal health services to traditional and small-scale livestock keepers in Africa. This trend is expected to continue, with most countries foreseeing a greater role for para-professionals in the future.

One of the key concerns remains the quality of the services provided by para-professionals and the level of drug misuse that might arise through para-professionals. Most countries are limiting the risks associated with para-professional service delivery by creating legislation that requires para-professionals to operate under the supervision of a veterinarian.

So, it seems that things are starting to change. It is difficult to be sure how much can be attributed to the policy influence role of CAHW projects, and how much is due to the general decline in livestock service budgets and the pressure to privatize services. However, there is no doubt in Dr Untung Sulistiyo's mind. He is the District Veterinary Officer in Minahasa District in North Sulawesi who worked with the DELIVERI Project to set up a CAHW programme in his district:

> *Community Animal Health Workers, or Tonkeswan as they are known in Minahasa, are a very important element in the delivery of services by the District Livestock Service. Before there were only a few livestock service staff with a background in animal health; only one veterinarian and two paravets. It was impossible to deliver animal health services effectively. But since we trained the Tonkeswan, our animal health service is faster and more appropriate. Also, the farmers actually pay for the service immediately. These are the benefits of real empowerment, where services are provided by farmers, for farmers.*

CHAPTER

9

Sharing experiences and networking

Stephen Blakeway

CONTENTS

9.1 Introduction

The experience of individuals is a vital part of developing our knowledge of the world, and personal experience provides a context against which to compare or empathize with the experiences of other people. Similarly, the many community groups and small projects around the world represent a mass of important accumulated experience.

This chapter is about networking. Networking involves sharing ideas, information and experiences, and working together with people who may be widely dispersed, in very different situations, possibly in different organizations or countries.

The chapter looks at the benefits of networking. It considers who might want to network and why, and looks at different ways to do so, including recording and writing up experiences or activities. It considers the range of ways that people work with animals, and the range of different community projects that address animal health and welfare issues. Lastly, it looks at some current or emerging areas in community animal health and welfare where networking could be helpful, and reviews some relevant groups or networks that already exist. It is written for a variety of people, for example:

- people starting or involved in community animal health projects and looking for practical guidance;
- people wanting to share the lessons they are learning in their work;
- people wanting to explore links between their work and other sectors;
- people wanting to debate issues arising from their work, or needing support.

The chapter also provides some ideas for people wishing to facilitate networking for others. It assumes there are benefits from networking that come through, for example:

- sharing information and experiences between projects that provide animal-related services;
- discussing ideas and approaches that guide different types of projects;
- discussing the connections between the welfare of people, animals and the environment;
- involving and empowering stakeholders;
- increasing effectiveness and impact of work beyond the immediate boundaries of a project;
- feeding field experience to policy makers.

The chapter does not cover sharing disease intelligence because this is discussed in Chapter 7.

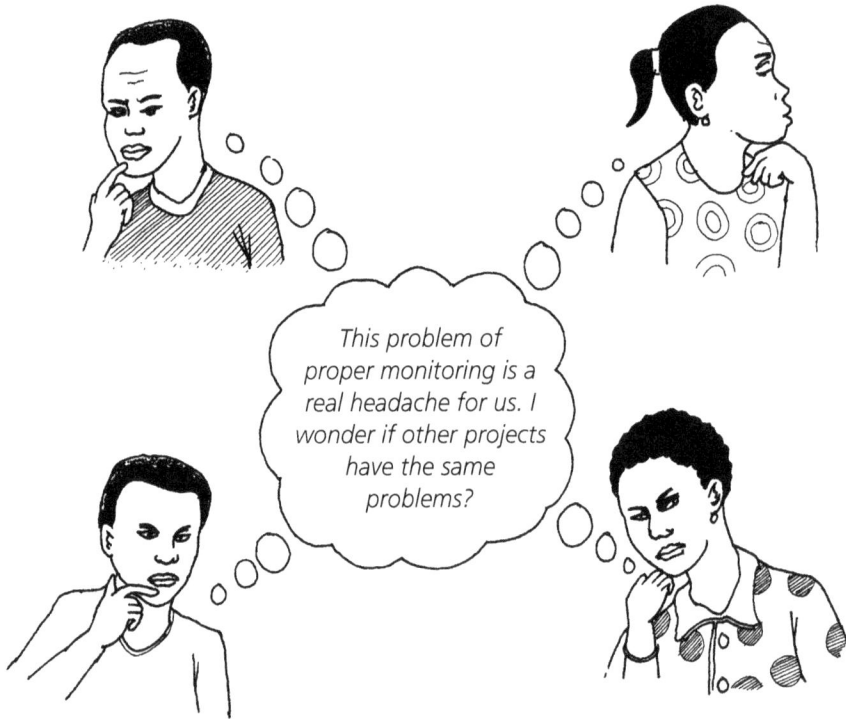

This problem of proper monitoring is a real headache for us. I wonder if other projects have the same problems?

9.2 Networking

Why network?

Reasons for networking include:

- ◆ reducing feelings of isolation in your work;
- ◆ finding out what is going on;
- ◆ accessing balanced information;
- ◆ learning from the experience of others;
- ◆ collaborating with others involved in similar or complementary work;
- ◆ helping develop confidence locally as a step towards empowerment;
- ◆ lobbying and influencing policy more effectively;
- ◆ and, in places where change is not likely to occur quickly, bearing witness to the lives and aspirations of animal keepers who might otherwise not have a voice.

Benefits of networking

Effective networking benefits individuals, projects, communities, groups and society as a whole.

Individuals become better known through sharing their work and experience.

This can help them to obtain information, to influence decision making, to access funds, and to help in finding employment and developing a career.

Projects also become better known through sharing experience and can improve by learning from others. This can improve success in fundraising. Increasingly, community animal health and welfare projects are competing with each other for limited sources of funds. It helps if donors have heard something good about a project.

Communities and other groups can learn better how to defend their interests and rights; can get ideas for projects which might work for them or for ways of working which might suit them and help them deal with specific challenges; and can help find funding. Ultimately, networking can be a tool for empowerment.

Society gains if people, projects, communities and groups network effectively. Improved knowledge and understanding help to break down barriers and to overcome prejudices. Effective networking can ensure that diverse interests are properly represented so that they can be balanced, and conflicts can be resolved fairly and openly.

The power of networking

Throughout this book there are many examples reflecting experiences from different community animal health and welfare projects. In addition to these, Boxes 9.1 and 9.2 show in two brief examples the power of networking.

The first illustrates the value of networking around a subject, in this case ethnoveterinary knowledge (EVK) in Kenya in the early 1990s. The second from the Arid Lands Information Network (ALIN) illustrates the direct impact of sharing practical information between remote village groups.

Box 9.1 Ethnoveterinary knowledge in Kenya in the early 1990s

The early 1990s saw an increase in interest in ethnoveterinary knowledge (EVK). This broad field of knowledge encompasses husbandry and herding practices; the use of veterinary medicinal plants; traditional surgery, bone-setting and birthing techniques; integration between traditional and new methods; and anything else that people do to keep their animals healthy.

In Kenya in the early 1990s, different groups and projects were approaching this field from various directions. ITDG-Kenya (Intermediate Technology Development Group, Kenya), through its involvement in community animal health projects, made contact with many other projects and organizations, and had itself been contacted by individuals or community groups, who were doing innovative work supporting the use and development of local knowledge and wanted to network more widely.

ITDG-Kenya has a stated aim of facilitating the sharing of information, and therefore had money budgeted for workshops. In 1993, the ITDG-Kenya Rural Agriculture and Pastoral Programme (RAPP) organized a workshop to bring together the various people and organizations doing work in this field. These included:

◆ Individuals and representatives from local community or church projects in Kenya and Tanzania (e.g. Olkiramatian and Shompole Community Development Project);
◆ Kenyan NGOs (e.g. ACTS; KENGO; KIFCON; Manor House Agricultural Centre, Kitale; PINEP, Pastoral Information Network Programme);
◆ Kenyan government bodies (e.g. East African Herbarium; Social Forestry Division, Kenyan Forestry Research Institute; Kibwezi Dryland Field Station, University of Nairobi, Department of Range Management; National Animal Health Research Centre; National Veterinary Research Centre, Kenya Agricultural Research Institute; Veterinary Office, Kilgoris; District Veterinary Office, Kajiado; University of Nairobi, Radio Lecturer; Department of Adult Education);
◆ Collaborative projects, themselves the result of networking (e.g. the Indigenous Food Plant Programme – a joint project by Kenya National Museums, Kenya Freedom from Hunger Council, and World View International; Marimanti Sheep and Goat Station – a collaboration between Government of Kenya and the Embu-Meru-Isiolo Programme of the UK Overseas Development Administration (now DFID));
◆ International organizations (e.g. ActionAid; Africa 2000; African Wildlife Foundation; ARUNET; Bellerive Foundation; Environment Liaison Centre International; International Centre for Research in Agro-Forestry; International Board for Plant and Genetic Resources; International Bureau for the Preservation of Genetic Resources; Oxfam; PARC; Plan International; UNEP; World Neighbors).

The workshop allowed this diverse group of people to meet and exchange experiences. Various collaborations were arranged, for example on policy work, on identification and validation of veterinary medicinal plants, and on fundraising. As well as these benefits, many participants gained confidence in the value of the work they were doing. RAPP made a greater commitment to EVK in its future work, which has continued to the present day.

EVK has had a higher profile around the world over the last decade, something that many participants of the 1993 ITDG-Kenya workshop have continued to contribute towards.

(contributed by Bob Wagner)

The current state of networking

Around the world there are many ideas about animal health and welfare and services related to animals. The ideas are being explored and services provided in many different ways (see Boxes 9.5 and 9.6). A few projects have been described in great

Box 9.2 The power of networking: how salt-lick blocks for ruminants spread

This case illustrates what happens when good (simple, useful, replicable) information is picked up by a network, and transferred to a place where it 'takes root'.

The Arid Lands Information Network (ALIN) operated from a small secretariat in Dakar, Senegal for over ten years. It published the popular networking magazine *Baobab*, in French and English. The magazine appeared three times a year, and was specifically aimed at meeting the under-served information needs of community development workers in dryland regions of Africa.

A majority of the material printed in the 40-page gazette came from those same community development workers. In 1996, a brief article appeared showing how one animal health worker in Benin, West Africa, made his own salt-lick blocks from readily obtainable materials. The *Baobab* editors, with help from their talented artist Sidy Drame, transformed the basic French text into the universal language of drawings.

Some Kenyan members of the network read the article and got excited. They were just starting a community-based animal health project at the time, and decided to use the simple recipe in their initial training workshops. Local women were shown how to make their own salt-lick blocks. They quickly saw that all the materials they needed were within easy reach, mostly for free except the salt and small quantity of cement/lime for binder. They also quickly discovered that their livestock appreciated the blocks, and stopped behaviour due to mineral deficiency, such as chewing soapy laundry.

They selected this 'new' technique as an activity for their self-help groups to raise income, by making and selling the blocks in local village markets. The idea spread both spontaneously and through the structured training activities of the ITDG-supported animal healthcare project in the District.

Although the larger international network (ALIN) was essential for making this technique known across the vast distance from West to East Africa, it was ultimately the *local* network of NGO project workers and village-based self-help groups that made the rapid and successful spread of this valuable technique happen. ALIN commissioned a follow-up study a year or so later to document the extent of spread, finding it in surprisingly wide use in Kitui District, Western Kenya, being made in more than 35 villages, being sold at several major markets, and moving beyond the area of the original project.

The moral: allocate more resources to help *field-based* innovators to document their own innovations. These are the ones that work best. Promote the 'farmer-first' or 'bottom-up' approach to information exchange and networking, and let the impact be seen.

detail, written up in books or on internet sites. ITDG-Kenya, for example, has a community animal health (CAH) programme in which sharing of information is a stated aim, and has broadcast its experiences widely. Some projects are less well-known because no time or money has been available to broadcast information, yet formally or informally these projects may be sharing information and experience locally in a variety of ways. Other projects may be geographically isolated and little known beyond the boundaries of their own communities, despite the valuable work they do.

Opportunities and constraints

All experiences from projects working in animal health and welfare, whether successful or not, are a useful resource and provide useful lessons. All projects should therefore be encouraged to reflect on their work, to record it and share it in some way. Donors should be encouraged to value sharing experience from the projects they fund, and therefore to allocate resources specifically for this activity.

Methods of networking will be discussed in greater detail later (see section 9.4) but electronic communication is providing new opportunities for dissemination of information. These opportunities are currently constrained by inequalities of access, the value of the communication being limited by a bias towards wealthier users. (see *Electronic media, e-mail and the internet*).

The case study of the DELIVERI Project in Indonesia (see Chapter 8) illustrates how changes in politics or in policies may provide unexpected opportunities for diversification of projects and for networking and spreading ideas.

Experience indicates that CAH projects are often poor at disseminating information and sharing experiences. Some reasons why this might be the case are summarized in Box 9.3.

Box 9.3 Some constraints to sharing information and experiences

Remoteness of CAH services

Many CAH projects are located in remote areas with poor infrastructure and communications. Contacting people and sharing ideas can be frustrating when telephones are absent or don't work, there are no fax or e-mail facilities, and the postal service is slow and expensive. The process of sending draft papers or articles to colleagues or editors for feedback can be a long and arduous business, and enthusiasm can wane when documents get mislaid.

Organizational management

In some organizations, centrally located managers try to control all the information that leaves or enters field-level projects. This inhibits information flow by either delaying the time taken to release news from a project or by inappropriate editing of reports and

---

articles produced by field staff. All this discourages field staff from writing up their experiences.

Donor dependency

Many CAH projects are dependent on donor funding. In this situation, there is a tendency for people to over-report positive lessons and under-report negative lessons. However, mistakes and mishaps are often very useful experiences for other people to learn from.

Project bias

Projects tend to value their own work and approaches, and may not be able to see a wider context, different perspectives, or alternative approaches beyond these.

Competition between agencies

When then are many agencies present in a given area they can compete for funding and therefore tend not to want other organizations to know too much about their work.

CAHW work is not 'scientific'

In veterinary medicine there are many journals that publish technical information on livestock diseases, but relatively few publications that present experiences of service delivery. Scientific journals tend to support conventional papers based on 'objective' data.

The lack of formal recognition of CAHWs

In those countries where CAHWs have no formal status, projects can be reluctant to publicize experiences in the fear that this might attract unwanted attention from government authorities.

The general political environment does not encourage the free flow of information

Many countries have experienced political systems that discourage free speech and open discussion. Even when these systems are replaced, it can take many years for people to feel confident about talking or writing freely.

Project staff are too busy

Many people involved in CAH are busy people. They also have to write reports (sometimes too many reports) and therefore writing even more can become a chore.

Resource constraints

Particularly lack of funding.

9.3   Who wants to network?

Stakeholders

Many people have a stake or interest in community-level animal health and welfare projects. They include:

◆ animal owners;
◆ people who care for animals they do not own;
◆ other people dependent on animals for food, transport, social interaction, sport, pleasure or companionship;
◆ animal health and welfare workers of all types, 'traditional' and 'modern';
◆ other people in the community who may be affected by the activities of animals or animal owners;
◆ students of different disciplines;
◆ local authorities and government at all levels;
◆ the international community;
◆ donors and funders;
◆ pharmaceutical companies;
◆ animal food and supply companies.

Other projects

In addition, networking is useful between specific projects or services. The design of animal health services at whatever level is affected partly by the relationships people have with their animals, the reasons why animals are being cared for, and the social situation. These points are discussed further in Box 9.4. For this reason, a wide range of different types of animal health and welfare service are already operating or have been tried. These are listed in Box 9.5, with greater detail in Box 9.6. Although these services are sometimes seen to exist in completely different sectors (e.g. CAHW projects for ruminants in semi-arid rangelands and birth control projects for dogs in cities) there are many common challenges (e.g. on community involvement, ownership and education) which make networking between these projects fruitful.

Box 9.4 How and why people look after animals: the impact on animal health service design

The design of an animal health service depends partly on the relationships people have with the animals in their community.

People keep animals for one or more of a variety of reasons. These include production of food, wool, hair or other by-products; carrying or pulling things; hunting; security;

318

racing; conservation or education; their value in sale, exchange or gifts; social, aesthetic or spiritual functions; and simple companionship. Also, many human communities are intimately involved with wild animals which may from time to time come under their care. There are various theories put forward to explain the attachments that people have to animals, and the strong desire many people in many cultures have to share their lives with animals in some way but, whatever the reasons, people have been living closely with animals in a variety of roles for many thousands of years.

People with animals usually try to keep them healthy as far as possible, either using their own means or using the advice or services of others in their communities who have specialized knowledge or skills. The services available within a community vary. A community with a long history of animal keeping may have considerable knowledge and experience to draw on, and individuals with specialized knowledge of husbandry, diagnosis, cures for illnesses, surgery or birthing interventions. For example, many pastoralist societies have highly sophisticated animal health and welfare practices with various individuals who are recognized as specialists; Chinese medicine has developed specializations in a number of different disciplines including the use of herbs and acupuncture; and western veterinary services have become increasingly specialized with diagnostic laboratories, referral centres and the development of various cadres of animal husbandry, animal behaviour, and animal health workers. A community going through rapid change, or with a shorter history of animal keeping, may have less experience and knowledge to draw on and less sophisticated services. Draft animals and companion animals in cities are often owned by people with no previous experience of keeping animals, and the health and welfare of these animals may suffer as a result. Even within a community, access to the available services may vary, affected by understanding of need, ability to pay, and physical (e.g. distance) or social (e.g. gender, tradition) factors.

The complexity of services also varies. In most pastoralist societies the organization of animal health and welfare practice is simple without specific regulatory institutions. In European societies it has become organizationally complex with much regulation.

While obviously important to animal keepers, animal health and welfare are increasingly of society-wide, even worldwide, interest. World trade in animals and animal products is growing. Countries and regions need to monitor and control the health status of their animals if they are to be able to join in this trade. Conservation legislation is tightening around trade in rare or endangered animals. There is also increasing knowledge about and concern for the welfare and just treatment of animals as sentient beings capable of suffering. There is now international debate about what is and what is not acceptable to do to animals. This debate is in its infancy and needs to be extended to all animal keepers in all cultures.

New animal health projects are usually driven by at least two things. First is recognition that changes in the wider world bring new challenges to keeping animals healthy, and growing knowledge and technology in animal health and welfare can benefit even cultures with sophisticated animal health and welfare structures already in place. Second is recognition that existing models of animal health and welfare service – the means by which people should be able to access new knowledge – are not reaching an acceptable proportion of the population of animal keepers and their animals and that we need therefore to re-examine the structure of these services.

Community animal health and welfare projects, as described in this book, are therefore often underpinned by reflection on the social context of existing services and the relationships between people and animals. This process may be started by an outsider to the community, or by an individual within the community with a specific vision of change. The diversity of cultures makes it unlikely that a single model of service will suit every situation equally well. Community animal health and welfare projects need to be processes, not fixed plans. In discussing networking, therefore, we are not talking about circulating standard models, but about sharing ideas, understanding how some things work within one cultural context while other things work in another, and allowing communities to develop animal health services that best serve their own needs.

Box 9.5 The range of community-level animal health and welfare services

Chapter 1 in this book discusses the history of community animal health and welfare projects, and the other chapters concentrate mostly on projects in which community animal health workers are trained to serve their communities. However, these are not the only projects working within communities to improve animal health and welfare. As mentioned above, human communities are involved with animals in widely different ways, with animals often taking a variety of different roles. Animal health services tend to limit their focus to specific groups of animals. Yet many useful lessons can be learnt across these different services or projects. With government and private veterinary clinics, the following illustrate a range of approaches to animal healthcare provision at community level. Even within the type of service or project there are many differences, reflecting how each place is unique with a different starting point. Projects should anyway draw on local resources and develop organically as far as possible. Different approaches will be appropriate for different situations.

The range of animal health and welfare services operating at community level includes:

◆ local specialists with local (ethnoveterinary) knowledge;
◆ ethnoveterinary knowledge (EVK) projects;
◆ farmer/herder education projects;
◆ community vaccinators;
◆ community-based animal health workers;

- people's committees animal health workers (PCAHWs);
- alternative medicine services;
- donkey and draft animal projects;
- animal birth control (ABC) projects;
- charity clinics;
- subsidized animal health services;
- community and public dialogue or education projects;
- community wildlife management projects.

Box 9.6 provides more detail about these types of service.

Box 9.6 The range of community-level animal health and welfare services: details

This box looks in greater detail at the types of service and project listed in Box 9.5.

Local specialists with local knowledge

In many places, people still rely almost exclusively on local knowledge and local specialists, with no outside inputs at all. Local knowledge may include use of some drugs, vaccines and other exogenous husbandry practices as well as traditional practices or treatments. New projects need to ensure they do not undermine this existing local knowledge.

Ethnoveterinary knowledge (EVK) projects

Some projects have been set up specifically to support the continuation, propagation and verification of local 'traditional' veterinary treatments and knowledge. While EVK includes husbandry, spiritual and surgical practices as well as remedies, specific projects often focus on plant-based treatments. There are many EVK-based projects in India, some aiming to make the plant remedies commercially available, others giving greater emphasis to social factors affecting their use within the community. There are also examples from Africa. Heifer Project International was involved in establishing gardens of veterinary medicinal plants in Cameroon. ITDG-Kenya has a project in Samburu District investigating local treatments which are used with confidence and returning knowledge to the community with 'added value'. The Christian Veterinary Mission has a similar project in Karamoja, northern Uganda. In Tanzania there is a collaborative project between the Animal Disease Research Institute of Dar-es-Salaam and Vetaid, a British NGO, investigating local veterinary knowledge. In addition, many individuals and small community projects are collecting and dealing with their own local knowledge either informally or as part of their other work. Increasingly, it is being recognized that EVK should provide the starting point for all CAHW projects – an approach advocated in this book.

Farmer/herder education projects

Projects which aim to increase farmer or herder knowledge labour under the name of extension projects and have a long and chequered history. When done well, direct work with farmers and herders can address problems identified by the farmers and herders themselves, possibly in response to changing demands from the market, and can help develop practical solutions. When done badly, messages from a centrally planned agriculture policy are broadcast unasked and unwanted to farmers who remain unreceptive to the advice they are being given.

Farmer/herder education is useful for things which farmers or herders do for themselves. What is appropriate for pastoralists who do most things to their animals themselves may not be appropriate for a settled farmer who pays someone else to do specialized tasks.

Successful examples of direct farmer training often involve an investigative phase (which may come from the working experience of a local vet or animal healthcare worker); an understanding of why things are being done the way they are, including time and financial constraints for the farmer/herder; and timing of interventions at appropriate and convenient times of the day, season and year. They will usually have simple, specific aims such as teaching good birthing practices and neo-natal care, or teaching the correct and timely use of wormers.

Examples of less useful projects include those which aim to teach donkey owners better harnessing practices using harnesses too expensive for owners to afford.

In East Sepik Province of Papua New Guinea in the late 1980s, the Provincial Livestock Officer saw that the existing veterinary services (town-based, with a ruminant bias, and designed around the operational needs of veterinary service staff) had fallen out of line with the needs of village livestock owners who mostly keep pigs and poultry. During informal meetings, villagers identified internal parasites as the health problem of greatest concern, so simple in-village training was given on parasite control.

Community-based animal health workers

Most of this book is about community-based animal health workers. These people tend to operate as private business men and women, selling their services and drugs within their own communities after a short, locally appropriate training course.

People's committees animal health workers (PCAHWs)

Under communist regimes, for example in Ethiopia in the 1980s and in Vietnam up to the present, PCAHWs have been part of the local administration infrastructure throughout the country. In some ways these are similar to CAHWs and the experience of these programmes might be useful for those considering the 'scaling-up' of CAHW projects. At this scale, it is more difficult to ensure that communities have a say in choosing the person who is to become the PCAHW, a central tenet of the sort of projects described in this book. It is also difficult to ensure consistent quality from so numerous a group of service providers. It is unclear whether local communities have any influence on whether ineffective PCAHWs can be replaced and deprived of their licences to work. It is unclear what formal relationship exists between PCAHWs and other levels of animal health workers such as AHAs and vets.

Alternative medicine services

In addition to traditional or western animal health services, other forms of therapy are becoming popular. For example homeopathy is popular in various parts of the world (e.g. India, Europe) and different 'physical' therapies – including physiotherapy, massage, shiatsu, reiki – are used by animal keepers. Usually these are provided on a commercial basis by private practitioners.

Donkey and draft animal projects

A number of charitable projects target horses, donkeys and mules used for transport, because they often suffer terribly. This suffering is particularly prevalent in rapidly changing urban and peri-urban areas where there is little tradition of their use and care, and where both animals and owners survive on increasingly insecure short-term livelihoods. In various places, charities are providing veterinary, foot care and harnessing services. The approaches used vary and include static hospitals, mobile clinics, owner open days, training of local farriers and other specialists. Some services are entirely free; others attempt some recovery of costs by charging for the service. ILPH (International League for the Protection of Horses), Brooke Hospital, IDPT (International Donkey Protection Trust), SPANA (Society for the Protection of Animals Abroad) and TAWS (Transport Animal Welfare Society) are British charities which work almost exclusively in this sector. Some of these are now investigating the same participative approaches used by CAHW projects.

Animal birth control (ABC) projects

Town councils and similar local authorities often consider all cats and dogs that are not obviously owned to be strays. Strays are considered to be a health risk especially when rabies is endemic, a hygiene risk because of faeces, and a danger because they can bite and scratch. In the past it was often thought that the best way to deal with strays was by mass killing, even if this involved terrible means.

Recent studies have shown a number of errors in the above views. Even if cats and dogs are not obviously owned, they may have a place in the affections of the local community, and they may be fed and cared for by local people. Local cat and dog populations are often quite settled and static and their numbers are at the level they are because of human support (which implies a responsibility to control them humanely). Mass killing alone does little to control numbers in the long term because other animals soon move into an area that has been cleared. And, by destabilizing populations and encouraging the movement of animals, control by slaughter has been found to increase the chances of dog bites and the spread of rabies. Surprisingly, bites from pet dogs have been found to be generally more serious than those from strays. Also mass killing has become less acceptable for humanitarian reasons.

As a result of these findings, guidelines for the control of urban cat and dog populations have been drawn up by WHO (World Health Organization), involved primarily because of rabies control. By advocating control by surgical neutering, these guidelines throw ABC programmes into the veterinary arena.

There is still much scope for improvement to these programmes based on behavioural studies of the animals themselves and social studies among the communities in which the animals are living. Many programmes are already appreciating the value of community involvement, in much the same way that CAHW programmes have learnt the value of community involvement, and are considering the role of community education in taking their work forward.

Town councils often have the statutory duty to deal with 'stray' animals but local animal welfare charities may also become involved, usually attempting to raise welfare standards by doing so. These animal welfare charities can be numerous and are good models of local self-organization offering opportunities for direct collaboration with western charities and funding agencies. Some western welfare charities such as WSPA (World Society for the Protection of Animals) already operate at least partly through collaborations of this sort.

Charity clinics

In some places, charities provide free or heavily subsidized veterinary services to certain sections of society through static or mobile clinics. Equine clinics, as mentioned above, are one example of this. Companion animal clinics in the UK operated by the People's Dispensary for Sick Animals (PDSA, which provides free treatment to the pets of people on government means-tested benefits), or by the Blue Cross or Royal Society for the Prevention of Cruelty to Animals (RSPCA) are other examples.

Some of the charities running these clinics have been operating for nearly 100 years. Within their own frame of reference, these services are proving quite sustainable.

Subsidized animal health services

Government veterinary services are generally subsidized. Donors (e.g. IMF, World Bank) are trying to restrict the range of subsidized services to cut costs. Services which primarily benefit the animal owner ('private good services') are supposed to be handed over to the private sector, while government can continue to pay for services which primarily benefit the country ('public good services'). Payment by government to the private sector for performing public good services can, to a certain extent, continue to subsidize private good work.

Directly subsidized government veterinary services remain in place in some parts of western Europe, for example in the Highlands and Islands Scheme in Scotland, and for the same political reasons that many aid recipient countries are trying to resist having to privatize all their veterinary services. These reasons can include maintaining the viability of rural communities, or levelling costs across the country to make services equally accessible to the whole population.

Community and public dialogue or education projects

Community education projects are appropriate where improved understanding or changes in attitudes and behaviour patterns across a community can lead to improvements in human and animal health and welfare. Community education, through school teaching, leaflets, newsletters, radio, television or whatever, works primarily by raising awareness about issues and encouraging public debate. Many projects come to realize the usefulness of including some community education activities, even though it can be difficult both to do and to evaluate. Draft donkey health and welfare projects in Ethiopia have circulated books around many of the primary schools in the country which illustrate in story form the ways that community-identified 'good donkey owners' look after their animals. Animal birth control projects in India have learnt that involving and informing communities increases the effectiveness and acceptability of their work.

Some sort of dialogue with a community is necessary if community education is to be successful. This is not easy because communities are complex, and community leaders often feel they speak for their communities even when there are distinct groups within the community who are clearly un- or under-represented. These processes require time and willingness to learn from the community, things which projects on tight funding schedules do not always have much of. Yet without them, 'community dialogue' can too easily become 'community monologue'.

Community wildlife management projects

Views on wildlife vary between those who believe that it has a value independent from human interest and that it should be left alone, and those who believe that its survival now will depend on how valuable it is to human society. In the latter camp, there is increasing interest in projects that involve local communities in the care and management of local wildlife. This interest is based on a view that such involvement provides the most realistic hope of ensuring survival of wildlife. Such projects now often include some facility for the care and rehabilitation of sick, injured or orphaned wild animals and the development of health services for domestic animals. This is partly because of the risk of disease spread between wild and domestic animal populations, but also because such an approach seems balanced and sensible.

9.4 How to network

The section on *Opportunities and Constraints* and Box 9.3 looked at some of the constraints to networking. Constructive reflection on constraints can help to identify ways these might be overcome. The following are some methods of networking.

Conversation and local groups

In daily life, direct sharing of information between people in conversation, at markets, in local meetings and in local organizations such as farmers' groups is the most vital form of networking. Local organizations and farmers' groups are 'networks' formed around common interests.

Where local common interest groups do not exist, it can be useful to form them. These work best when the purpose is clear to the community members involved – for example to set up and run a community drugstore, to organize vaccination of village chickens against Newcastle disease, to cooperate in the processing or marketing of animals or animal products, to represent the interests of local farmers in local government, or to lobby at a national level.

Workshops and conferences

Workshops and conferences bring together people who would not normally meet. A workshop is a small conference but usually less formal, with fewer participants, fewer official presentations, and more opportunities for participants to interact and share ideas. Sometimes the word is qualified, for example in 'training workshop' (which implies a more participative training style than 'training course'). Workshops have for several years been a favourite development tool and, until recently, few questions have been asked about their value. Now, however, they have to justify their often comparatively high costs with clear, realistic and definable outcomes. Unless they are seen to be part of a clear process, it is getting more difficult to raise the funds to run them.

Visits

Organized, formal visits are another way people can share information face to face. Letters, telephone or e-mail allow personal links to continue after such visits.

One person calling in on a neighbour is making a visit. They will chat and share some information, and possibly one will see how the other is doing something. Formal visits work on the same principle. Organizing a formal visit for a group of people takes a lot of work. Careful planning increases the likelihood of it being successful. Organized visits should have definite aims. The description of a training visit in Chapter 4 applies equally well to a formal visit between different projects. Visitors need to be clear in advance about what they want to learn from the visit and, if possible, the hosts should be informed of this beforehand. If there are cultural differences between the groups (e.g. dietary restrictions), these should be sorted out in advance also. Sometimes two projects will arrange that each will visit the other, in which case the term 'exchange visit' is used.

> **Experience in the field**
>
> *When Save the Children Fund staff started community animal health projects in Ethiopia in the mid-1990s, they realized they could gain from the skills and experience of organizations that were running similar projects already. They therefore arranged for their project staff to attend a training course on participative training techniques run by Intermediate Technology Development Group, Kenya (ITDG-Kenya), and to visit some ITDG-Kenya CAHW projects at the same time. During these visits they were able to ask CAHWs what they thought of the training they had received, and to hear from community members how effective these CAHWs were being.*

Recorded information

Apart from person-to-person contacts, information is shared using a range of other recorded methods. These include publicity materials, newsletters, magazines, technical or academic journals, books, databases, tapes, videos, radio and television programmes.

Some development magazines have occasional articles or whole editions on community animal health and welfare. *Appropriate Technology, Footsteps, PLA Notes, Baobab* and *IKM (Indigenous Knowledge Monitor)* are examples.

Some of these media are using the internet to stay up to date. While books can only be updated by producing a new edition, publishing on the internet allows more regular updating. The internet is now the preferred method of maintaining and publishing databases for this reason. Information can be entered directly into an internet database and become immediately available to anyone with internet access. The Prelude database on veterinary medicinal plants from across Africa is a good example of such a database (see Further reading for the internet address for this and other databases). Increasingly, magazines are published on the internet as well as in paper copy. They can then be printed out anywhere and distributed locally. This is one way in which the internet can be useful even in places with a poor telephone infrastructure.

Radio and television

Some projects have discovered the networking potential of radio or even television. International radio stations such as the BBC World Service (particularly the local language services), and national or local radio stations are constantly looking for good stories, and they may be willing to make a feature of a project. CAHW projects are interesting from a number of angles – agriculture, development, food, human interest – and programmes can be in the form of documentaries, educational stories or educational soap operas. 'The Archers', one of the longest running radio serials on

British radio, is a fictional story of life in a farming community and was started as a way of keeping farmers informed of agricultural news. This model is being used in other situations now.

Visual media, including cameras (often disposable) or video equipment, are increasingly common and accessible. With training and skilled use, these media produce graphic images of people's lives or project work that can be valuable in putting over messages or telling stories.

Electronic media, e-mail and the internet

Electronic media include three main resources: CD-ROMs, e-mail and the internet.

CD-ROMs (and other similar file storage systems) are information disks that you put into a compatible computer (i.e. one with a CD drive, the correct operating system and the correct software) and which contain enormous amounts of information. This can be in the form of articles, pictures, interactive diagrams or video clips. One CD-ROM can contain the equivalent of many books worth of information. As CD writers for personal computers are becoming available, CD-ROMs of development resources are becoming more common.

E-mail is a cross between letters and the telephone and is sent between computers connected by telephone lines. E-mail can be a fast, efficient and cheap way to network. Messages are sent very quickly, so phone time can be much cheaper than for a telephone conversation. Good practice (or 'netiquette') for polite and efficient use of e-mail is evolving. Box 9.7 shows some 'netiquette' guidelines based on those circulated by Phytomedica (an e-mail discussion forum about medicinal plants).

The internet (or world wide web) is the place with vast amounts of information – it is like a huge virtual library spread across millions of computers around the world. Although modern 'search engines' are effectively part of all internet

---

Box 9.7 Guidelines on the use of an e-mail discussion forum

As many of us know, in this age of electronic communication, if we choose to, it is now possible to spend our entire days (and nights) 'speaking' to others via e-mail. While many of us would still prefer to speak to people face to face, we are blessed with the ability to develop 'communities' with those who we would otherwise have no contact with. Being a new phenomenon, electronic communities are still defining their rules. There are some that are obvious, however, yet can easily be forgotten due to the newness of this mode of conversation.

One important rule is to consider the unequal resources distributed throughout the community. Many members have infrequent and costly access to e-mail. While the beauty of an international 'listserv' is to develop a truly diverse community of like-minded people, the challenge is to respect where each member is coming from. While

---

it is exciting for an American researcher to speak to a colleague in Cameroon, she can imagine what it must be like for her colleague, who is only able to access e-mail once a week at most (due to unreliable phone lines and cost) to log on to find 100 messages. Some e-mail services do not mark personal e-mails as different from listserv e-mails, which makes the task of sorting through and deleting that much more difficult. These colleagues may never 'meet' if the researcher from Cameroon has to unsubscribe due to an overloaded mailbox.

What can be done to maintain a community like our own? The following are some basic rules to abide by:

Messages to the entire list *should* include:

◆ announcements about conferences, meetings, and other events of interest to the community;
◆ requests for help with one's own and/or colleague's work;
◆ discussion about a major news story relevant to Phytomedica;
◆ carefully crafted thought-pieces on a topic when you want input from potentially 300 people.

Messages to entire list *should not* include:

◆ responses to an individual person's query when it is sufficient to respond only to that person;
◆ messages that basically say 'I agree' or 'I disagree' with someone, especially with the whole text of previous discussion attached (remember words can be/always are expensive). If you feel the need to agree/disagree with a statement, think about sending individually to the person;
◆ the body of the original text in your replies, except as absolutely necessary. Please keep only relevant and necessary pieces of the original text in your replies;
◆ large attachments. Not all users have access to the same decoding software. Instead, please give a brief summary and ask those interested in receiving it to contact you directly.

REMINDER: Look at the address you are sending e-mail to before you hit the send key. With many e-mail services, hitting 'Reply' will send your message to the whole list. If your intention is to reply to one or two people on the list, make sure only their addresses appear on the 'To:' line.

We don't want to silence this new and exciting community but we want to remind you to be mindful of the realities of a large international, electronic community.

(Adapted from Phytomedica e-mail discussion forum (Phytomedica-subscribe@egroups.com) as quoted in a message on the Ethno-Veterinary Medicine e-mail discussion forum (join-EVM@lyris.nuffic.nl)) systems and easy to use, searching for information on the internet can be time-consuming. The sheer volume of information available can make it time-consuming to sort through what is useful. Some websites require increasingly sophisticated software to read, although it is possible to make very simple websites with minimal knowledge and very basic computer software. Projects that have internet access may also be able to create their own internet website and so become part of this world wide web. This can be a way of becoming better known, assuming the site is well-designed and promoted in some way.

It is possible to request web pages and perform simple web searches by e-mail and for free (see Box 9.8). This can be the best way to use the internet when resources are limited, where telephone connections are unreliable, or when computer equipment cannot receive or read some of the more complicated internet sites.

Box 9.8 Accessing internet websites by e-mail

If you do not have full internet access, websites can be accessed easily by e-mail, by using:

Web to e-mail servers

Web to e-mail servers are computers which fetch documents from the world wide web, and send them to the user as e-mail messages, either in plain text or html (hyper text mark-up language – a bit of coding which allows computer files to be read on the web).

◆ To use the system, simply send an e-mail message addressed to one of the web to e-mail servers listed below:
   – www4mail@web.bellanet.org (Canada)
   – www4mail@unganisha.idrc.ca (Canada)
   – www4mail@wm.ictp.trieste.it (Italy)
   – www4mail@ftp.uni-stuttgart.de (Germany)

(For best results, use the server closest to you.)

◆ Leave the subject line blank.
◆ In the body of the e-mail message, type: 'GET http://....'(i.e. the URL, the web address beginning with http://, of the web page you want to read). (Omit the 'GET' command to receive the page as an html attachment.)

Alternatively

◆ Use the kfs service which is very similar, but this one uses the subject line or the body of the message.
◆ Send an e-mail to: www@kfs.org

- In the subject line (or the message line) put the full address of the web page file name (e.g. http://www.vetwork.org.uk/index.html).
- You will receive a message back quickly with the web page you asked for. The message will also list the full file names of all the subsidiary pages to the website and explain how to get them all too.

Searching the web

It is also possible to search the Web by e-mail.
- Send an e-mail to: www@kfs.org
- In the subject line or the message put the words: 'search animal health' (where 'animal health' are the words you want to search).

Remember: Things can change quickly on the web so the above services may stop working (sometimes only temporarily). Ask around for current web to e-mail servers.

At present computers and access to electronic communication are unequally spread around the world. This limits their value for networking because many people cannot take part in the networking process. This is very noticeable in the many 'electronic conferences' that are being conducted. Most of the participants are academics or development workers based in central offices of large organizations, and few community-level workers are aware of the conferences or able to take part.

Nevertheless, access to electronic media is increasing, with development projects specifically aiming to provide computers with e-mail access in remote locations. Where there are no phone lines, a few projects are even distributing satellite phones. E-mail and the internet can be accessed with surprisingly basic computer equipment and software, including laptop computers. These can often be powered from solar panels. The second-hand computer market is growing and computers will inevitably become cheaper. One computer can serve many people and, if organized efficiently, information downloaded through e-mail or the internet can be printed out onto paper and distributed locally in the form of newsletters. Larger projects can facilitate this process, especially if they already run a resource centre of some sort.

9.5   Developing networking skills and activities

Networking encompasses wide-ranging activities that include everything from everyday conversation to specific and directed dissemination of knowledge and experience. The development of networking skills and activities will require personal (and project) commitment, allocation of time and other resources, and possibly training.

Self-belief and personal commitment

Many people feel shy about their own work and experiences, feel perhaps that what they do is just some small and insignificant thing. Because of this, much good experience and many good ideas are lost. The experiences of individuals form the basis of much accumulated knowledge. Personal experience also provides a context against which to compare or empathize with the experiences of other people. Effective networking requires that we have confidence in the value of our own personal experience and that we recognize the value of other people's experiences.

A first step towards overcoming a lack of confidence is to talk with friends and colleagues, or to establish an informal relationship with someone in the same field, in order to bounce ideas around. A solid support network provides strength while we are working through our ideas and, by providing feedback on these ideas, can help us to weigh their value. It is best if these friends and colleagues provide constructive criticism, and feel able to say when they disagree with something or feel more work is needed in order to clarify the message.

Developing communication skills

As well as having confidence in the value of our own experience, effective networking also benefits from good communication skills. These skills help when encouraging others to offer their own experiences, and when structuring reports of our own work to draw out lessons that could have wider value. These can be learnt and developed.

The listening skills described in Chapter 4 apply equally to situations outside training, and provide a useful basis for ensuring that we get the most out of our exchanges with other people. This can be particularly true when meeting new people for a short time, for example in workshops, conferences or project visits.

The principles of good presentation apply equally whether the presentation is written or verbal and are summarized in Box 9.9. Effective presentation relies on clear structure. This applies whether the presentation is in the form of an article for a magazine or a talk at a conference.

The expansion of electronic media makes it important that a wide spectrum of people have access to training in how to use it effectively. Even where the technology is not widely available, it is useful if there are people around who understand something about it so that advantage can be taken of whatever access is available.

Personal contacts

Personal contacts are invaluable to effective networking. Much of the value of conferences and workshops comes from talking to colleagues and getting to meet new people. Visits also provide opportunities to meet new people. However, not everyone has the opportunity to attend such events. Personal contacts can be made by writing to people. Articles in newsletters, magazines or journals often provide contact

---

Box 9.9 Presentation skills: writing articles and giving talks

---

Say what you are going to say; say it; then say what you said.

The following basic points apply whatever the presentation, whether writing an article or giving a talk:

1. Make your presentation appropriate to your audience. Keep it clear and concise. Keep your language as simple as possible.
2. Try to draw out just one or two strong lessons or points and try to stick to them. If you try to include too much, people may get confused. If you have a lot to say or describe, it may be better to find a different medium (e.g. by writing a booklet case study divided into short specific chapters).
3. Always follow the guidelines given. For a talk stick to time limits and to the subject that you were asked to speak about. For a written article, follow any outline or structure set down by the magazine or journal.
4. Always start with an introduction ('say what you are going to say'). If you are sending a written article to a magazine in the hope it will be published, the magazine may be able to publish your introductory paragraph as a summary, so make it self-contained as far as possible. The introduction should be lively enough that people want to read the rest of the article.
5. Then describe more fully what you want to say ('say it'). Describe the background or context; describe what you or your project did; describe the result; then discuss what this might mean. Mention why this could be relevant to other situations because people generally find something interesting if they can relate it to their own work or some other wider context.
6. Provide a conclusion or summary ('say what you said'). The conclusion should contain no new information. It should briefly repeat the main points of the article or talk.
7. If it is a talk, practise it by yourself and in front of friends. If it is an article, ask a friend or colleague to read it. Ask for support but also constructive criticism.
8. Afterwards reflect on what you have done; think what you did well and also what you could do better next time.

---

addresses for authors, or for people referred to in the text. Referenced articles provide further possible contacts through other journals. Not everyone will reply to unsolicited letters or electronic mail but many people will be interested to receive unexpected comments and feedback, particularly if these are unusual, constructive and relevant.

Time and money

Networking takes time and money. These need to be planned and budgeted for. The most basic resource is time. It takes time to talk to people, to write articles or prepare for workshops. It also takes time to reflect on work. This is a very different activity from the 'doing' that most project work involves. Ideally, time for these activities should to be built into work plans.

Networking can also require financial commitment. This can be for paper or presentation media, for communications (post or telephone), for communication equipment (phones, faxes, computers), or for attending meetings or paying for visits. Again, realistic figures should be included in project funding proposals.

Incorporating networking into project planning

In order for project staff to feel confident about networking, and for them to do it effectively, project plans should include networking as a stated activity with time and resources budgeted for it. These resources should include money for training staff in the skills needed for effective communication. Many projects assume that staff are just born with these skills. It is useful if the project plan includes some funding for a workshop, or attendance at a workshop by key personnel, at the end of specific periods of the project in order to share the lessons learnt.

Workers involved in projects relying on external funding usually worry about how to present their experience. It would be constructive if donors valued an honest report that explains how a project intends to move forward in the light of problems as well as successes; and made this clear to the projects it funds. Selective reports which concentrate only on successes and deny problems lose much of the value of project experience.

Projects which have a range of staff and beneficiaries need to consider how to include all viewpoints in their reports. Including these viewpoints leads to a rounded (and believable) description of the work, and also gives motivation across the spectrum. It will usually not be practical for everyone to attend meetings or to write articles, although individuals with a particular interest and aptitude can be encouraged. Some organizations have employed professional writers to visit the work, interview staff and beneficiaries, and then write articles. Reports and articles should be made available within the project so that everyone can see the results of their work.

Resource centres

Some organizations will find it useful and practical to start a resource centre within the framework of their project activities. A resource centre can be just a bookshelf or trunk; it does not have to be a large thing. It should be a place where project personnel can find information. It should contain all project documentation and as many relevant external books, documents, audio-visual aids and other resources as possible. Many of the larger organizations will send copies of reports on request. There are also sometimes offers of free book tokens from NGOs in conjunction with publishers of development books (e.g. ITDG Publishing). Some development journals are free to organizations within developing countries. It is always worth asking. The articles, magazines, books and other resources in the centre need to be catalogued and tracked in some way so that they do not all get lost.

A resource centre is an ideal place to install a computer linked to the internet if this is practical in terms of electricity and telephone connections. Though this may seem unlikely, there are already several donor projects that aim specifically to increase access to the internet. These may provide much or all of the equipment needed. Information can be downloaded from e-mail or the internet, printed onto paper and posted or distributed in local newsletters.

Resource centres can be made available to other projects in the area. This will add value to a project, increasing the range of beneficiaries and therefore making the project more attractive to donors.

Donor attitude

Many donors already recognize the value of networking, if only so that successful projects they have funded become more widely known. If this is the case, they should publicize their willingness to fund networking as a specific activity within a project. Many project workers are unaware that these activities can be funded and therefore do not consider applying for funds specifically for them.

Donors who do not see the value of networking need to be presented with evidence of the benefits it can bring to a project.

9.6   Finding out what is going on: networking issues

So far this chapter has looked at the benefits of networking, who might be interested to network, and some ways to do it. This section looks at some of the things people involved in CAHW projects might want to network about.

Background and trends

Animal keepers have always shared information relating to their animals. Obvious examples include information about food (appropriate foods, grazing and food availability, preservation and preparation of foodstuffs), health (disease avoidance strategies, quarantine, treatments for sick animals, techniques for surgery, sources of good advice about health), husbandry (when to move or do certain things) and marketing (barter values or prices in different places and at different times).

Globalization has widened the range of things that directly affect our lives. Information technology has not only facilitated this process but has also vastly widened the range of things we can find out about. There can be pressure to do things similarly when before there may have been greater cultural diversity. Small ethnic groups have become submerged within nation states. These trends have been accompanied by changes directly affecting animal keeping. Small-scale animal herding livelihoods are disappearing under the pressure of industrialized food production. People who were pastoralists with their own herds may now be herding for city-based business people. Meanwhile, small-scale subsistence animal keeping is becoming established within urban areas. The need for modern drugs (and other modern services such as education) has forced people away from barter into monetization of their animals. The knowledge of traditional healers has lost status at local level in the face of powerful new drugs and vaccines yet, paradoxically their knowledge of plants is recognized but not rewarded in the development of these new drugs. Globalization has seen a quickening of the trend for wealth and power to end up concentrated in the hands of a smaller proportion of the population.

In the face of these changes, it is becoming more important for people to access information that will help them preserve, adapt or defend their livelihoods. While modern communication technology makes information flow faster than ever before, this technology remains poorly distributed, and people in rural areas have little access to most information. Increasing a meaningful flow of information between animal keepers around the world remains a challenge.

Sharing information is, of course, an active process involving choice. Many factors affect whether people wish to share information or not, and choosing not to share information can be a valid and sensible choice. Patenting and intellectual

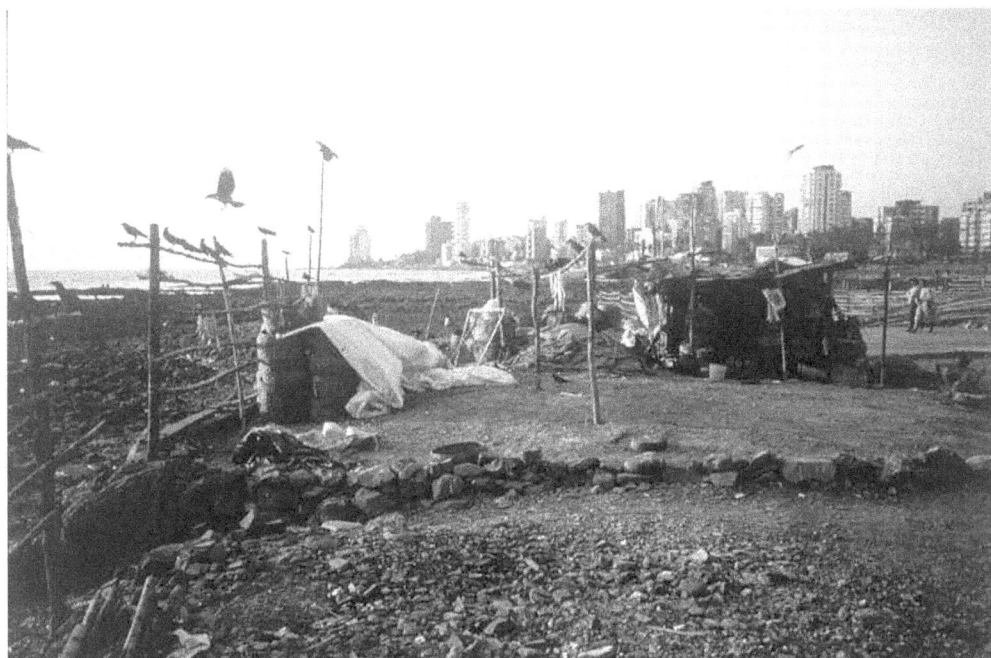

Plate 9.1 In a changing world with rapid urbanization, information and networking helps people to preserve, adapt or defend their livelihoods. (*Stephen Blakeway*)

336

property rights, and prosecution for infringements of patents and intellectual property rights, have focused interest on how to register knowledge, particularly that which has arisen from knowledge systems other than western reductionist scientific enquiry. Any network dealing with the knowledge, experience and traditions of small-scale farmers needs to consider these issues carefully, although the legal situation is complex and rapidly evolving, and so needs specialist advice.

Areas of networking activity

There are several different aspects of community animal health and welfare work that people network about. These include:

- technical information, for example vaccines, drugs, traditional treatments, surgical practices that have proven effective in CAHW projects (with safety, stability, ease of use, cost etc. all important factors);
- project planning information, for example lessons that have been learnt in community planning (see Chapter 2), models of community ownership, gender and equality, practical training (see Chapter 4), monitoring and evaluation (see Chapter 6);
- policy-level information, for example how different countries have dealt with 'quality control', 'consumer protection' or 'national interest' issues (see Chapter 8);
- campaigning information, for example policy issues affecting minority groups or rural producers, debate over intellectual property rights, how other groups in similar situations have defended their interests;
- ethical debate, for example how what we think or believe about animals affects the way we look after them.

These are discussed briefly below. Some specific current and emerging issues in animal health and welfare which require wider debate and possible action – including some raised in other chapters of this book – are given in Box 9.10.

Box 9.10 Some current and emerging issues in community animal health and welfare

This box shows some current issues in community-based animal health and welfare. Debate about all these issues needs to be based on recorded practical experience.

Modernization, technology and biotechnology

The social impact of new bio-technologies will soon be felt as much by animal keepers around the world as by people in other sectors. New technologies may not yield the benefits claimed for them, and can tie producers into high-input systems which they

---

may not be able to afford. Genetic manipulation of animals will continue to compromise their welfare both as a result of greater burdens of production and from unforeseen side effects. Plant manipulation will also affect animal keepers. For example, further manipulation of the genes controlling plant height will continue to reduce stem biomass often used as animal food. Other results of genetic modernization – such as development of substitutes for palm oil that can be grown in western countries – could have both macro- and micro-economic impact by reducing national export income and reducing availability of palm cake where this is used for animal food. Access to debate about these issues is particularly important for those whose livelihoods are already precarious. Past failures – such as group ranches, many grade animal projects, and many vaccination programmes – suggest caution when introducing new technologies.

Ethnoveterinary knowledge and intellectual property rights

Multinational pharmaceutical and life sciences companies are actively searching for new drugs among plants growing in developing countries ('bio-prospecting'). They are interested not only in finding new cures, but in isolating the genes that code for the compounds involved. To identify plants with potentially useful genes and chemicals, companies often draw on knowledge held in communities about traditional medicines and treatments. Without acknowledging the community knowledge that led them to the plant in the first place, the company may claim to have invented the chemicals, genes and plants and their uses, and try to patent them. Profits from any drugs produced stay with the company. The community receives no money for its knowledge and may find itself having to pay high costs for a drug it was instrumental in developing.

There is an urgent need to identify when such 'bio-piracy' has taken place and to find alternative means of protecting the intellectual property of local communities. Networking has been vital in alerting people to claims made in developed countries for patents for plants and medicines taken from developing countries. These networks have made possible successful challenges to, for example the *Quinoa* patent, and have ensured that the voices of those working at a community level are heard internationally.

The International Convention on Biodiversity is supposed to set rules for bio-prospecting but there is controversy over interpretation of the guidelines. Patents are awarded using evidence from 'scientific' testing with definitions about what is 'new' that favour the pharmaceutical and life science companies. It is difficult for communities to collect strong enough evidence to protect their own knowledge by patents. Nevertheless the judgements that have gone in favour of existing knowledge show the value of recording traditional usage.

Sustainability: privatization and subsidy (see Chapter 3)

Is privatization the only way to provide animal health services or is there still a role for subsidized or free services? What factors need to be taken into consideration? What do private and public good mean in real terms?

Technical information and project planning

Technical problems are usually the most easily solved because information is often available through books, magazines or other methods of specific enquiry. Where there are unsolved technical problems (e.g. the problem of *liei* or wasting in cattle in southern Sudan which has a multi-factorial aetiology that makes specific advice about treatment difficult) it may be necessary to seek the assistance of diagnostic laboratories or research institutes.

Information about project planning is also growing. An increasing body of literature deals with different stages of project cycles, particularly the use of participative processes in, for example, planning, training, monitoring and evaluation. However, much project literature is written partly with a thought to future funding. It therefore tends to ignore areas that have not gone according to plan, which are often the areas in which learning and progress have most usefully been made. Direct contact with other projects, with visits or personal contacts, will help to get a more realistic idea of how things actually work in practice.

Policy and campaigning

Networking is central to policy work and campaigning. Human society is a complicated thing. Most of us are not sure how it is that things get decided, how it is that some people seem to be able to influence decisions while others do not. Many people do not realize that their actions can make a difference and that, by working with others, they can influence the way things turn out. Most issues do not have a right or wrong, but there are opportunities to make things a bit better or a bit worse. One of the challenges for all community-level projects is to make their voices heard in debates about policy issues that will affect them. Policy makers have a very different perspective to small-scale animal owners. While policy makers portray their decision making as balanced in the interests of the majority, in fact they are often shaped more to the needs of those closer to government, often those with a greater interest in power and money. This may be because they do not hear the voices of those far from them.

In policy and campaigning work, the key to success is in framing the issue effectively. When raising funds or lobbying for animal health projects, different aspects of the project may need to be highlighted at different times. Outside the world of animal keepers, animals may be seen only as items of food and their wider role in human welfare may be missed. You may have to remind people of the many ways that animals are important. Where livestock keeping is appropriate, animals contribute to the robustness of local livelihoods, have a role in maintaining the well-being of the local environment (both of these in the light of increasingly severe recent environmental disasters) and support local economies where the alternative may be a drift into urban poverty. From local barter to international trade, animals are financially important. For a significant proportion of the human population, animals enrich and add quality to life. In rural communities, especially among pastoral societies, animals are central to culture. In urban environments also, animals have a vital role. Contrary to previous perceptions, street dogs living around urban settlements are valued and actively cared for even by the poorest human populations; in post-industrial urban cultures where increasing numbers of people live alone, animal companionship has proven health benefits. There is evidence to suggest that humane treatment of animals is linked to humane treatment of fellow human beings (although this needs further investigation particularly across cultures). These different benefits can be highlighted in different ways at different times.

Effective networking can protect community interests and defend the value of community involvement. Grassroots lobbying and action played a vital part in successful challenges to the patenting of *quinoa* and *neem* (plants with traditionally recognized qualities for which food or biotechnology companies have recently tried to take out patents). These are landmark cases in defence of local knowledge. The worldwide challenge to the biotechnology industry over genetic modification has been through a network of small organizations working together. The gradual acceptance of CAHWs as a part of rural animal health services has come about through small projects around the world sharing their experiences and ideas, and working together to make their successes known to policy makers within the veterinary establishment. By persistent presentation of evidence, veterinary epidemiologists are having to accept that local disease knowledge can be as useful as 'formal' surveys when investigating disease patterns (see Chapter 7).

Ethical debate

Discussion about the way we treat animals is an essential part of animal health and welfare work. Many cultures have animal husbandry practices that protect animals from abuse. Samburu pastoralists in northern Kenya make herding sticks from softer woods in order to protect their animals from damage. In many places, maximum loads for donkeys and camels are respected. Turkana pastoralists in northern Kenya and Dinka pastoralists in southern Sudan have refused to use their cattle for ploughing because it is disrespectful.

In many communities and cultures, animals are treated with compassion and respect. But will these attitudes change in the face of commercialization and globalization?

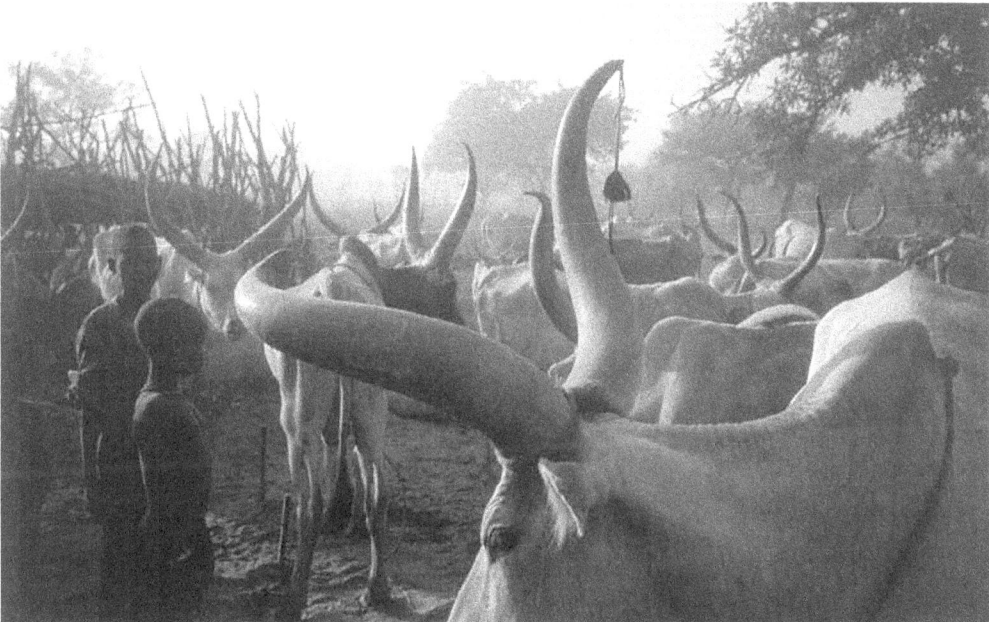

Plate 9.2 *(Stephen Blakeway)*

However, as the world changes, animals are increasingly being kept in new situations where there is no traditional guidance on good husbandry. Some similar patterns of change are being seen in many different places. The poor condition of draft animals in cities, the rising numbers of urban ruminants (and with them the rise in rumenal impaction from plastic bags), intensive poultry units, and the rising numbers of community dogs, are common to many cities now. It is vitally important that knowledge of good practice in these situations is shared between projects. Part of this good practice is understanding the beliefs of the animal owners and how these can be used to encourage better welfare practices. Local religious leaders can play a part in this by teaching animal-friendly texts.

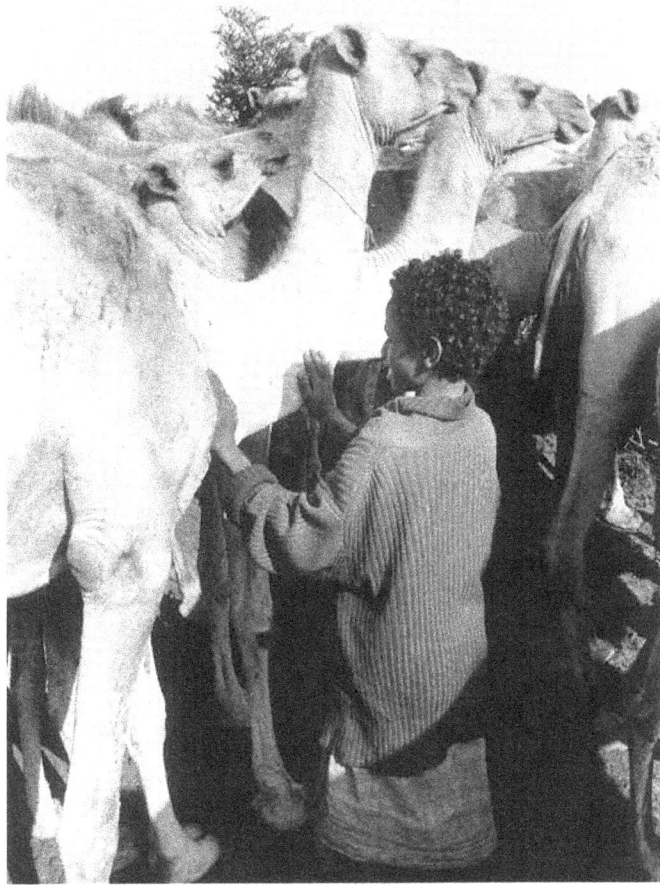

Plate 9.3 *(Andy Catley)*

9.7 Summary

Networking brings benefits to individuals, community groups and society as a whole. As shown by the many good experiences that have come out of effective networking, it has important roles at both the human level and at the level of policy debate. CAHW projects, like many projects on short-term funding, and funding agencies themselves, often undervalue networking and fail to allocate adequate resources (particularly time, but money also). There are many ways to network but all rely on effective communication skills whether through speech, writing or visual presentation. The wide variety of animal health and welfare projects in the world make networking in this field a rich and rewarding activity. All CAHW projects should be encouraged to share their experiences. Ideally, the project should create an environment that helps all stakeholders (project staff and beneficiaries) to feel valued so that they feel comfortable sharing and discussing their ideas and experiences.

Contributors

Stephen Blakeway is a veterinarian and co-founder of Vetwork UK. He is interested in the ways people relate to animals, in animal welfare, and in the range of animal health and welfare services available to communities.

Andy Catley is a veterinarian working for the Feinstein International Famine Centre, Tufts University, USA and is seconded to the Organisation of African Unity/Interafrican Bureau for Animal Resources. He is a former Associate Researcher with the International Institute for Environment and Development and has been working on community-based animal healthcare in Africa since 1991, focussing in Horn of Africa countries. He is a co-founder of Vetwork UK.

David Hadrill has worked in 19 developing countries. He has been involved with community-based animal health services since 1981 when he researched the need for decentralized veterinary services for ITDG. He then managed ITDG's pilot animal health project in India and did feasibility studies in Kenya to prepare for their animal health project there. He currently works as a veterinary consultant.

Karen Iles is a consultant based in UK, with a background in livestock husbandry and agriculture, as well as participatory approaches to training, surveys, project design, monitoring and evaluation. She has been working with community-based animal health projects in Africa and Asia, with multilateral agencies and NGOs, since 1988.

Boniface K. Kaberia is a veterinarian working with FARM-Africa. He has worked in private practice and has extensive experience in the establishment of community-based animal health systems in Meru, Kenya, with FARM-Africa, including community development work, community mobilization skills and microenterprise development. He has also worked with a United Nations project, Child Health Nutrition and School Participation and the Government of Kenya as a veterinarian for seven years.

Tim Leyland is a veterinarian who has worked in private practice and overseas development since 1984. He has specialized knowledge of community-based animal health issues from his work in Africa, Asia and the Pacific Region. He is currently working for the Feinstein International Famine Centre, Tufts University, USA and is seconded to Organisation of African Unity/Interafrican Bureau for Animal Resources.

Jeff Mariner is a veterinarian who has been active in the development of appropriate methods for surveillance and control of infectious disease in extensive production systems since 1987. He is currently working as a consultant on veterinary epidemiology and participatory development for RDP Livestock Services.

John Woodford is a veterinarian who has spent much of his professional career working on the development of animal health service delivery systems targeting pastoralist and smallholder farming systems in less developed countries. Currently, he is the Chief Technical Adviser to the DFID funded Animal Health Services Project which aims to influence policy and institutional frameworks governing the delivery of animal health services in Tanzania.

John Young worked as a veterinarian in the United Kingdom and Sri Lanka before moving to Kenya in 1986 to establish ITDG's paravet programmes with marginal farmers and pastoralists, and support other programmes in India and Nepal. He recently returned to the UK after five years in Indonesia managing the DFID-funded Decentralised Livestock Services in the Eastern Regions of Indonesia project and is now a Research Fellow at the Overseas Development Institute working on policy processes, livelihoods and information systems.

Further reading

General books and reports

Participatory learning, approaches and methods

IIED and ActionAid Ethiopia (1992) *Look Who's Talking: Report of a Training of Trainers course in participatory rural appraisal in Dalocha, southern Shewa, Ethiopia*, Sustainable Agriculture Programme, IIED, London.

IIED and Ethiopian Red Cross Society (1991) *Rapid Rural Appraisal for Local Level Planning, Wollo Province, Ethiopia*, Sustainable Agriculture Programme, IIED, London.

IIED and Farm Africa (1991) *Farmer Participatory Research in North Omo, Ethiopia: report of a training course in rapid rural appraisal*, IIED, London.

Leurs, R. (1993) *A Resource Manual for Trainers and Practitioners of Participatory Rural Appraisal*, Papers in the Administration of Development No. 49, Development Administration Group, University of Birmingham.

McCracken, J.A., Pretty, J.N. and Conway, G.R. (1988) *An Introduction to Rapid Rural Appraisal for Agricultural Development*, IIED, London.

Pretty, J., Guijt, I., Thompson, J. and Scoones, I. (1995) *A Trainer's Guide for Participatory Learning and Action*, Sustainable Agriculture Programme, International Institute for Environment and Development (IIED), London. ISBN 1899825002.

Scoones, I. and McCracken, J. (eds) (1989) *Participatory Rapid Rural Appraisal in Wollo, Ethiopia: Peasant association planning for natural resource management*, Ethiopian Red Cross and IIED, London.

Waters-Bayer, A. and Bayer, W. (1994) *Planning with Pastoralists: PRA and more. A review of methods focused on Africa*, Deutsche Gessellschaft für Technische Zusammenarbeit (GTZ), Eschborn.

Wajir Pastoral Steering Committee (2001) *Supporting Pastoral Associations in Wajir: A manual for development practitioners*. Oxfam UK/Ireland, Nairobi, Kenya.

Training and learning

Stewart, S., Stoufer, K., Shoemaker, J. and Lindquist, B.J. *Learning Together: The Agricultural Worker's Participatory Sourcebook*. ISBN 1-886532-10-9. Available through: Heifer Project, PO Box 808, Little Rock, AR 72202, USA (also available from Women Inc).

Werner, D. and Bower, B. (1982) *Helping Health Workers Learn: A book of methods, aids and ideas for instructors at the village level*, Hesperian Foundation, California. ISBN 0942364104.

Monitoring, impact assessment and evaluation

Feuerstein, M. (1983) *Partners in Evaluation*. TALC, PO Box 49, St Albans, Herts AL1 4XA, UK. ISBN 0333422619.

Gosling, L. and Edwards, M. (1998) *Toolkits: A practical guide to assessment, monitoring, review and evaluation*, Development Manual 5, Save the Children, London. ISBN 1870322932.

Guijt, I. (1998) *Participatory Monitoring and Impact Assessment of Sustainable Agriculture Initiatives*, SARL Discussion Paper No. 1, IIED, London. ISSN 15602192.

Rifkin, S.B., Muller, F. and Bichmann, W. 'Primary Healthcare: On measuring participation', *Social Science and Medicine*, 26 (9), 1988, pp. 931-40.

Roche, C. (1999) *Impact Assessment for Development Agencies: Learning to value change*, Oxfam GB, Oxford. ISBN 085598418X.

Participation and policy

Blackburn, J. and Holland, J. (eds) (1998) *Who Changes? Institutionalizing participation in development*, Intermediate Technology Publications, London. ISBN 1853394203.

Holland, J. and Blackbum, J. (1998) *Whose Voice? Participatory research and policy change*, Intermediate Technology Publications, London. ISBN 185539419X.

Books and reports related to community-based animal healthcare

General

Anon (2000) *Community-based Animal Healthcare in East Africa: Experiences and case-studies with particular reference to Kenya*, Intermediate Technology Development Group (East Africa), Nairobi. ISBN 996693104X.

Appropriate Technology 19 (4), 1993, Intermediate Technology Publications, London. (Now available from Research Information Limited, Hemel Hempstead.)

Catley, A. and Leyland, T.J. 'Community Participation and the Delivery of Veterinary Services in Africa', *Preventive Veterinary Medicine*, 49, 2001, pp. 95-113.

Grandin, B., Thampy, R. and Young, J. (1991) *Village Animal Healthcare: A community-based approach to livestock development in Kenya*, Intermediate Technology Publications, London. ISBN 1853390925.

Hadrill, D. (1989) 'Vets in Nepal and India: The provision of barefoot animal health services' in *The Barefoot Book: Economically appropriate services for the rural poor*, Carr, M. (ed.), Intermediate Technology Publications, London.

Halpin, B. (1981) *Vets: Barefoot and otherwise*, Pastoral Development Network Paper 11 c, Overseas Development Institute, London.

Holden, S. and Peeling, D. (eds) *Community-based Animal Health Workers: Threat or Opportunity?* Department for International Development. Due for publication 2001.

Jones, B.A., Deemer, B., Leyland, T.J., Mogga, W., Stem, E. (1998) 'Community-based Animal Health Services in Southern Sudan: The experience and future', Proceedings of the ninth International Conference of Association of Institutes of Tropical Veterinary Medicine (AITVM), 14-18 September 1998, Harare.

Leidl, K. (1996) 'Development of Primary Animal Healthcare Systems: Examples based on the animal health project in north-east Thailand and basic animal health service project in northern Malawi' in: Zimmerman, W., Pfeiffer, D.U. and Zessin, K.H. (eds) *Primary Animal Health Activities in Southern Africa*. Proceedings of an International Seminar held in Mzuzu, Malawi, 26 February to 8 March 1996, German Foundation for International Development, Food and Agriculture Centre, Feldafing.

Leyland, T. (1996) 'The Case for a Community-based Approach with Reference to Southern Sudan' in *The World Without Rinderpest*, FAO Animal Health and Production Paper 129, pp. 109-120.

Mariner, J.C. (1996) 'The World Without Rinderpest: Outreach to marginalised communities' in *The World Without Rinderpest*, FAO Animal Health and Production Paper 129, pp. 97-107.

Quesenberry, P. and Birmingham, M. (2000) *Where There Is No Animal Doctor*, Christian Veterinary Mission, Seattle.

Sandford, D. (1981) *Pastoralists as Animal Health Workers: The Range Development Project in Ethiopia*, Pastoral Development Network Paper 12c, Overseas Development Institute, London.

Participatory methods and veterinary epidemiology

Baumann, M.P.O. (1990) 'The Nomadic Animal Health System (NARA System) in Pastoral Areas of Central Somalia and its Usefulness in Epidemiological Surveillance', MPVM thesis, University of California, Davis School of Veterinary Medicine.

Catley, A. (1999) *Methods on the Move: A review of veterinary uses of participatory approaches and methods focusing on experiences in dryland Africa*, IIED, London.

Mariner, J.C. (2001) *Manual on Participatory Epidemiology: Methods for the collection of action-oriented epidemiological intelligence*, FAO Animal Health Manual No. 10, Food and Agriculture Organization, Rome. ISBN 9251045232.

RRA Notes (1994). Special Issue on Livestock, No. 20. IIED, London.

Sollod, A.E. and Stern, C. (1991) 'Appropriate Animal Health Information Systems for Nomadic and Transhumant Livestock Populations in Africa', *Office Internationale des Epizooties Revue Scientifique et Technique,* 10(1), pp. 89–101.

Indigenous veterinary skills and knowledge

Bizimana, N. (1994) *Traditional Veterinary Practice in Africa*, Deutsche Gessellschaft für Technische Zusammenarbeit (GTZ), Eschborn. ISBN 3880855021.

Martin, M., Mathias, E. and McCorkle, C.M. (2001) *Ethnoveterinary Medicine: An annotated bibliography of community animal healthcare*, ITDG Publishing, London. ISBN 1853395226.

Mathias-Mundy, E. and McCorkle, C.M. (1989) *Ethnoveterinary Medicine: An annotated bibliography*, Bibliographies in Technology and Social Change Series No. 6, Iowa State University, Ames. ISBN 0945271166.

McCorkle, C.M., Mathias, E. and Schillhorn van Veen, T.W. (eds) (1996) *Ethnoveterinary Research and Development*, Intermediate Technology Publications, London. ISBN 1853393266.

Training manuals for community-based animal health programmes

UNDP (1994) *Practical Handbook for Veterinary Field Units*, United Nations Development Programme, Office for Project Services, Afghanistan Rural Rehabilitation Programme Office.

United Mission to Nepal (1998) *Textbook for Village Animal Health Workers*, Rural Development Centre, United Mission to Nepal, PO Box 126, Kathmandu, Nepal.

UNICEF-Operation Lifeline Sudan (1997) *A Training Manual for Community Animal Health Workers in Southern Sudan*, available from Livestock Projects Officer, UNICEF-OLS Livestock Programme, PO Box 41445, Nairobi, Kenya.

The economics of veterinary services

Holden, S. (1999) 'The Economics of the Delivery of Veterinary Services', *Office Internationale des Epizooties Revue Scientifique et Technique,* 18(2), pp. 425-39.

Holden, S., Ashley, S. and Bazeley, P. (1996) *Improving the Delivery of Animal Health Services in Developing Countries: A literature review*, Livestock in Development, PO Box 20, Crewkeme, Somerset TA18 7YW, United Kingdom.

Leonard, D.K., Koma, L.M.P.K., Ly, C. and Woods, P.S.A (1999) 'The New Institutional Economics of Privatizing Veterinary Services in Africa', *Office Internationale des Epizooties Revue Scientifique et Technique,* 18(2), pp. 544-61.

Reviews and evaluations

Catley, A. (1996) *Pastoralists, Paravets and Privatization: Experiences in the Sanaag region of Somaliland*, Pastoral Development Network Paper 39d, Overseas Development Institute, London.

Hanks, J., Oakeley, R., Opuku, H., Dasebu, S. and Asaga, J. (1999) *Assessing the Impact of Community Animal Healthcare Programmes: Some experiences from Ghana*, Veterinary

Epidemiology and Economics Research Unit, University of Reading and Ministry of Food and Agriculture, Republic of Ghana.

Iles, K. (1998) *Community Animal Health Workers in Karamoja: A report for PARC Uganda*, Livestock in Development, Crewkerne.

Mariner, J.C. (1999) *Review of Community-based Animal Healthcare in the Northern Communal Areas of Namibia*, FAO, Rome.

Moorhouse, P. and Ayelew Tolossa (1997) *Consultancy Report on Cost Recovery in Delivery of Animal Health Services*, Pan African Rinderpest Campaign, Addis Ababa, Ethiopia.

Participatory monitoring and assessment

ActionAid Somaliland (1993) *Programme Review by Sanaag Community-based organization*, ActionAid, Hamlyn House, Macdonald Road, London NI9 5PG, United Kingdom.

Catley, A. (1999) *Monitoring and Impact Assessment of Community-based Animal Health Projects in Southern Sudan: Towards participatory approaches and methods*, Report for Vétérinaires sans Frontières Belgium and Vétérinaires sans Frontières Switzerland, Vetwork UK, Musselburgh.

Young, J., Stoufer, K., Ojha, N. and Dijkema, H.P. (1994*) Animal Health Training: Case study of animal health improvement training programme*, IT Publications, London.

Some useful internet and other contact addresses

This list includes some useful internet and other contact addresses. Please note that these addresses can change and may become inaccessible (particularly internet addresses). They are included partly to demonstrate the range of organizations that exist. The addresses are listed under the following headings:

- ◆ Magazines or publications;
- ◆ Organizations involved in community animal health;
- ◆ Ethnoveterinary, ethnobotany and other indigenous knowledge;
- ◆ Animal welfare and animal rights;
- ◆ Veterinary;
- ◆ Livestock and agriculture;
- ◆ Development;
- ◆ Downloading electronic pictures and diagrams;
- ◆ Miscellaneous.

Magazines or publications
Baobab
Arid Lands Information Network (ALIN) / Resau d'Information des Terres Arides (RITA) CP 3, Dakar-Fann, Senegal
PLA Notes
International Institute for Environment and Development (IIED), 3 Endsleigh Street, London WC1H 0DD, UK: http://www.iied.org/resource/

Organizations involved in community animal health
Vetwork UK home page: http://www.vetwork.org.uk
Intermediate Technology Development Group: http://www.itdg.org
   A British NGO which has been involved in projects exploring approaches to decentralized animal health services for the last 15 years.
Vetaid (UK): http://www.vetaid.org

Veterinaires sans Frontieres: http://www.vsf-france.org

Veterinarios sin Frontieras: http://tau.uab.es/associacions/vetersf/index.eng.html
> European NGOs implementing CAHW and other animal health-related projects. All part of: VSF Europa: http://www.vsfeuropa.org

DELIVERI, Indonesia: http://www.deliveri.org
> A British Government funded project providing decentralized animal health services in Suluwezi, Indonesia.

Community-based Animal Health and Participatory Epidemiology (CAPE) Unit: http://www.ids.ac.uk/eldis/pastoralism/cape
> CAPE works in the Horn of Africa region and links field experience to policy and legislative reform to support community-based veterinary services.

Ethnoveterinary, ethnobotany and other indigenous knowledge

Prelude Database of Veterinary Medicinal Plants of Africa: http://pc4.sisc.ucl.ac.be/prelude.html

Proceedings of International Ethnonoveterinary Conference, Pune, India, November 1997 (Volume 2): http://www.vetwork.org.uk/pune20.htm

Indigenous Knowledge and Development Monitor: http://www.nuffic.nl/ciran/ikdm/index.html

Royal Botanical Gardens, Kew, UK: http://www.kew.org/ceb/ebinfo

Directory of Ethnobotany Resources on the www: http://www.cieer.org/directory.html

Plants Toxic To Animals: http://www.library.uiuc.edu/vex/toxic/intro.htm

Biodiversity Links: http://biodiversity.uno.edu/

Animal welfare and animal rights

The NORINA database of audio-visual alternatives to the use of animals in education: http://oslovet.veths.no/norina/
> Contributes towards reduction, refinement and replacement of animals in scientific procedures.

Animal Rights Resource Site: http://www.envirolink.org/arrs/

Veterinary

Office International des Epizooties: http://www.oie.int/

Centre for Tropical Veterinary Medicine, UK: http://www.vet.ed.ac.uk/ctvm/

Livestock and agriculture

SLAP (Sustainable Livestock and Animal Production Newsletter):http://www.geocities.com/RainForest/Canopy/3770/

GeneWatch: http://www.genewatch.org
> An independent organization facilitating informed, precautionary public debate about the use of genetic modification technologies.

International Livestock Research Institute, Nairobi, Kenya: http://www.cgiar.org/ilri/

New Agriculturalist On Line: http://www.new-agri.co.uk/

Development

Monitoring and Evaluation News: http://www.mande.co.uk/news.htm (Download MandE News by e-mail, by sending the message 'http://www.shimbir.demon.co.uk/news.htm' (only) in an e-mail to 'www@kfs.org')

Intellectual Property Rights Site: http://www.vita.org/technet/iprs/

Institute of Development Studies, UK: http://www.ids.ac.uk/ids
World Bank: http://www.worldbank.org
International Development Research Centre (IDRC): http://www.idrc.ca
Development Media Resources Web Site: http://www.devmedia.org/

Downloading electronic pictures and diagrams
Dev Art: http://www.geocities.com/The Tropics/cove/1003

Miscellaneous
New Scientist magazine: http://www.nsplus.com/
CABI, Scientific Abstracting Service: http://www.cabi.org

Humanity Libraries Project

The objective of the Humanity Libraries Project (formerly known as Humanity CD-ROM Project) is to provide all persons involved in development, well-being and basic needs, access to a complete library containing most solutions, know-how and ideas they need to tackle poverty and increase the human potential.

Contents: The Humanity Development Library 2.0 edition (September 1998) contains the equivalent of 160 000 pages/340 kg/US$20 000 of useful books/reports and newsletters on one single CDROM of 25 grammes. The publications are those of the 70 participating organizations and cover 23 major subjects; with each 20 to 50 books. There are about 30 000 linked images in Gif, PNG and jpg format.

System requirements: Win 3.1, Win 3.11 or Windows 95/98/NT, preferably minimum 486 processor, 12 Mb free space on hard-disk is required. The CD-ROM library runs on PowerMacs which are Windows compatible but is not compatible with earlier Apple Macintosh computers. The CD-ROM works on some 386 PCs.

User-friendly: The CD-ROM library is very user-friendly and uses the powerful Greenstone search engine from the NZDL. It requires the latest version of Netscape 4.04 or Explorer 4.0 browser. This latest Netscape version is available for installation on the CD-ROM.

Prices for direct orders: US$13 rapid airmail delivery included for developing countries; US$30 rapid airmail delivery included for developed countries.

For non-profit distribution in developing countries, prices get as low as US$6 per CD-ROM plus delivery costs from 40 to 50 CD-ROMs on. This means US$240 plus delivery costs for 40 CD-ROM Libraries. But for wider non-profit redistribution of at least 300 CD-ROMs or more, the costs are about US$2.50 per CD-ROM plus about US$0.50–1.00 delivery costs per CD-ROM.

For further information or for ordering CD-ROMs, contact:
Humanity Libraries Project
c/o Global Help Projects vzw & HumanityCD Ltd
Oosterveldlaan 196
B-2610 Antwerp, BELGIUM
Tel: +32-3-448.05.54 - Fax: +32-3-449.75.74
General e-mail: humanity@globalprojects.org
Humanity Libraries Project websites
http://www.oneworld.org/globalprojects/humcdrom
http://www.oneworld.org/globalprojects
http://www.humanitylibraries.net/

Index

www.ingramcontent.com/pod-product-compliance
Lightning Source LLC
Chambersburg PA
CBHW051611030426
42334CB00035B/3483